MRI of Rectal Cancer

Arnd-Oliver Schäfer
Mathias Langer

MRI of Rectal Cancer

Clinical Atlas

Springer

Prof. Dr. Arnd-Oliver Schäfer
Department of Diagnostic Radiology
Freiburg University Hospital
Hugstetter Straße 55
79106 Freiburg
Germany
arnd-oliver.schaefer@uniklinik-freiburg.de

Prof. Dr. Mathias Langer
Department of Diagnostic Radiology
Freiburg University Hospital
Hugstetter Str. 55
79106 Freiburg
Germany
mathias.langer@uniklinik-freiburg.de

Additional material to this book can be downloaded from http://extras.springer.com

ISBN 978-3-662-50135-1 ISBN 978-3-540-72833-7 (eBook)

DOI 10.1007/978-3-540-72833-7

Springer Heidelberg Dordrecht London New York

Softcover reprint of the hardcover 1st edition 2010

Cover design: eStudio Calamar Figueres/Berlin

Printed on acid-free paper

Springer is part of Springer Science+Business Media (www.springer.com)

Preface

Oncology in general has seen vast advancements over recent years. Improved understanding of tumor biology, multidisciplinary team decisions and an individualized therapy are cornerstones of treatment planning for cancer patients today. These developments have challenged the imaging community with ever more specific questions on tumor detection, staging and therapy control. Whereas this evolution applies to many tumor entities, rectal cancer takes an outstanding role, as it was the recognition of certain anatomical and pathological features of the disease, with the help of magnetic resonance imaging (MRI), that induced radiology not only to aid in disease management, but in fact to be a powerful engine for new concepts in rectal cancer treatment.

The continuous improvement of highly specialized MRI and the groundbreaking scientific contributions of radiologists all over the world have paved the way for substantial refinements of this technique during the last decade.

Consequently, dedicated imaging protocols for routine diagnostic work-up of rectal cancer patients are now available, which can guide multidisciplinary team decisions and, in combination with optimized surgery and chemoradiotherapy, lead to longer survival and a better quality of life.

Besides the scientific advances, the enduring clinical success of MRI in the field of rectal cancer is highly contingent upon expertise. To this end, ongoing education and continuous training are vital.

MRI of Rectal Cancer – Clinical Atlas is a comprehensive yet streamlined synopsis reflecting current clinical opinions and case-based imaging features of rectal cancer. We hope it will aid radiologists and clinicians in understanding the essential aspects of rectal cancer and in incorporating this knowledge into their daily practice.

Arnd-Oliver Schäfer
Freiburg, Germany Matthias Langer

Contents

Contributors

Tobias Baumann, MD Department of Diagnostic Radiology, Freiburg University Hospital, Hugstetter Strasse 55, 79106 Freiburg, Germany
tobias.baumann@uniklinik-freiburg.de

Ulrich Theodor Hopt, MD Department of General and Visceral Surgery, Freiburg University Hospital, Hugstetter Strasse 55, 79106 Freiburg, Germany
ulrich.hopt@uniklinik-freiburg.de

Mathias Langer, MD, MBA Department of Diagnostic Radiology, Freiburg University Hospital, Hugstetter Strasse 55 79106 Freiburg, Germany
mathias.langer@uniklinik-freiburg.de

Arnd-Oliver Schäfer, MD Department of Diagnostic Radiology, Freiburg University Hospital, Hugstetter Strasse 55, 79106 Freiburg, Germany
arnd-oliver.schaefer@uniklinik-freiburg.de

Martin Werner, MD Institute of Pathology, Freiburg University Hospital, Breisacher Strasse 115a, 79106 Freiburg, Germany
martin.werner@uniklinik-freiburg.de

Thorsten Wiech, MD Institute of Pathology, Freiburg University Hospital, Breisacher Strasse 115a, 79106 Freiburg, Germany
thorsten.wiech@uniklinik-freiburg.de

Introduction: From a Surgeon's Point of View 1

Surgical therapy of rectal carcinoma: Value of imaging

Ulrich Theodor Hopt

Surgical therapy of rectal carcinoma has advanced enormously since the 1990s. However, not only the surgical technique itself has improved; first and foremost has been the effort to adapt the radicality of the surgical approach to the individual patient. The objective is to avoid therapies that are either too aggressive or too conservative, while taking the patient's unique situation into account. A surgery that is too radical may not further increase the chance of cure, but may ultimately result in a long-lasting and severe reduction in quality of life. If the therapy regimen is too conservative, an increased rate of recurrence will result and the patient's long-term survival will be unavoidably reduced.

1.1 Therapeutic Options

Surgical therapy in rectal carcinoma ranges from local transanal excision to multivisceral resection (Bretagnol et al. 2007). Modern imaging procedures allow physicians to determine which surgical procedure is best-suited for the individual patient and whether multimodal therapy is also necessary. The central goal of surgical therapy for rectal carcinoma is the prevention of local recurrence. Local recurrence results in fatal consequences for many patients and is directly linked to markedly reduced survival. Advanced rectal carcinoma frequently extends dorsally into the sacral plexus, causing severe pain. Ventral expansion may result in infiltration of the urinary bladder, seminal vesicles, prostate, uterus, and vagina; provoke the formation of a fecal fistula; or, at worst, lead to the formation of a cloaca, which is almost impossible to treat. Since total mesorectal excision was introduced as the standard surgical procedure for rectal resection, the risk of local recurrence has decreased considerably (Wibe et al. 2002). Nevertheless, in some large series, the recurrence rate ranged from 5 to 15%, depending on the location of the primary tumor (Kapiteijn et al. 2001; Sauer et al. 2004). This high rate of local recurrence also determines whether multimodal therapy is warranted in certain groups of patients.

The decision as to which surgical procedure should be applied for a given patient strongly depends on a number of patient-specific factors, such as age, general condition, and competence of the sphincter apparatus. Various tumor-specific parameters are also of central importance. In addition to the histological classification of the tumor, exact oncological staging is a major prerequisite to evidence-based therapeutic decision making, including the stage of the primary tumor (T), the presence of lymph node metastasis (N), and the presence of distant metastasis (M). The evaluation of the so-called circumferential resection margin (CRM) is also of crucial importance.

Today, a number of imaging procedures are available for staging purposes, which exhibit different degrees of accuracy for each aspect of rectal cancer staging. The current role of imaging for therapy decision making is discussed in this chapter.

1.2 Local Excision of a Rectal Carcinoma

Local transanal excision can be performed in cases of T1 (low-risk) rectal cancers. Because magnetic resonance imaging (MRI) is not yet deemed accurate

U. T. Hopt
Department of General and Visceral Surgery, Freiburg University Hospital, Hugstetter Strasse 55, 79106, Freiburg, Germany
e-mail: ulrich.hopt@uniklinik-freiburg.de

A-O. Schäfer, M. Langer, *MRI of Rectal Cancer*,
DOI: 10.1007/978-3-540-72833-7_1, © Springer-Verlag Berlin Heidelberg 2010

enough to consistently distinguish between T1 and T2 tumors, endorectal ultrasound is presently the best-suited technique. Although an oncologically adequate resection with respect to the rectal wall is possible by local tumor excision in most patients with early-stage tumors, the underlying problem of lymph node metastasis still remains. Because nodal metastases in T1 carcinomas are usually micrometastases, the affected lymph nodes are usually not enlarged. Therefore, imaging alone is not enough to determine the nodal spread. Consequently, the histologic grading of the tumor itself is used as an indicator to differentiate between low- and high-risk tumors (Idrees and Paty 2006; Merkel et al. 2001). Criteria for a low-risk T1 tumor are submucosal infiltration grade 1 or 2, no lymphatic vessel invasion, no venous invasion, histologic grade 1, and size ≤3 cm. Because high-risk T1 tumors show nodal metastasis in more than 10% of cases, rectal resection is usually recommended. If staging indicates a tumor eligible for local excision, the transanal endoscopic microsurgery can be used to resect tumors up to the peritoneal fold. Because local excision is less stressful than rectal resection or even rectal exstirpation, it is a suitable procedure for patients in a reduced general condition.

1.3 Primary Transabdominal Resection

Primary transabdominal rectal resection with total mesorectal excision is the method of choice for high-risk T1N0 and T2N0 tumors. The role of primary resection for T3N0 carcinomas is currently under debate. Whereas tumors that deeply invade the mesorectal fat are candidates for preoperative treatment, there is evidence that T3 tumors with only minimal invasion of the mesorectal tissue exhibit recurrence rates similar to T2 tumors and should therefore be primarily resected if no signs of lymph node involvement are present (Merkel et al. 2001). Although MRI is ideal for measuring the depth of tumor invasion beyond the rectal wall, the cutoff value that best divides the T3 group according to the risk of recurrence is still unclear. Patients with histopathology that reveals lymph node metastasis despite negative imaging should undergo postoperative chemoradiation. However, in the majority of patients classified preoperatively as N0, no lymph node metastasis can be found by histopathology. Thus, primary surgical resection can protect these patients from oncologically nonindicated overtherapy.

1.4 Multimodal Therapy of Rectal Carcinoma

There is strong evidence that multimodal treatment of advanced rectal carcinoma is superior to surgery alone. It has been shown that neoadjuvant radiochemotherapy has advantages over adjuvant radiochemotherapy in terms of toxicity and oncological effectiveness (Kapiteijn et al. 2001; Sauer et al. 2004). The exact determination of T stage and N stage, as well as the precise evaluation of the CRM, are crucial for deciding whether neoadjuvant radiochemotherapy is indicated. T4 tumors should, in principle, be pretreated. This approach is also still recommended for T3 tumors. There is general agreement that all patients with suspected mesorectal lymph node metastasis in cross-sectional imaging should undergo neoadjuvant therapy, independent of T stage; however, the accuracy of imaging for prediction of nodal disease is still limited.

1.5 Importance of the Circumferential Resection Margin

The rectum and mesorectum are enveloped by a thin fascia, the so-called mesorectal fascia, which can be excellently visualized on MRI. In perimesorectal excision, the mesorectal fascia forms the outermost layer. For this reason, it is called the CRM. A histopathologically proven R0 resection is only possible if the CRM is tumor free. Most local recurrences result from a tumor-ridden CRM (Quirke et al. 1986). Several studies have shown that the local recurrence rate increases provided that the tumor extends to 1 mm of the CRM (Glynne-Jones et al. 2007). The distance between the tumor or involved lymph nodes and the mesorectal fascia can be precisely determined on MRI. This has two important implications. First, if the CRM is positive or questionably positive in MRI, neoadjuvant radiochemotherapy is always indicated. Second, during total mesorectal excision, the surgeon can change the plane of dissection more laterally towards the pelvic sidewall in areas where the mesorectal fascia is threatened by tumor.

1.6 Lymph Node Metastasis Outside the Mesorectum

The main pathway of lymphatic drainage, and thus potential lymph node metastases in rectal carcinoma, are found in the mesorectum and further cranial along the trunk of the inferior mesenteric artery. In approximately 10 to 15% of patients, however, there is nodal spread along the iliac vessels. For this reason, bilateral iliac lymphadenectomy is part of the standard procedure for rectal cancer surgery in Japan. However, this is not the case in Europe and the United States because of the low rate of iliac lymph node metastasis in rectal cancer. In addition, radical bilateral iliac lymphadenectomy largely destroys nerval functions with serious consequences. Two-thirds of patients develop persistent problems with bladder evacuation, and impotence and retrograde ejaculation occur in 80 to 90% of male patients (Hida et al. 1997). When bilateral lymphadenectomy is performed, between 80 and 90% of patients are subject to the serious adverse effects of this procedure without having additional lymph node metastases excised. MRI is of particular importance with respect to this problem. If suspicious iliac lymph nodes are detected, the surgeon can specifically excise them. Extramesorectal lymphadenectomy can, in most cases, be limited to one side. The fact that the rate of local recurrence in Europe is slightly lower than in Japan indicates that this concept is correct.

1.7 Surgical Consequences of a Stage T4 Rectal Carcinoma

The question of whether a T4 tumor is present in a patient with rectal carcinoma must be unequivocally answered during preoperative imaging. Such patients should undergo neoadjuvant radiochemotherapy. After neoadjuvant therapy, imaging should again be employed to decide whether a curative surgical procedure can be performed. In the majority of cases, multivisceral resection offers the only possibility to achieve this goal, but it requires detailed presurgical planning. Additional diagnostic procedures, such as separate-side renal clearance, are often necessary. Furthermore, the cooperation of various surgical teams (e.g., colorectal surgeons, urologists, gynecologists, plastic surgeons) is mandatory to successfully manage these complex cases.

1.8 Ultralow Sphincter Preserving Anterior Resection vs. Abdominoperineal Resection

The frequency of abdominoperineal resection with definitive colostomy has decreased dramatically since the 1990s. Because of refinements and further developments of the surgical technique, the dissection of the rectum can now be performed into the intersphincteric space while maintaining natural continence (Ross et al. 2005). However, only a colorectal surgeon with special experience in the treatment of rectal carcinoma can decide whether such an ultralow anterior rectal resection is preferred over abdominoperineal resection. Digital rectal examination, rectoscopy, rectal ultrasound, and digital (and possibly manometric) examination of the sphincter function are required. Additionally, the classification of the rectal carcinoma has a major impact on the final decision. MRI is of limited value with respect to this surgical decision making. However, the findings obtained by the surgeon may be confirmed by MRI, which offers additional confidence.

1.9 Summary

Surgical therapy of rectal carcinoma has become very complex. The therapeutic options differ primarily with respect to their oncological radicality and their invasiveness. A rational decision for the therapy of choice strongly relies on the results of imaging procedures, mainly MRI. The surgeon referring rectal cancer patients for imaging should obtain the following information:

- Differentiation between T1 and T2 tumors
- Differentiation between T3 and T4 tumors
- Depth of mesorectal invasion
- Lymph node involvement inside and outside the mesorectum

In the future, surgeons expect cross-sectional imaging to provide more information on the effects of neoadjuvant therapy. Early detection of nonresponsive tumors and the differentiation between scar and viable tumor after completion of treatment are of high clinical relevance. Surgeons are eagerly awaiting new developments in this field.

In conclusion, only the close cooperation of an experienced multidisciplinary team of surgeons and radiologists will allow for the successful treatment of patients with rectal cancer. This clinical atlas will help the reader to detect and define decisive imaging features of rectal cancer.

References

Bretagnol F, Rullier E, George B et al (2007) Local therapy for rectal cancer: still controversial? Dis Colon Rectum 50:523–533

Glynne-Jones R, Mawdley S, Novell JR (2007) The clinical significance of the circumferential resection margin following preoperative chemo-radiotherapy in rectal cancer: why we need a common language. Colorectal Dis 8:800–807

Hida J, Yasutomi M, Fujimoto K et al (1997) Does lateral lymph node dissection improve survival in rectal carcinoma? Examination of node metastases by the clearing method. J Am Coll Surg 184:475–480

Idrees K, Paty PB (2006) Early rectal cancer: transanal excision or radical surgery? Adv Surg 40:239–248

Kapiteijn E, Marijnen CA, Nagtegaal ID et al (2001) Preoperative radiotherapy combined with total mesorectal excision for resectable rectal cancer. N Engl J Med 345:638–646

Merkel S, Mansmann U, Siassi M et al (2001) The prognostic inhomogeneity in pT3 rectal carcinomas. Int J Colorectal Dis 16:298–304

Quirke P, Durdey P, Dixon MF et al (1986) Local recurrence of rectal adenocarcinoma due to inadequate surgical resection. Histopathological study of lateral tumour spread and surgical excision Lancet 2:996–999

Ross HM, Mahmoud N, Fry RD (2005) The current management of rectal cancer. Curr Probl Surg 42:72–131

Sauer R, Becker H, Hohenberger W et al (2004) Preoperative versus postoperative chemoradiotherapy for rectal cancer. N Engl J Med 351:1731–1740

Wibe A, Moller B, Norstein J et al (2002) A national strategic change in treatment policy for rectal cancer – implementation of total mesorectal excision as routine treatment in Norway. A national audit. Dis Colon Rectum 45:857–866

Anorectal Anatomy

Clinical implications for the MR radiologist

Arnd-Oliver Schäfer

2

2.1 Introduction

Detailed knowledge of the anatomy of the rectum and its fascial relationships is one major prerequisite for both accurate diagnostic imaging and successful treatment. The rectum, interposed between the sigmoid colon and the anal canal, has a curved shape in humans and occupies the sacral hollow from the level of the promontory down to the coccyx (Moran and Jackson 1992). The rectum and anal canal are responsible for the storage and controlled evacuation of feces through sophisticated neuromuscular sphincter mechanisms (Salerno et al. 2006).

2.2 Anatomy and Embryology of the Rectum and the Perirectal Tissues

The upper rectum develops from the embryological hindgut (Williams and Warwick 1980). The lower part, derived from the cloaca, is surrounded by condensed extraperitoneal connective tissue (Bharucha 2006). The primitive gut tube is suspended dorsally by a mesentery throughout its length, which persists in the hindgut as the mesorectum (Heald and Moran 1998). During early prenatal life, the muscular layers of the rectum and anal canal derive from the mesenchyme that accompanies the endodermal part of the anorectum. The inner circular layer of the rectum precedes the outer longitudinal layer in the seventh week of human embryonic development.

The anlage of the levator ani muscle and the external anal sphincter muscle occur within the surrounding mesenchyme. They are clearly separated from each other. In the eighth week of development, they both show signs of proliferation activity when they get in contact with bundles of smooth muscle cells deriving from the outer longitudinal layer of the rectal wall. As a result, the levator ani muscle and external sphincter muscle grow larger and get in contact. A layer of undifferentiated mesenchyme separates the rectal muscular layers from the levator ani muscle as well as the muscular layer of the future anal canal from the external sphincter muscle (Aigner et al. 2007). The precise locations of both the proximal and distal end of the rectum are debatable. The rectosigmoid junction is considered to be at the level of S3 by anatomists, and at the sacral promontory by surgeons. The distal limit is regarded as the muscular anorectal ring by surgeons and as the dentate line by anatomists (Jorge and Wexner 1997). The rectum is 15- to 20-cm long and can be divided into three parts: the upper, middle, and lower rectum. From the anal verge, these three parts are defined as follows: the lower rectum, 0 to 6 cm; the middle rectum, 7 to 11 cm; and the upper rectum, 12 to 15 cm (Salerno et al. 2006).

Although not anatomically distinct, delineating the sections of the rectum is of great importance to the surgeon for the surgical treatment of rectal cancer. Anatomically, the sigmoid colon is differentiated from the rectum by the segmentation of the complete longitudinal muscle layer to form the taenia coli. Most parts of the rectum are extraperitoneal, although anteriorly the upper rectum is covered by a thin layer of visceral peritoneum around the front and sides down to the peritoneal reflection (Heald and Moran 1998).

A-O. Schäfer
Department of Diagnostic Radiology, Freiburg University Hospital, Hugstetter Strasse 55, 79106, Freiburg, Germany
e-mail: arnd-oliver.schaefer@uniklinik-freiburg.de

A-O. Schäfer, M. Langer, *MRI of Rectal Cancer,*
DOI: 10.1007/978-3-540-72833-7_2, © Springer-Verlag Berlin Heidelberg 2010

The peritoneal reflection is normally found between 7 and 9 cm from the anal verge. In women it may be lower, at 7.5 to 5 cm from the anal verge (Jorge and Wexner 1997). At its lower end, the rectum is angled forward by the puborectalis sling, forming the anorectal junction. Anteriorly, in women, the rectum is related to the posterior vaginal wall; in men, the rectum lies behind the prostate, seminal vesicles, vas deferens, and urinary bladder. The rectum exhibits lateral curves, which correspond on the intraluminal aspect to Houston's valves. There are usually three: two on the left side (at 7 to 8 cm and 12 to 13 cm) and one at 9 to 11 cm on the right side. The middle valve, termed Kohlrausch's valve, is the most consistent (Jorge and Wexner 1997).

2.2.1 Blood Supply

The rectum, which is part of the distal portion of the hindgut, is mainly supplied by the superior rectal artery, arising as a main branch from the inferior mesenteric artery (IMA). Similarly, the venous drainage of the hindgut, and therefore of the rectum, is to the inferior mesenteric vein into the portal system (Heald and Moran 1998). Veins from the upper two-thirds of the rectum are drained by the superior rectal vein. Veins from the lower third of the rectum are drained by the middle and inferior rectal veins into the internal iliac veins. The venous rectal drainage may explain why tumors of the lower rectum and anal canal can directly establish pulmonary metastases without hepatic metastases (Sakorafas et al. 2006). The relationship of the ureters to the IMA and superior rectal artery is of particular importance to the colorectal surgeon. Because the trunk deviates to the left, it passes close to the left ureter and left spermatic vessels, which are in danger during ligation of the IMA (Goligher 1967). The rectum is additionally supplied by the middle and inferior rectal arteries.

2.2.1.1 Superior Rectal Artery

The superior rectal artery (Fig. 2.1) typically continues in the same downward course as the IMA to reach the back of the upper third of the rectum. At this point, it bifurcates into two vessels, adjacent to the inferior portion of the pouch of Douglas and opposite the level of

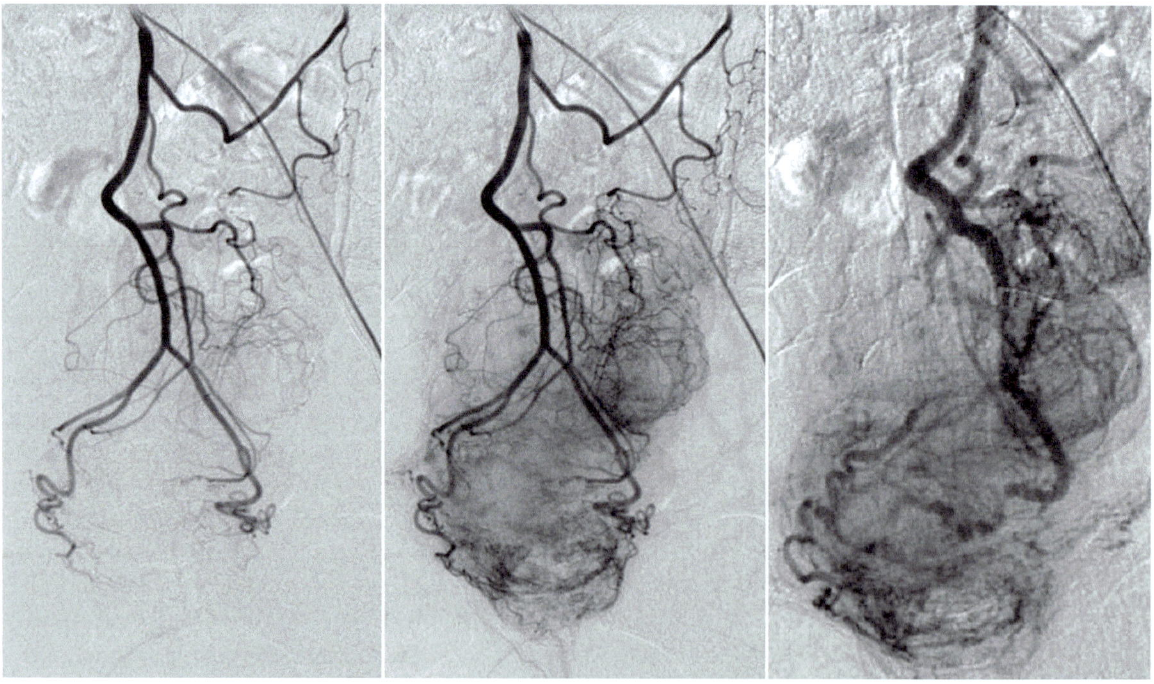

Fig. 2.1 DSA of the superior rectal artery and its branches and the accompanying superior rectal vein

S3 (Goligher 1967). The larger right branch supplies the posterior and lateral surface of the rectum. It divides into two main branches, which run down to the right anterior and posterior aspects of the rectum. The smaller left branch supplies the anterior surface of the rectum and continues undivided down the left lateral aspect of the rectum. These branches generally break up into smaller vessels that finally penetrate the muscle layer to reach the submucosa. Here they proceed downward as straight vessels, which run in the columns of Morgagni and terminate usually above the anal valves as a capillary plexus (Lin and Chaikof 2000; Sakorafas et al. 2006).

2.2.1.2 Middle Rectal Artery

The middle rectal arteries originate from the anterior divisions of the internal iliac arteries or from their inferior vesical branches. They proceed medially and forward below the pelvic peritoneum, in the tissue of the lateral ligaments, to reach the rectal wall. Here they anastomose with the branches of the superior and inferior rectal arteries. However, their arrangement is variable and the middle rectal artery may be absent (Goligher 1967; Lin and Chaikof 2000).

2.2.1.3 Inferior Rectal Artery

The inferior rectal arteries spring from the internal pudendal arteries in Alcock's canal in the fascia of the outer walls of the ischiorectal fossa. They run medially and slightly forward, dividing into branches that penetrate the external and internal anal sphincters, and finally reach the submucosa and subcutaneous tissue of the anal canal. These terminal branches communicate with arterial branches of the opposite side and possibly from the middle rectal arteries (Vogel and Klosterhalfen 1988).

2.2.2 Lymphatic Drainage

The disposition of lymph nodes tends to be relatively uniform throughout the entire gastrointestinal tract. Numerous small nodes are located adjacent to—or even on—the bowel wall. They drain to the larger nodes along the mesenteric vessels and subsequently to clustered nodes around the origins of the main arterial trunks (Heald and Moran 1998).

2.2.2.1 Intramural Lymphatics

In the submucous and subserous layer of the rectal wall, there are continuous lymphatic plexuses, which drain into the extramural lymphatics.

2.2.2.2 Extramural Lymphatics

The extramural lymphatics follow the blood vessels supplying the rectum and anal canal. Lymph from the parts of the rectum that receive blood supply from the superior rectal artery drains to superior rectal nodes after transversing pararectal nodes. From superior rectal nodes, lymph passes to inferior mesenteric nodes. The lymphatic drainage of the remainder of the rectum and anal canal is dependent on its relationship to the mucocutaneous junction. The area proximal to the mucocutaneous junction either drains superiorly (parallel to the middle rectal arteries on the corresponding pelvic sidewall) or traverses the levator ani muscle to follow the inferior rectal arteries. These two possible pathways lead to internal iliac nodes, common iliac nodes, and the lumbar trunk. Lymphatic drainage below the mucocutaneous junction does not parallel blood vessels. The collecting ducts pass anteriorly and superiorly in the perineum. Together with lymphatic channels from perianal skin, they pass to superficial inguinal nodes (Sakorafas et al. 2006).

2.2.3 Mesorectum and Fascial Structures

The pelvis is supported by the endopelvic fascia, which has two components: a visceral and a parietal layer. The visceral layer of the endopelvic fascia (fascia propria of the rectum) lines the rectum. It is a thin, transparent layer that maintains the integrity of the mesorectum. The parietal layer of the endopelvic fascia (presacral fascia) covers the sacrum. Violation of this layer exposes the sacral veins and is a potential source of severe bleeding during the mobilization of the rectum (Church et al. 1987; Kaiser and Ortega 2002). The mesorectum represents the enveloping mesentery of the rectum and is derived from the dorsal mesentery. This perirectal tissue compartment consists of adipose tissue that is subdivided by septa of connective tissue in adults. The mesorectum extends from the level of the peritoneal reflection down to the puborectalis muscle sling. Its outermost connective tissue lamella forms the rectal fascia and fuses with the superior fascia of the pelvic diaphragm, which is the covering fascia of the levator ani muscle. The perirectal tissue sheath is formed by a condensation of loose mesenchymal tissue surrounding the rectum in the early fetal stages (by the 9th week post conception). It develops along the terminal branches of the superior rectal artery containing the rectal nerves and lymphatics. During the later fetal stages (by the 16th week postconception), the mesenchymal tissue is replaced by dense connective tissue lamellae, forming the mesorectal fascia proper. This connective tissue layer gets thinner in the craniocaudal direction, completely vanishing beyond puborectalis muscle sling, beyond which there are virtually no perirectal lymphatic tissue or lymph nodes (Aigner et al. 2007).

The key concept of modern rectal surgery is to remain on the mesorectal fascia. The posterior surgical plane lies between this fascial layer of the mesorectum (visceral fascia) and the presacral fascia (parietal fascia), which covers the sacrum, coccyx, middle sacral artery, and presacral veins. Inferiorly, at the fourth sacral vertebra (S4 level), the visceral and the parietal fascia condense and form the rectosacral fascia, which represents a thick fascial reflection that runs anteroinferior to the presacral fascia, known as Waldeyer's fascia. The result of this fascial arrangement is a relatively avascular areolar tissue plane between the mesorectal fascia and the parietal pelvic fascia. Posteriorly to this "holy plane" of rectal surgery (the perimesorectal plane) is the presacral venous plexus, which is a structure at risk of damage during surgical procedures. Distal condensations of the mesorectal fascia form the lateral ligaments of the rectum, which may contain branches of the middle rectal arteries. These ligaments attach the rectum to the lateral pelvic sidewall (Jorge and Wexner 1997; Kaiser and Ortega 2002; Heald and Moran 1998).

2.2.3.1 Denonvillier's Fascia

The Denonvillier's fascia, the anterior surface of the mesorectum, is easier to identify in male patients. It is formed by the fusion of two layers of the primitive coelomic cavity during embryology. In males, a distinct plane separates the Denonvillier's fascia from the seminal vesicles in front. More distally, this fascia fuses with the fascia on the posterior surface of the prostate. Adjacent to its lateral aspects, the neurovascular bundles and inferior hypogastric plexuses pass medially. In females, the Denonvillier's fascia is less obvious and the anterior mesorectum less substantial (Heald and Moran 1998).

2.2.3.2 Pelvic Diaphragm

The pelvic floor (or diaphragm) is a musculotendineous termination of the pelvic outlet and allows the anorectal and urogenital viscera to pass through two hiatal openings (Strohbehn 1998). The levator ani muscle, which forms a symmetrical array of paired striated muscles (puborectalis; pubococcygeus; ileococcygeus; and the variable fourth component, the ischiococcygeus or coccygeus muscle), can be distinguished in the early fetal period (Fritsch and Froehlich 1994). These muscles are attached to the pubic body, the ischial spine, and the arcus tendinus—a condensation of the obturator fascia. The anococcygeal raphe is a fibrous condensation of the iliococcygeus muscle in the posterior midline. The important puborectalis muscle forms a strong, U-shaped sling of striated muscle that pulls the anorectal junction anteriorly to the posterior aspect of the pubis. The resulting effect is an angulation between the rectum and anal canal (the anorectal angle). The puborectalis sling relaxes during defecation, thereby widening the anorectal angle and straightening the rectum (Jorge and Wexner 1997; Kaiser and Ortega 2002).

2.2.4 Anal Canal

In adults, the rectal wall is composed of the mucosa, submucosa, and muscularis propria. The muscularis propria has an inner circular layer and an outer longitudinal layer. The longitudinal muscle of the rectum fuses with striated fibers of the levator ani and puborectalis muscle at the level of the anorectal ring, forming the conjoined longitudinal muscle. At the level of the puborectalis portion of the levator ani muscle, the rectal adventitia constitutes a thin, microscopic layer that is interposed between the outer longitudinal muscular layer and the inner fascia of the levator ani muscle. The wall of the anal canal is composed of the mucosa, submucosa, and muscularis. The muscularis is composed of a thick inner circular layer (the inner sphincter) and an outer longitudinal layer that is composed of a small layer of connective tissue (the intersphincteric space). The latter separates the longitudinal layer from the striated external sphincter (Aigner et al. 2007). The sphincter muscles form an anteroposterior slit, which is the anal canal. The anal valves and the distal end of the ampullary part of the rectum mark the proximal margin of the anal canal. The proximal 10 mm of the anal canal are lined by columnar, rectal-type mucosa. The following 15 mm, including the valves, are lined by stratified epithelium. Distal to that is approximately 10 mm of thick, non-hairy stratified epithelium. The most distal 5 to 10 mm are lined by hairy skin (Bharucha 2006). Histological measurements of the length of the surgical anal canal (anorectal ring to anal verge) demonstrated an average length of 4.2 cm. The average length of the anal canal from the dentate line to the anal verge (anatomical anal canal) is about 2.1 cm (Salerno et al. 2006).

2.2.5 *Pararectal and Para-Anal Spaces*

The anorectum comprises clinically relevant spaces, including the ischiorectal, perianal, intersphincteric, submucous, superficial postanal, deep postanal, supralevator, and retrorectal spaces. The ischiorectal fossa is subdivided by a thin horizontal fascia into two spaces: the perianal and the ischiorectal space. The ischiorectal space occupies the upper two-thirds of the ischiorectal fossa. It forms a pyramid-shaped space between the anal canal and the lower part of the rectum medially and the pelvic sidewall laterally. The ischiorectal fossa includes fat, the inferior rectal vessels, and nerves. The perianal space envelops the lower portion of the anal canal. It runs laterally with the subcutaneous fat of the buttocks and extends medially into the intersphincteric space. The intersphincteric space is a potential space between the internal and external anal sphincter muscles. The superficial postanal space is between the anococcygeal ligament and the skin, and the deep postanal space lies between the anococcygeal ligament and the anococcygeal raphe. The supralevator spaces are between the peritoneum superiorly and the levator ani muscle inferiorly. These bilateral spaces are medial to the rectum and lateral to the obturator fascia. The retrorectal space is located between the fascia propria of the rectum anteriorly and the presacral fascia posteriorly. The lateral rectal ligaments are laterally located and the rectosacral ligament is inferiorly located; above, the retrorectal space is continuous with the retroperitoneum (Jorge and Wexner 1997).

2.3 MRI of Rectal Anatomy: Important Landmarks

According to the work of Brown and colleagues (2004) thin-section magnetic resonance imaging (MRI) performed with a pelvic phased-array coil provides sufficient accuracy to depict fine details of the rectal wall, the anal sphincter, the mesorectum, and the pelvic sidewall. Fourth branches of the IMA and lymph nodes as small as 2 mm can be consistently identified.

2.3.1 *Parietal Fascia*

On MRI, the parietal fascia appears isointense relative to the signal intensity of muscle. It is often not detectable as a separate structure except anterolaterally, where it appears as a separate layer overlying the internal obturator muscle.

2.3.2 *Retrorectal Space*

The retrorectal space is limited anteriorly by the mesorectal fascia and posteriorly by the presacral parietal fascia. The presacral fascia is best visualized on sagittal MRI as a low-intensity linear structure covering the presacral vessels (Fig. 2.2).

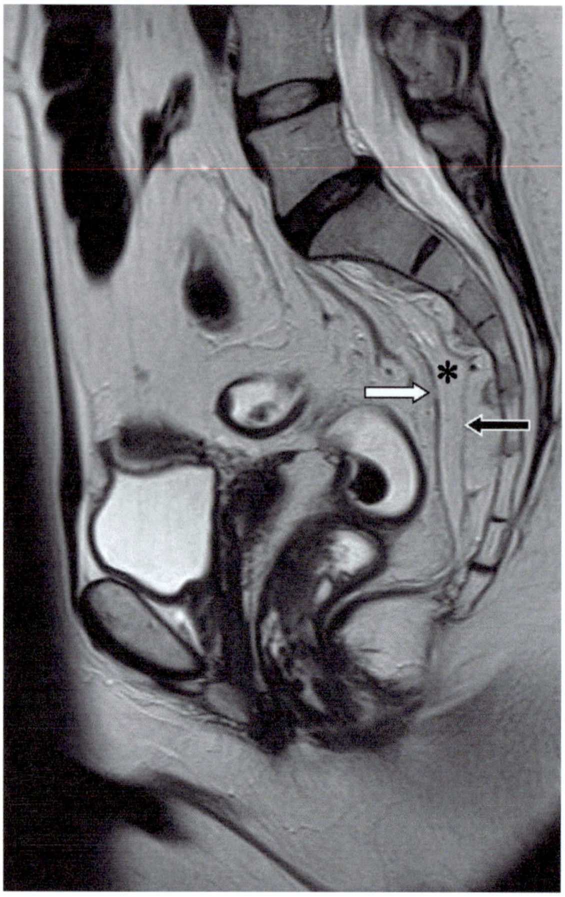

Fig. 2.2 Retrorectal space. On the sagittal T2-TSE image, the retrorectal space is clearly outlined in this obese rectal cancer patient (*asterisk*) delimited by the presacral fascia dorsally and the mesorectal fascia ventrally (*arrows*)

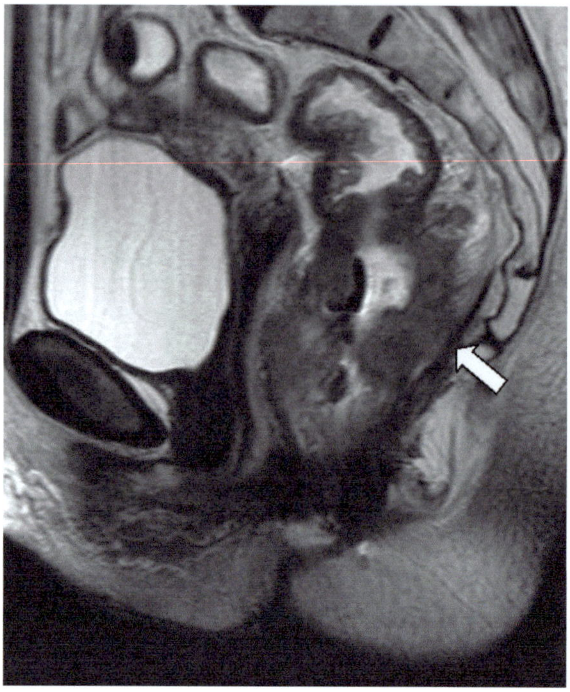

Fig. 2.3 Rectosacral fascia. Sagittal T2-TSE image displays Waldeyer's fascia in a patient with a locally advanced rectal cancer (*arrow*)

2.3.3 Rectosacral Fascia

The rectosacral fascia represents an inconstantly visible fascial band of variable thickness on MRI, running from the sacrum to the mesorectal fascia at the S4 level (Fig. 2.3).

2.3.4 Peritoneal Reflection

From the uppermost part of the posterior surface of the bladder, the peritoneum extends posteriorly to the junction of the upper two-thirds and lower one-third of the rectum in males. In females, the site of attachment in the lower one-third of the rectum is more varied. The peritoneum-lined recess between the rectum and the posterior aspect of the bladder is the rectovesical pouch. On sagittal MRI, the peritoneal reflection appears as a low-signal-intensity linear structure (Fig. 2.4). The peritoneum attaches in a V-shaped manner onto the anterior aspect of the rectum—the "seagull" sign (Fig. 2.5).

2.3.5 Denonvillier's Fascia

Current MRI is capable of distinctly visualizing the anterior surface of the mesorectum (Denonvillier's fascia), which has a low signal intensity and can be traced up to peritoneum in the sagittal plane (Fig. 2.6).

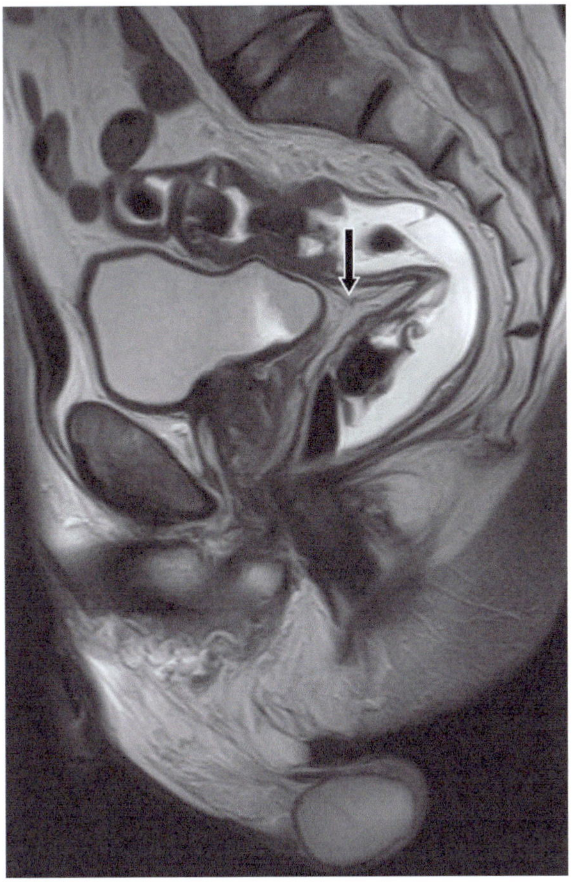

Fig. 2.4 Peritoneal reflection. The peritoneal reflection appears as a thin linear structure attached to the anterior aspect of the midrectum (*arrow*)

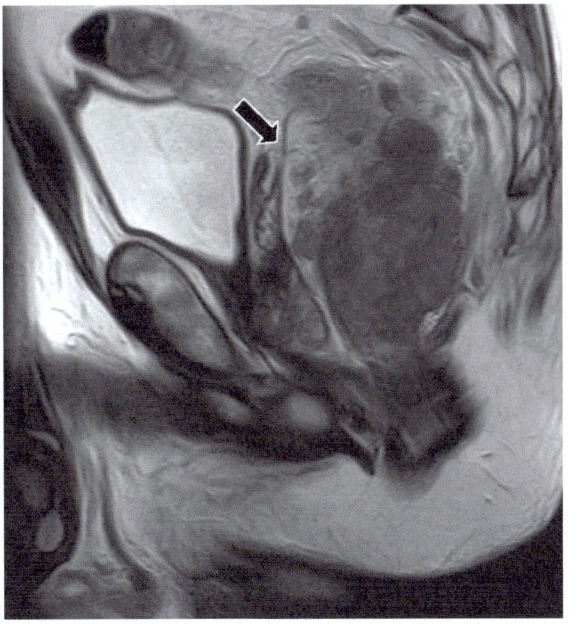

Fig. 2.6 Denonvillier's fascia. Delineation of the anterior surface of the mesoractal fascia om the sagittal T2-TSE image of a patient with advanced rectal cancer (*arrow*)

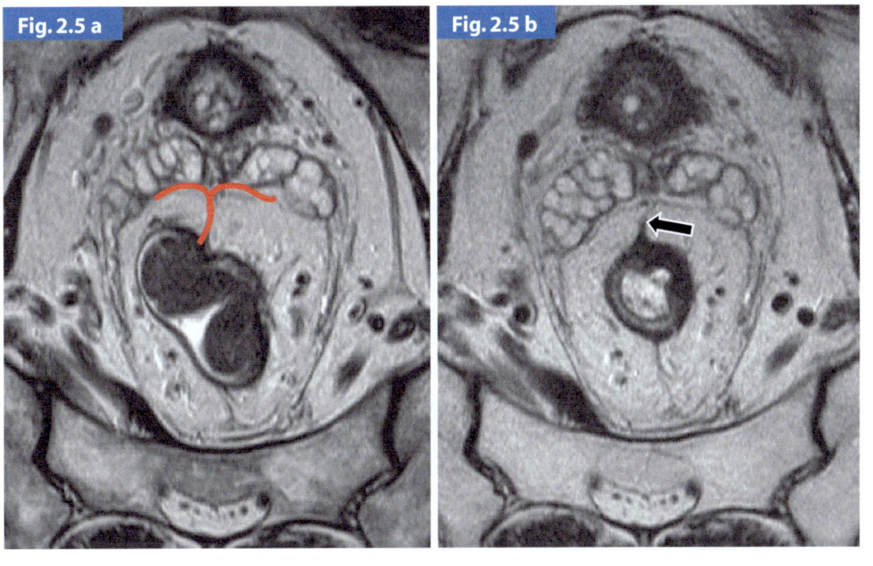

Fig. 2.5 Peritoneal reflection. The corresponding para-axial T2-TSE images of a rectal cancer patient before (**a**) and after (**b**) neoadjuvant chemoradiation reveal the relationship of the peritoneal reflection at the anterior rectal wall. The peritoneal attachment forms the seagull sing (indicated as *red lines* in (**a**), *arrow* in (**b**))

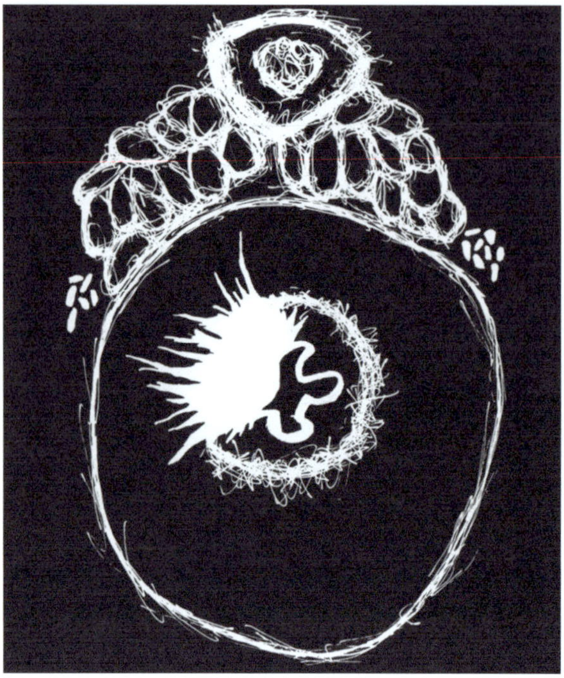

Fig. 2.7 Ink drawing: mesorectum and mesorectal fasia

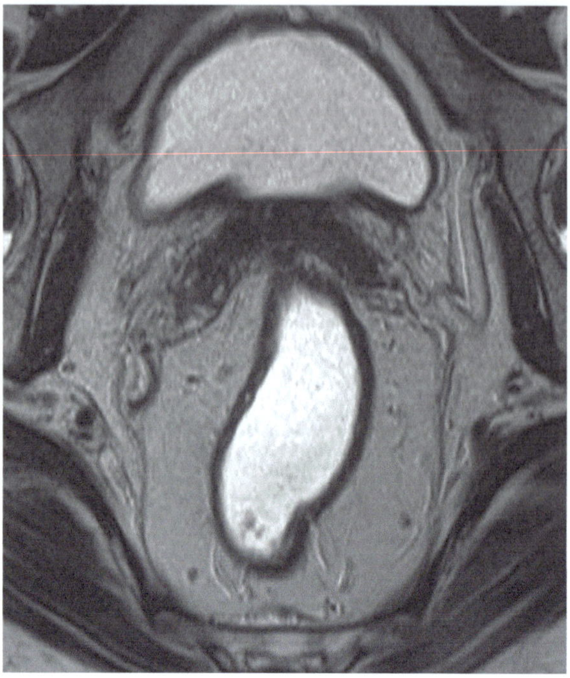

Fig. 2.8 Mesorectum and mesorectal fascia. Para-axial view of a T2-TSE sequence clearly displays the boders of the mesorectum which is surrounded by a thin low-signal band corresponding to the mesorectal fascia

2.3.6 Mesorectal Fascia and Mesorectum

The mesorectal fascia is best seen on axial images. It appears as a fine low-signal-intensity structure enveloping the mesorectum. The mesorectum contains fatty tissue, vessels, and lymphatics. It is of high signal intensity on T2-weighted MRI with fast spin-echo sequences (Figs. 2.7 and 2.8).

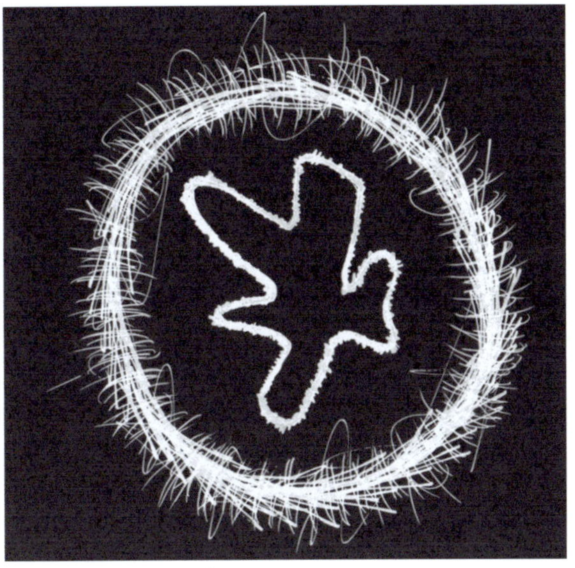

Fig. 2.9 Ink drawing: rectal wall layers

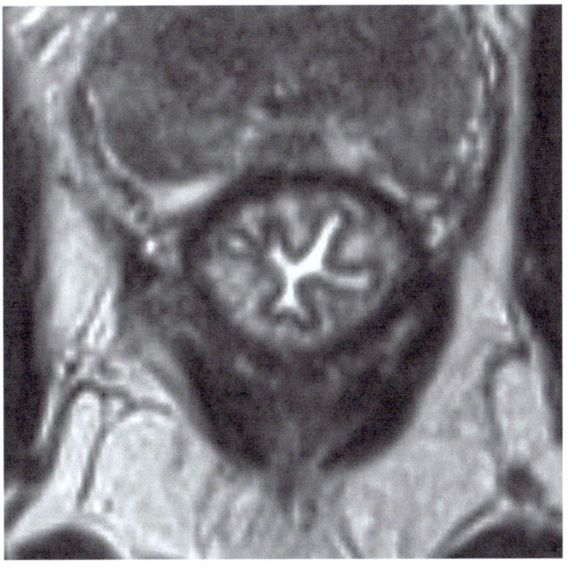

Fig. 2.10 Rectal wall layers. Typical signal behavior and architecture of the rectal wall components on the para-axial heavily T2-weighted TSE image

2.3.7 Rectal Wall

Histologically, the rectal wall consists of three layers that are of utmost importance for cross-sectional tumor staging: the mucosa, the submucosa, and the muscularis propria. They can be identified on axial T2-weighted MRI. The rectal lumen is surrounded by the mucosa, which is detectable as a thin hypointense line. It is followed by the submucosa, which appears as a thicker band of higher signal. The muscularis propria forms the outer low-signal-intensity layer (Figs. 2.9 and 2.10).

References

Aigner F, Trieb T, Öfner D et al (2007) Anatomical considerations in TNM staging and therapeutical procedures for low rectal cancer. Int J Colorectal Dis 22:1339–1342

Bharucha AE (2006). Pelvic floor: anatomy and function. Neurogastroenterol Motil 18:507–519

Brown G, Kirkham A, Williams GT et al (2004) High-resolution MRI of the anatomy important in total mesorectal excision of the rectum. AJR Am J Roentgenol 182:431–439

Church JM, Raudkivi PJ, Hill GL (1987) The surgical anatomy of the rectum – a review with particular relevance to the hazards of rectal mobilisation. Int J Colorectal Dis 2:158–166

Fritsch H, Froehlich B (1994) Development of the levator ani muscle in human fetuses. Early Hum Dev 37:15–25

Goligher JC (ed) (1967) Surgical anatomy and physiology of the colon, rectum, and anus. In: Surgery of the Anus, Rectum, and Colon, 2nd edn. Bailliere, Tindall & Cassell, London, pp 1–54

Heald RJ, Moran BJ (1998) Embryology and anatomy of the rectum. Semin Surg Oncol 15:66–71

Jorge JM, Wexner SD (1997) Anatomy and physiology of the rectum and anus. Eur J Surg 163:723–731

Kaiser AM, Ortega AE (2002) Anorectal anatomy. Surg Clin North Am 82:1125–1138

Lin PH, Chaikof EL (2000) Embryology, anatomy, and surgical exposure of the great abdominal vessels. Surg Clin North Am 80:417–433

Moran BJ, Jackson AA (1992) Function of the human colon. Br J Surg 79:1132–1137

Sakorafas GH, Zouros E, Peros G (2006) Applied vascular anatomy of the colon and rectum: clinical implications for the surgical oncologist. Surg Oncol 15:243–255

Salerno G, Sinnatambi C, Branagan G et al (2006) Defining the rectum: surgically, radiologically and anatomically. Colorectal Dis 8:5–9

Strohbehn K (1998) Normal pelvic floor anatomy. Obstet Gynecol Clin North Am 25:683–705

Vogel P, Klosterhalfen B (1988) The surgical anatomy of the rectal and anal blood vessels. Langenbecks Arch Chir 373:264–269

Williams PL, Warwick R (eds) (1980) Splanchnology. In: Gray's Anatomy, 36th edn. Churchill Livingstone, London, pp 1356–1364

3 Pathology of Rectal Cancer

Thorsten Wiech and Martin Werner

3.1 Introduction

Treatment of rectal cancer requires an interdisciplinary approach, with imaging techniques and morphological examination playing important roles. The pathologist is involved in several steps of diagnostics and treatment planning for patients with rectal tumors. Starting with the preoperative biopsy, the pathologist confirms the diagnosis of cancer and estimates the biological behavior of the tumor by classification and grading. Intraoperative diagnostics ensure the completeness of resection and postoperative examinations provide final histopathological and pTNM-classification. Additionally, information about the therapeutic response to neoadjuvant strategies is provided by the assessment of tumor regression. By including molecular pathological methods, the pathologist can evaluate predictive markers (e.g., *KRAS* mutation analysis for antibody therapy) and contribute to the diagnosis of hereditary nonpolyposis colorectal cancer (HNPCC) by analyzing microsatellite instability. This chapter describes the role of pathology in the management of rectal cancer.

3.2 Preoperative Biopsy

Endoscopically visualized carcinomas must be confirmed by biopsy and histopathological examination in order to exclude lesions that may grossly resemble carcinoma, such as solitary rectal ulcers due to prolapse. Rectal ulcers with reactive hyperplasia in the everted edge, which mimic adjacent adenoma, can be particularly difficult to distinguish macroscopically from ulcerating adenocarcinoma arising in an adenoma. Other differential diagnoses include scarring after diverticulitis. For a high level of diagnostic accuracy, at least five to six biopsies should be taken from the center and the margin of the lesion. If a biopsy is taken from the outer periphery, it will likely show noninvasive adenomatous characteristics. In contrast, if the biopsy is taken from the very center of the lesion, it may consist exclusively of necrotic tissue. Thus, several biopsies should be taken to ensure that enough malignant tissue is present to confirm the diagnosis (Fig. 3.1).

3.2.1 Histologic Classification

Histopathologic classification is performed according to the *World Health Organization Classification of Tumours* (Hamilton et al. 2000). Rectal carcinoma is defined as a malignant epithelial tumor of the rectum that has invaded through the muscularis mucosae. In contrast, adenomas, representing precursor lesions of colorectal carcinoma, are noninvasive but show cellular dysplasia (i.e., intraepithelial neoplasia). Most adenomas have hyperchromatic and stratified spindle-shaped nuclei with varying degrees of loss of polarity and cellular atypia (i.e., low-grade and high-grade intraepithelial neoplasia). The typical invasive adenocarcinoma, accounting for the vast majority of rectal cancer, consists of epithelial columnar cells arranged in a glandular pattern. These tumor glands, or tubules, range in size and shape from small round tubules to large irregular glands; they occasionally exhibit papillary

T. Wiech (✉)
Institute of Pathology, Freiburg University Hospital, Breisacher Strasse 115a, 79106 Freiburg, Germany
e-mail: thorsten.wiech@uniklinik-freiburg.de

A-O. Schäfer, M. Langer, *MRI of Rectal Cancer*,
DOI: 10.1007/978-3-540-72833-7_3, © Springer-Verlag Berlin Heidelberg 2010

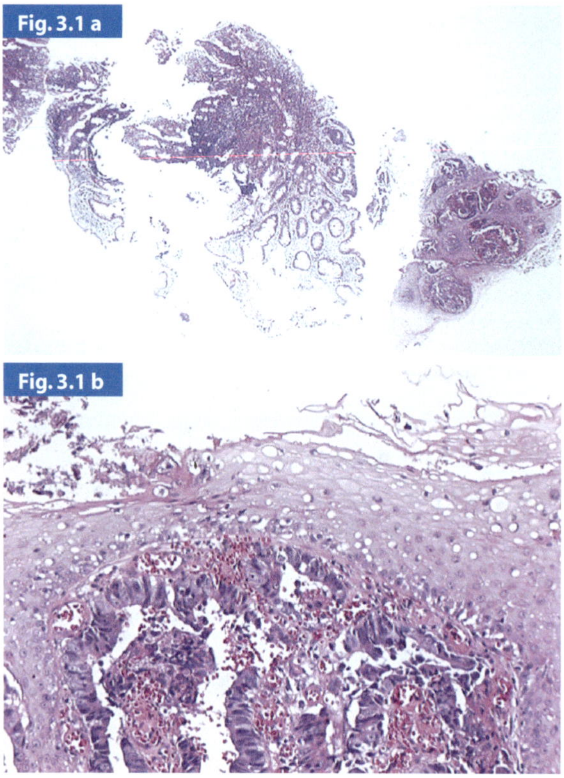

Fig. 3.1 Microphotographs of a preoperative biopsy: (**a**) overview of the particles (H&E, ×10), (**b**) adenocarcinoma glands as subepithelial infiltrates beneath the anal squamous epithelium (H&E, ×100)

configured epithelium. Intraglandular cellular debris is typically present, and the tumor glands are usually surrounded by desmoplastic stroma with some T-lymphocytic infiltrates. Mucin production can be demonstrated by periodic acid Schiff staining. If more than 50% of the lesion consists of mucin, the tumor is classified as mucinous adenocarcinoma, which is one of the subtypes associated with microsatellite instability. Another variant, consisting of more than 50% tumor cells which show intracytoplasmic mucin vacuoles, displacing the nuclei, is the signet-ring carcinoma, often showing diffuse infiltration and worse prognosis. However, because the biopsy might not be representative of the entire tumor, a final histopathological classification should be made using the resection specimen.

Several types of benign or malignant nonepithelial tumors may occur in the rectum, including lipomas, leiomyomas, gastrointestinal stromal tumors, sarcomas, melanomas, and lymphomas. Because some of these tumor types may endoscopically and radiologically resemble the much more frequent adenocarcinoma but require distinctly different treatment strategies, rectal tumors should be classified histopathologically by preoperative biopsy. Moreover, rectal metastases that are secondary tumors from other sites (e.g., breast or lung cancer) and the direct invasion of tumors from neighboring organs (e.g., gynecologic or urologic carcinomas) must be distinguished from primary rectal tumors.

An overview of the histologic types of epithelial tumors of the colon and rectum is shown in Table 3.1 (Fig. 3.2).

Table 3.1 WHO classification of epithelial tumors of the colon and rectum (Hamilton et al. 2000)

Adenoma	Tubular Villous Tubulovillous Serrated
Intraepithelial neoplasia associated with chronic inflammatory diseases	Low grade High grade
Carcinoma	Adenocarcinoma Mucinous adenocarcinoma Signet-ring cell carcinoma Small cell carcinoma Squamous cell carcinoma Adenosquamous carcinoma Medullary carcinoma Undifferentiated carcinoma
Carcinoid	
Mixed carcinoid-adenocarcinoma	
Others	

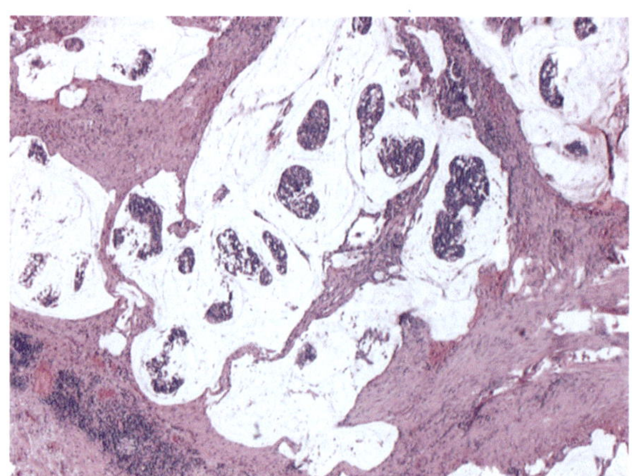

Fig. 3.2 Mucinous adenocarcinoma (H&E, ×25)

3.2.2 Grading

Adenocarcinomas are graded as well-differentiated (grade 1), moderately differentiated (grade 2), poorly differentiated (grade 3), and undifferentiated (grade 4) tumors. The major criteria for grading adenocarcinomas are the proportions of gland formation (see Table 3.2) and mucin production of the tumor cells. As an exception, mucinous adenocarcinomas and signet-ring cell carcinomas are, per definition, graded as poorly differentiated (grade 3). Because many adenocarcinomas show heterogeneity with different growth patterns and grades of cellular differentiation in different areas, grading should be re-evaluated on numerous sections of the resection specimen (Fig. 3.3).

3.2.3 Tumor Spread

The histopathologic report of the biopsy includes a statement about the portion of tissue being infiltrated by the tumor. In addition, the report documents whether the deeper layers of the rectum are included in the biopsy and, if so, whether tumor infiltrates are present. Because carcinoma cells that are confined to the mucosa virtually never show metastases, the most important feature of rectal adenocarcinoma is the infiltration of the muscularis mucosae into the submucosa. Thus, pure carcinomas of the epithelium or mucosa can be classified as high-grade intraepithelial neoplasia or intramucosal neoplasia instead of adenocarcinoma in situ or intramucosal adenocarcinoma, respectively. Finally, the report includes information about the possibility of tumor invasion into blood or lymphatic vessels.

Table 3.2 Grading of adenocarcinomas of the colon and rectum (Hamilton et al. 2000)

Histologic grade	Differentiation	Percent glandular structures
Grade 1	Well differentiated	>95%
Grade 2	Moderately differentiated	50–95%
Grade 3	Poorly differentiated	5–50%
Grade 4	Undifferentiated	<5%

3.3 Intraoperative Diagnostics

Intraoperative pathologic examination is performed particularly when involvement of the oral and aboral resection margins is suspected. Sufficient fixation is required for definitive staging. Formalin-fixed tissue can be cut into thinner slices without artificial changes, allowing for better determination of the deepest portion of tumor.

3.3.1 Macroscopy of the Fresh Specimen

The resected specimen is first inspected macroscopically and the length of the segment is recorded. The quality of the total mesorectal excision, which is performed for carcinomas of the middle and lower third,

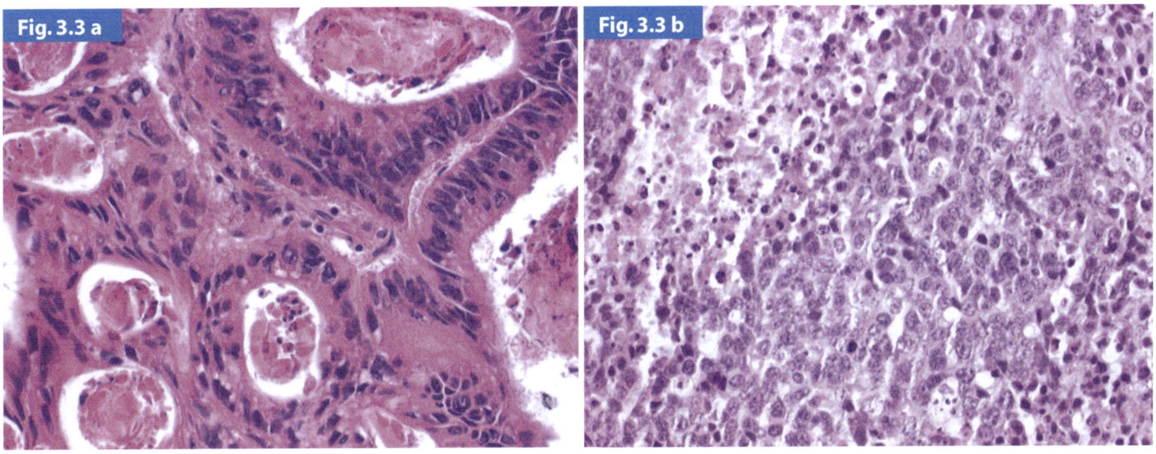

Fig. 3.3 (**a**) Moderately differentiated adenocarcinoma (G2; H&E, ×200). (**b**) Undifferentiated carcinoma (G4; H&E, ×200)

Table 3.3 Grading of quality and completeness of the mesorectum in a total mesorectal excision specimen (Parfitt and Driman 2007)

	Mesorectum	Defects	Coning	CRM
Complete	Intact, smooth	Not deeper than 5 mm	None	Smooth, regular
Nearly complete	Moderate bulk, irregular	No visible muscularis propria	Moderate	Irregular
Incomplete	Little bulk	Down to muscularis propria	Moderate – marked	Irregular

CRM, circumferential resection margin

is then evaluated. After opening the segment, the tumor appearance (e.g., polypoid or ulcerative) and the localization with regard to the enteral resection margins are documented. Additionally, for the purpose of documentation, the exact tumor size may be recorded in three dimensions. Although it has no effect on the clinical outcome (Compton et al. 2000), these measurements can be correlated with the size determined by imaging modalities for quality control or with other parameters for research purposes.

3.3.2 Mesorectum

Before the specimen is opened, the quality of the mesorectal excision is assessed by visual inspection of the fresh specimen. The completeness of resection can be ranked by evaluation of different parameters, such as the depth of eventual defects, coning of the mesorectum, and the regularity of the circumferential resection margin (see Table 3.3).

Because the quality of the mesorectum seems to be related to the involvement of the circumferential resection margin, its assessment is of high importance in estimating the risk of local recurrence. Additionally, this will provide feedback to the surgeon on the quality and completeness of the procedure (Fig. 3.4).

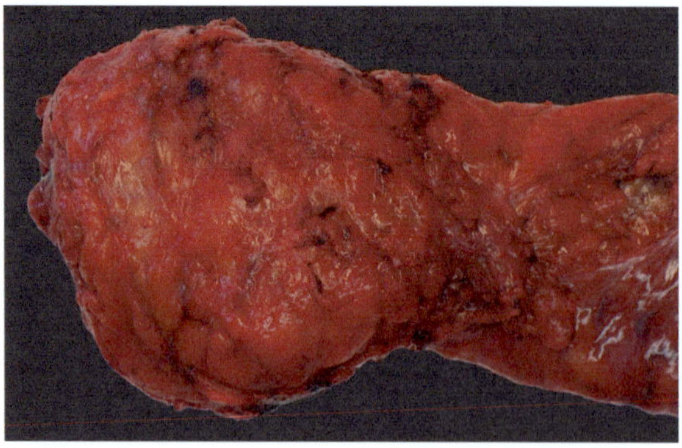

Fig. 3.4 Gross appearance of a complete mesorectal excision

3.3.3 Resection Margins

Tumor involvement of the resection margins is associated with local recurrence. For this reason, the enteral oral (proximal) and the enteral aboral (distal) margins should be assessed by frozen sections to determine whether the margins must be extended. However, tumor infiltration of the oral margin is extremely rare, and the aboral margin is infiltrated in less than 2% of cases. In contrast, the circumferential resection margin is infiltrated by tumor cells in nearly 20% of cases (Nagtedaal and van Krieken 2002; Wang et al. 2005).

The circumferential margin is one of the most important prognostic factors because it predicts the risk of local tumor recurrence. The margin should be carefully assessed after inking and sufficient fixation of the specimen.

3.4 Postoperative Diagnostics

For appropriate fixation, the fresh specimen should be pinned on a corkboard with an underlying soaked piece of cellulose or gauze to facilitate formalin diffusion into the perimuscular soft tissue. The specimen is usually placed in formalin at least 24 hours prior to fixation (Fig. 3.5).

3.4.1 Macroscopy of the Fixed Specimen

In addition to recording the tumor size in three dimensions and the distance to the three resection margins (oral, aboral, deep/circumferential), the gross appearance is also described. Most adenocarcinomas of the rectum are centrally ulcerating with a raised, everted edge. A small percentage of tumors appear as either as polypoid tumors without central ulceration or as flat, depressed tumors that show no evidence of originating from adenoma. Circumferential growth of the tumor

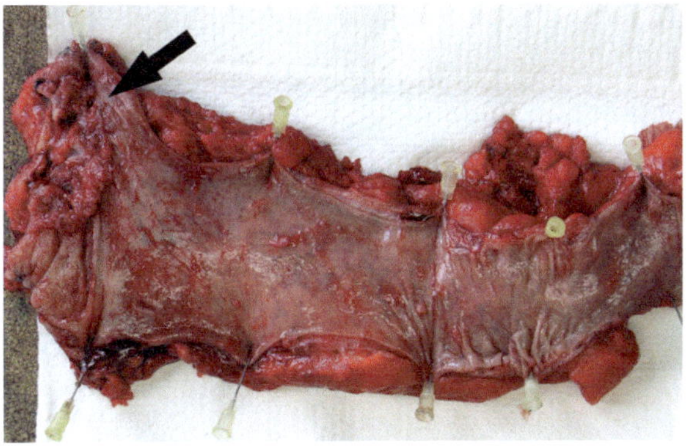

Fig. 3.5 Opened fresh resection specimen pinned on a corkboard before formalin fixation. *Arrow*: deep rectal carcinoma close at the aboral resection margin

may cause stenosis with dilatation of the oral portion of the segment. On the cross cut, the normally white to grayish tumor tissue infiltrates the bowel wall and may contain yellow (necrotic) and/or gelatinous (mucinous) areas. There may be relatively well-demarcated edges or finger-like infiltrations. Veins are examined for possible intraluminal tumor masses. All lymph nodes are removed for histologic evaluation after the size of the largest node is recorded. The entire mucosa is inspected for further changes, such as diverticula, erosions, polyps, or other carcinomas.

3.4.1.1 Tumor Spread

For TNM classification, the primary tumor is lamellated into 3- to 5-mm slices with regard to the inked deep/circumferential resection margin. The deepest intramural extension of the tumor and eventual transmural infiltration of the perirectal soft tissue are recorded and re-evaluated histologically. All lymph nodes in the perirectal tissue should be prepared for histologic evaluation.

3.4.1.2 Block Selection

Probes from the oral and aboral enteral resection margins, which contain mucosa and perirectal soft tissue, should be embedded. At least three blocks of the tumor are taken, including the areas closest to the deep/circumferential margin, the deepest infiltration into the wall, grossly remarkable areas such as mucinous parts of the tumor, and luminal areas within the transition zone from adenoma or nonneoplastic mucosa. Moreover, all lymph nodes of the perimuscular soft tissue should be sampled. If an involved lymph node is close to the circumferential margin, it should be embedded, including the inked margin. Finally, all visible polyps, conspicuous mucosal areas, and veins that are grossly suspicious for tumor infiltrates should be taken for histology.

3.4.2 Histopathology

Histopathologic examination of tissue block sections is performed to establish definite classification, grading, staging, and evaluation of the resection status of the tumor. Although in many cases the classification and grading of these results are in accordance with the preoperative biopsy, the gross inspection of the specimen (staging) and the intraoperative diagnosis (resection status) can differ. These differences may be due to tumor heterogeneity according to the classification and grading, or small, macroscopically invisible tumor infiltrates, and may lead to a revision of staging, nodal status, or resection status. Thus, it is important to re-evaluate these features on tissue sections cut from the fixed specimen.

3.4.2.1 Histologic Classification and Grading

Histologic classification of the tumor is performed according to the World Health Organization scheme (Hamilton et al. 2000) as described for preoperative biopsies above (see Table 3.1). Most rectal carcinomas are gland-forming adenocarcinomas, but some special types have to be distinguished because they may exhibit different biologic behavior. A small biopsy may be insufficient for correct diagnosis because it may be not representative of the whole tumor due to heterogenous histology. This particularly applies to three tumor subtypes: (a) signet-ring carcinoma, as per definition it consists of more than 50% tumor cells with prominent cytoplasmic mucin; (b) mucinous adenocarcinoma that shows more than 50% extracellular mucin; and (c) adenosquamous carcinoma, which is defined as a carcinoma with more than occasional small foci of squamous differentiation together with a gland-forming tumor part.

Grading of tumor differentiation is performed as described above, with the main criterion being the percentage of glandular tumor growth (Hamilton et al. 2000).

Regarding the possible heterogeneity of differentiation, grading is based on the tumor section with the highest grade corresponding to the least differentiation, unless this section is restricted to a small invasion of the tumor.

3.4.2.2 pTNM Classification

The TNM classification of rectal carcinomas, which replaced the Dukes classification, is based on the extension of the tumor into the wall as proposed by Dukes (Sobin and Wittekind 2002; Table 3.4). The prefix *p* in pTNM indicates the pathologic (postsurgical histopathologic) classification as compared with the clinical classification (i.e., TNM or cTNM). An important prognostic feature of the primary tumor (pT) is the invasion through the muscularis mucosae, because this increases the probability of lymphogenous and hematogenous metastases. Usually, 12 or more regional lymph nodes will be found in the perimuscular soft tissue for histologic examination (pN). Because only the primary tumor and not the distant metastases may be surgically removed, it is often difficult for the pathologist to exactly assess the pM-classification (Fig. 3.6).

3.4.2.3 Venous, Lymphatic Vessel, and Perineural Invasion

In addition to the TNM classification, the optional descriptors provide information about an eventual tumor invasion into venous (V) or lymphatic (L) vessels, or into nerve sheaths (Pn). These features are classified analogously to the TNM system, as shown in Table 3.5. Nodular infiltrates in the perirectal soft tissue without visible lymph node tissue are classified according to their contour. If they are smooth, they will be classified as lymph node metastasis. If they are irregular, they will be classified as a discontinuous part of the primary tumor (T) or as venous infiltration (V1 or V2) (Sobin and Wittekind 2002) (Fig. 3.7).

3.4.2.4 Resection Status

According to the general rules of the TNM system (Sobin and Wittekind 2002), the residual tumor is assessed by evaluation of the three resection margins: (a) the enteral oral, (b) the enteral aboral, and (c) the

Table 3.4 pTNM classification of carcinomas of the colon and rectum (Sobin and Wittekind 2002)

pT – Primary tumor	
pTX	Primary tumor cannot be assessed
pT0	No evidence of primary tumor
pTis	Carcinoma in situ: intraepithelial or invasion of lamina propria
pT1	Tumor invades submucosa
pT2	Tumor invades muscularis propria
pT3	Tumor invades through muscularis propria into subserosa or into nonperitonealized pericolic or perirectal tissues
pT4	Tumor directly invades other organs or structures and/or perforates visceral peritoneum
pN – Regional lymph nodes	
pNX	Regional lymph nodes cannot be assessed
pN0	No regional lymph node metastasis
pN1	Metastasis in 1–3 regional lymph nodes
pN2	Metastasis in four or more regional lymph nodes
pM – Distant metastasis	
pMX	Distant metastasis cannot be assessed
pM0	No distant metastasis
pM1	Distant metastasis

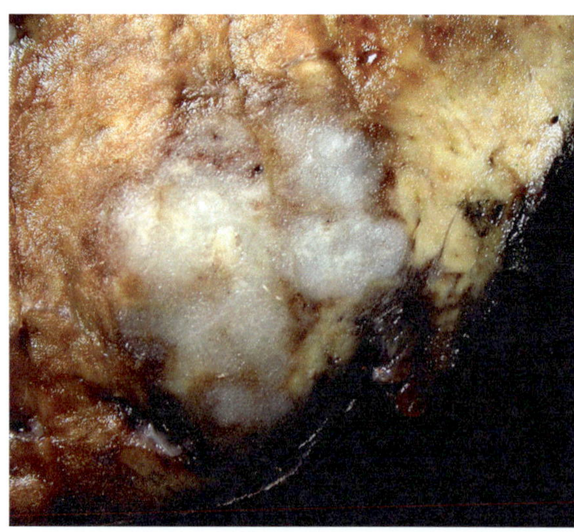

Fig. 3.6 Gross appearance of a section through a liver metastasis of a rectal adenocarcinoma (formalin-fixed)

Table 3.5 Optional descriptors (Sobin and Wittekind 2002)

V – Venous invasion	
VX	Venous invasion cannot be assessed
V0	No venous invasion
V1	Microscopic venous invasion
V2	Macroscopic venous invasion
L – Lymphatic invasion	
LX	Lymphatic invasion cannot be assessed
L0	No lymphatic invasion
L1	Lymphatic invasion
Pn – Perineural invasion	
PnX	Perineural invasion cannot be assessed
Pn0	No perineural invasion
Pn1	Perineural invasion

circumferential/deep resection margin. The presence or absence of residual tumor is described by the R classification (Table 3.6), which distinguishes whether the residual tumor on the resection margin is visible macroscopically (R2) or only microscopically (R1). There are two possible ways that tumor growth may involve the circumferential margin: direct infiltration or lymph node metastases in the resection margin. Both are classified as positive margins (R1) according to the International Union Against Cancer. However, direct infiltration appears to be more closely correlated to local tumor recurrence than the presence of lymph node metastases at the resection margin (Nagtegaal and Quirke 2008).

Table 3.6 Residual tumor classification (Sobin and Wittekind 2002)

R – Residual tumor	
RX	Presence of residual tumor cannot be assessed
R0	No residual tumor
R1	Microscopic residual tumor
R2	Macroscopic residual tumor

3.5 Tumor Regression

Assessment of tumor regression after neoadjuvant therapy is an important part of the pathologic examination because histologic regression grading has been shown to represent a prognostic factor in rectal cancer (Benzoni et al. 2006).

In contrast with pTNM, which is used for classification of the tumor before therapy, ypTNM is used for classification of the tumor after neoadjuvant therapy. The ypTNM classification reflects the tumor spread to vital tumor cells. If, for example, there is mucus without tumor cells in the perimuscular soft tissue, the tumor is classified as ypT2 rather than ypT3 (Wittekind and Tannapfel 2003). There is currently no international agreement regarding the histopathologic grading of colorectal carcinoma regression. Some proposals with only minor differences are shown in Table 3.7 (Fig. 3.8).

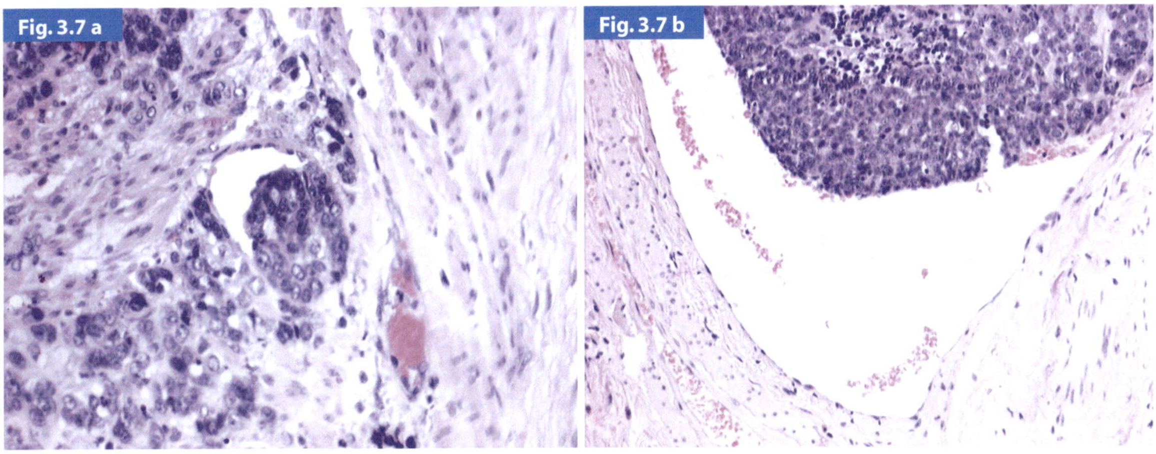

Fig. 3.7 (**a**) Tumor invasion into a small lymphatic vessel (L1; H&E, ×200), (**b**) Tumor invasion into a vein (V1; H&E, ×100)

Table 3.7 Proposals for histopathologic grading of tumor regression in colorectal/gastrointestinal carcinomas

	Dworak et al. 1997	Japanese Society for Cancer of the Colon and Rectum (JSCCR 1997)	Werner and Höfler 2000	Wittekind and Tannapfel 2003
No change	Grade 0: no regression	Grade 0: no regression	no regression	no regression
Minimal regression	Grade 1: dominant tumor mass with obvious fibrosis and/or vasculopathy	Grade 1a: <1/3 regression or only cellular or structural changes	<10% regression	≤25% regression
Low regression	Grade 2: dominantly fibrotic changes with few tumor cells or groups (easy to find)	Grade 1b: <2/3 regression, vital tumor cells present	10–50% regression	25–50% regression
Moderate regression	Grade 3: very few (difficult to find microscopically) tumor cells in fibrotic tissue with or without mucous substance	Grade 2: >2/3 regression, vital tumor cells present	>50% regression	>50% regression
High regression	Grade 4: no tumor cells, only a fibrotic mass (total regression or response)	Grade 3: complete regression, no vital tumor cells	complete regression	complete regression

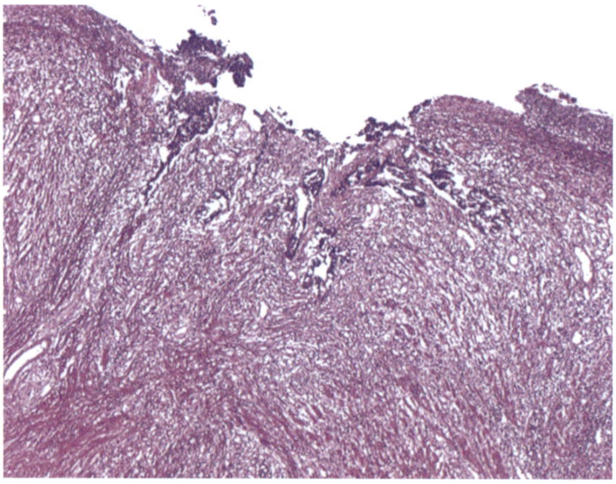

Fig. 3.8 Histomorphologic changes of a rectal adenocarcinoma after neoadjuvant therapy with only a few remaining tumor glands in the upper part of the ulcerative mucosa. Extensive vacuolization and karyorhexis of the cells is seen below (H&E, ×25)

3.6 Molecular Pathology

By application of additional techniques, the pathologist can provide useful information about genetic changes of the tumor that are associated with hereditary diseases, such as Lynch syndrome (HNPCC). Response to specific therapies, such as anti–epidermal growth factor receptor (EGFR) antibodies may also be discerned. HNPCC is an autosomal dominant syndrome that poses a high risk for cancer in the colon, rectum, endometrium, small intestine, ureter, and the renal pelvis. Among the colorectal cancers, there is a predominance of proximal colon cancers, but rectal cancer can also arise in HNPCC. Although the histopathologic pattern is nonspecific for HNPCC, some features may help diagnostically because they are seen less frequently in sporadic colorectal cancer, including mucinous carcinomas, poorly differentiated carcinomas, and a marked lymphocytic infiltration of the tumors.

HNPCC is associated with germline mutations of genes with DNA-mismatch repair functions, such as *MLH1, MSH2*, and *MSH6*. A loss of expression of these genes in the tumor can be detected in situ by immunohistochemistry, with adjacent nonneoplastic epithelium serving as an internal positive control. Furthermore, HNPCC tumors show high-level microsatellite (short tandem repeat sequences) instability (MSI-H). This can be diagnosed by polymerase chain reaction (PCR) analysis of five recommended markers from isolated genomic DNA of microdissected tumor or adenoma areas in comparison to adjacent nonneoplastic tissue. In a MSI-H cancer, bandshifts between tumor and normal tissue in two or more loci are seen. Nevertheless, microsatellite instability is not HNPCC specific, as it is detectable in 10 to 15% of sporadic tumors as well (Peltomäki et al. 2000).

Another example of the importance of molecular pathologic methods involves patients with metastatic colorectal cancer who are candidates for therapy with anti-EGFR-antibodies. KRAS (v-Ki-ras2 Kirsten rat sarcoma viral oncogene homolog) is a downstream intracellular protein of the EGFR signaling pathway, which is mutated in approximately 40% of colorectal cancer cases. Because mutation of *KRAS* induces auto-activation of the protein, blockade of EGFR by specific antibodies seems theoretically useless in these cases. Using allele-specific real-time PCR, seven somatic mutations located in codons 12 and 13 can be detected. Amado et al. (2008) demonstrated in a randomized study that *KRAS* mutation status should be considered when selecting candidates for anti-EGFR therapy with the antibody panitumumab.

3.7 Conclusion

As outlined in this chapter, pathologic examination of the preoperative biopsies and the resected specimens is an indispensable part of the interdisciplinary management of rectal cancer. Good communication between all involved departments and institutions is essential for optimal diagnostics, treatment, and postoperative care. Thus, tumor boards, in which individual cases are discussed by specialists, are an excellent option for patients with rectal cancer.

References

Amado RG, Wolf M, Peeters M et al (2008) Wild-type KRAS is required for panitumumab efficacy in patients with metastatic colorectal cancer. J Clin Oncol 26:1626–1634

Benzoni E, Intersimone D, Terrosu G et al (2006) Prognostic value of tumour regression grading and depth of neoplastic infiltration within the perirectal fat after combined neoadjuvant chemo-radiotherapy and surgery for rectal cancer. J Clin Pathol 59:505–512

Compton CC, Fielding LP, Burgart LJ et al (2000) Prognostic factors in colorectal cancer. College of American Pathologists Consensus Statement 1999. Arch Pathol Lab Med 124:979–994

Dworak O, Keilholz L, Hoffmann A (1997) Pathological features of rectal cancer after preoperative radiochemotherapy. Int J Colorectal Dis 12:19–23

Hamilton SR, Vogelstein B, Kudo S et al (2000) Carcinoma of the colon and rectum. In: Hamilton SR, Aaltonen LA (eds) World Health Organization Classification of Tumours Pathology and Genetics of Tumours of the Digestive System. IARC Press, Lyon

Japanese Society for Cancer of the Colon and Rectum (JSCCR) (1997) Japanese classification of colorectal carcinoma, 1st English edn. Kanehara, Tokyo

Nagtegaal ID, Quirke P (2008) What is the role for the circumferential margin in the modern treatment of rectal cancer? J Clin Oncol. 10;26:303–312

Nagtegaal ID, van Krieken JH (2002) The role of pathologists in the quality control of diagnosis and treatment of rectal cancer-an overview. Eur J Cancer 38:964–972

Parfitt JR, Driman DK (2007) The total mesorectal excision specimen for rectal cancer: a review of its pathological assessment. J Clin Pathol 60:849–855

Peltomäki P, Vasen H, Jass JR (2000) Hereditary nonpolyposis colorectal cancer. In: Hamilton SR, Aaltonen LA (eds) World Health Organization Classification of Tumours Pathology and Genetics of Tumours of the Digestive System. IARC Press, Lyon

Sobin LH, Wittekind C (2002) TNM Classification of Malignant Tumours, 6th edn. Wiley-Liss, New York

Wang Z, Zhou Z, Wang C (2005) Microscopic spread of low rectal cancer in regions of the mesorectum: detailed pathological assessment with whole-mount sections. Int J Colorectal Dis 20:231–237

Werner M, Höfler H (2000) Pathologie. In: Roder JD, Stein HJ, Fink U (eds) Therapie gastrointestinaler Tumoren. Prinzipien der Chirurgischen Klinik und Poliklinik der Technischen Universität München. Springer, New York, pp 45–53

Wittekind C, Tannapfel A (2003) Regression grading of colorectal carcinoma after preoperative radiochemotherapy. An inventory. Pathologe 24:61–65

4 Magnetic Resonance Imaging of Rectal Cancer

From Current Facts to Future Perspectives

Arnd-Oliver Schäfer

4.1 Introduction

Understanding the nature of rectal cancer is a dynamic process. The significance of imaging in relation to the interaction of treatment and individual prognosis is constantly evolving. Although specialized rectal cancer surgery offers the most probable chance of cure, the contribution of neoadjuvant chemoradiation to the reduction of local recurrence rates and improved patient survival is increasingly realized. To this end, magnetic resonance imaging (MRI) is frequently used to select patients for neoadjuvant chemoradiation and to predict a tumor-free circumferential resection plane at surgery.

Current state-of-the-art pelvic MRI consistently depicts the mesorectal fascia. By definition, if a tumor lies within 1 mm of this fascia, then the surgical resection margin is deemed to be involved. Hence, MRI strongly supports the identification of patients who are at high risk of oncologically incomplete resection. Selecting these patients prior to surgery allows for the addition of preoperative chemoradiation therapy (Koh et al. 2006). MRI for rectal cancer has emerged as the first-line imaging tool for multidisciplinary team (MDT) decisions. The adoption of new concepts such as moving-table MRI for the assessment of metastatic spread and diffusion-weighted imaging (DWI) will further strengthen the role of MRI as a "one-stop-shop" staging procedure. Although MRI can provide a broad overview of the extent of the disease, but it may also make diagnosis more complex. A radiologist who specializes in pelvic MRI must be familiar with the principles of recent imaging techniques, as well as with characteristic imaging findings associated with rectal cancer. This chapter provides a summary of current clinical practice regarding pelvic MRI at 1.5 T for staging of rectal cancer.

A-O. Schäfer
Department of Diagnostic Radiology, Freiburg University Hospital, Hugstetter Strasse 55, 79106, Freiburg, Germany
e-mail: arnd-oliver.schaefer@uniklinik-freiburg.de

4.2 Technical Aspects

4.2.1 The Basics of Rectal MRI for Local Staging Purposes

Optimal management of rectal cancer requires detailed preoperative planning that includes assessment of tumor extent and depth of invasion (van Lingen et al. 2003). A variety of examinations have been used for the preoperative planning of rectal cancer, including digital rectal examination, endorectal ultrasound (EUS), computed tomography (CT), and MRI (Mathur et al. 2003). However, thin-slice MRI is increasingly being employed because of its ability to show both tumor extent and depth of invasion (Brown et al. 1999). The principle of any published MRI protocol for local staging of rectal cancer using multichannel external phased-array coils is based on T2-weighted sequences, usually oriented in three planes.

There is some debate as to whether rectal cleansing and subsequent filling with a distension media in combination with antispasmodic agents increases accuracy. Various materials have been used to induce rectal distension, including barium enema, the superparamagnetic iron oxide contrast agent ferristene, methylcellulose, and warm water (Goh et al. 2002; Kim et al. 2008, b; Panaccione et al. 1991; Wallengren et al.

A-O. Schäfer, M. Langer, *MRI of Rectal Cancer,*
DOI: 10.1007/978-3-540-72833-7_4, © Springer-Verlag Berlin Heidelberg 2010

Table 4.1 MRI protocols for local staging of rectal cancer

Sequence	Freiburg protocol			Akasu 2005		Allen 2007				
	T2 sagittal	T2 axial, coronal	T1 VIBE axial fat-saturated	T2 sagittal	T2 axial	T1 axial	T2 axial	T2 coronal	T2 sagittal	T2 axial
Anatomical reference	Pelvis	Tumor-axis	Pelvis	Pelvis	Pelvis	Pelvis	Pelvis	Pelvis	Pelvis	Tumor-axis
FOV (mm)	250	150	250	150	150	350	350	200	200	200
Slice thickness (mm)	5	3	2	6	3	6	6	3	3	3
TR (ms)	6,000	9,500	4.11	4,000	9,500	500	6,000	4,500	6,500	7,000–7,500
TE (ms)	128	119	1.76	120	120	20	130	135	135	130
Signal averages (NEX)	4	4	3	4	4					
Matrix	320 × 240	192 × 192	384 × 240	166 × 256	166 × 256	256 × 512	256 × 512	292 × 512	292 × 512	318 × 512

VIBE, volumetric interpolated breath-hold examination

2000). The infusant should have both adequate viscosity and contrast to induce good distension and visualization on MRI. Ultrasound transmission gel is magnetically inert, semisolid, inexpensive, easy to handle, and is well tolerated by patients (Kim et al. 2008). In our experience, cleansing of the rectum ampulla with a microclyst is beneficial to avoid interference caused by feces. Antispasmodic agents help to reduce motion artifacts and thereby enhance image quality. To distend the rectum, 200 ml of a water and ultrasound transmission gel solution is routinely administered before examination in the supine, head-first position.

The application starts with a T2-weighted fast spin-echo sequence in the sagittal plane. The sagittal sequence serves as a scout view for correct planning of the thin-slice, high-resolution, T2-weighted fast spin-echo sequence in the axial plane. For the most important axial images, it is necessary to plan the slices strictly perpendicular to the tumor axis, resulting in para-axial or para-coronal imaging planes, dependent on the location of the rectal tumor. The coronal T2-weighted fast spin-echo sequence displays the relationship of the tumor and the levator muscles, helps to define the region of the anorectal junction, and is important for detecting metastatic iliac nodes, especially in locally advanced rectal carcinomas.

The use of an intravenous gadolinium-based contrast agent is not generally accepted as an adjunct to local staging of rectal cancer because different opinions exist about the value of contrast-enhanced MRI. Vliegen et al. (2005) reported that the addition of gadolinium-enhanced T1-weighted MRI sequences to T2-weighted fast spin-echo sequences did not significantly improve the diagnostic accuracy for the prediction of tumor penetration through the rectal wall. Okizuka et al. (1996) also found no improvement in T staging after addition of a gadolinium-enhanced fat-suppressed sequence to conventional T1- and T2-weighted MRI. In contrast, Maier et al. (2000) showed that the tumor could be better identified and delineated using a double-contrast technique of intravenous gadolinium-based contrast material combined with an enema of ferristene. In our experience, intravenous gadolinium helps to clarify the relationship of tumor margins and the anal sphincters in low-lying rectal cancers.

Contrast agents are also helpful in distinguishing tumor infiltration beyond the muscularis propria from penetrating vessels, which is sometimes confusing when relying on T2 imaging only. Because rectal adenocarcinoma typically presents as a hypovasacular mass, metastatic nodes may be identified more precisely when compared with T2 imaging alone. Table 4.1 provides an overview of currently proposed imaging protocols for local staging of rectal cancer.

4.2.2 Future Developments

4.2.2.1 Moving-Table MRI for Simultaneous Assessment of Metastatic Spread

Cancer belongs to the class of diseases with systemic character, often spreading metastases over a wide range (Stewart and Kleihues 2003). For this reason, a comprehensive diagnosis is definitely necessary prior to treatment planning. Whole-body MRI can be considered as a first-line diagnostic procedure capable of detecting and determining the extent of metastatic

Beets-Tan 2001				Brown 1999			MERCURY Study Group 2007			Kim 2008	
T1 axial	T2 sagittal	T2 axial, coronal	T1 axial, coronal postcontrast	T1 axial	T2 axial, sagittal	T2 axial	T2 sagittal	T2 axial	T2 axial, coronal	T1 axial, sagittal	T2 axial, sagittal
Pelvis	Pelvis	Tumor-axis	Pelvis	Pelvis	Pelvis	Tumor-axis	Pelvis	Pelvis	Tumor-axis	Pelvis	Pelvis
250	200	200	200	240	240	160	240	240	160	240	240
8	3	3	3	4	5	3	5	5	3	5	5
656	3,427	3,427	612	540	4,000	4,000	2,500–5,000	4,000	4,000	500–600	4,500
10	150	150	15	16	85	85	85	85	85	11	107.5
4	8	8	8	2	2	4		2	4	2	4
166 × 256	175 × 256	175 × 256	383 × 512	256 × 256	512 × 256	256 × 256		512 × 256	256 × 256	320 × 192	384 × 224

disease. This kind of application demands a large field of view, which cannot be realized by conventional MRI technology because the homogeneous main-field region is restricted in contemporary scanners. Clinical needs and the desire for increased patient comfort have led to the development of methods that virtually extend the actual field of view (FOV) of MRI systems (Börnert and Aldefeld 2008).

For whole-body imaging with currently available technology, the patient table must be moved to overcome the finite length of the magnet's homogeneity region. This method is commonly used to acquire the MRI data at a number of successive stations while the table is at rest (Leiner et al. 2004). Once all data have been acquired for a certain anatomical region, the system moves the table with the patient to the next location, and data acquisition is continued as soon as the table is halted. This multistation approach is based on the technique of conventional MRI, but all scanning parameters can easily be adjusted to the body part under examination and all available MRI contrasts can be generated. However, there is an alternative approach that is based on MRI data collection while the table moves continuously (Barkhausen et al. 2001; Fain et al. 2004; Johnson et al. 1997; Kruger et al. 2002; Ludwig et al. 2006; Shankaranarayanan et al. 2003; Sommer et al. 2006). This moving-table approach is technically challenging, but provides increased flexibility in monitoring dynamic processes, shortens scan times, and increases patient comfort.

Continuously moving-table (CMT) MRI may provide a new perspective in oncology—one in which it is important to assess the risk of each patient individually and to localize suspected tumors and their metastases (Schaefer and Schlemmer 2006). Besides the more common approach based on automated scanning using a constant table velocity, interactive real-time patient examination has been proposed, in which the physician freely decides which parts of the body are to be inspected in more detail (Sabati et al. 2006). To achieve adequate spatial resolution, whole-body scanning usually takes several minutes. With this timeframe, respiratory motion, especially in the thorax and abdomen, is a substantial source of artifacts. Hence, the implementation of gating and motion compensation is desirable for moving-table MRI (Börnert and Aldefeld 2008).

Another important issue related to the screening of patients with cancer involves diagnostic contrasts. Using axial multislice techniques, almost all MRI contrasts are achievable (Fautz and Kannengiesser 2006; Fautz et al. 2007; Ludwig et al. 2006; Sommer et al. 2006). However, axial moving-table techniques present three major challenges: (a) the minimization of artifacts due to gradient nonlinearity; (b) the optimization of scan efficiency to limit the total scan time; and (c) the acquisition of images during free breathing, because extended FOVs typically cannot be covered during a single breath-hold period.

Parallel acquisition techniques can be applied to axial moving-table imaging to address these issues. The goal is to reduce artifacts from gradient nonlinearity and breathing motion, as well as ghosting artifacts. One of the simplest approaches for reducing motion artifacts is averaging (Dixon et al. 1988). In this context, parallel imaging has been found to be particularly helpful because it can compensate for the increased scan time required for the repeated acquisition of each *k*-space line. Fautz et al. (2007) showed that a combination of generalized autocalibrating partially parallel acquisition (Griswold et al. 2002) and subsequent averaging is an effective method for artifact reduction in axial multislice moving-table imaging. The proposed method works on a conventional, fully sampled k-space with no need for additional scans or reference lines to estimate the coil sensitivities. It is based on the subdivision of k-space into multiple undersampled data sets from which multiple full FOV images can be reconstructed using parallel acquisition techniques.

As mentioned above, the goal of CMT MRI is to extend the FOV beyond an available scan region with a temporally (Kruger et al. 2002) and spatially seamless acquisition (Shankaranarayanan et al. 2003). One approach attempts to cover the extended FOV as quickly as possible. The other approach attempts to cover the extended FOV by using a minimum spatial window of data collection along the z-space. Sliding multislice (SMS) is an interleaved multislice acquisition technique for axial CMT imaging (Fautz and Kannengiesser 2006). Similar to stationary interleaved multislice imaging, a package of N parallel slices with distances d is acquired by successively performing $n \times N$ acquisition steps of duration ΔT, where n denotes the total number of acquisition steps required for the reconstruction of one image (Sommer et al. 2008). Hence, $TR = N \times \Delta T$ (the velocity of continuous table motion) is adjusted to traverse the table by the extension of a whole slice package during the time $(n \times TR)$. SMS divides k-space into N segments that are allocated to N scan positions prescribed by the slice positions of the multislice package in the coordinate system of the scanner. Each k-space segment comprises n/N acquisition steps that are recorded while a patient slice passes by the corresponding scan position. N parallel patient slices are addressed during the same TR, acquiring data from different k-space segments sequentially at different scan positions. After having passed all N scan positions, each patient slice is fully acquired as it exits the static acquisition window (Sommer et al. 2008).

As demonstrated by Fautz and Kannengiesser (2006), SMS has additional beneficial properties that encourage the application of the method to abdominal imaging. The SMS technique is based on the hypothesis that similar parts of the k-space (segments) should be acquired when each slice is in the same position. This requires the acquisition of similar k-space sections of different slices at different time points. Applied to CMT acquisitions, this slice phase-encoding reordering allows the acquisition of certain k-space segments to be allocated to specific scanner positions. In particular, all center k-space lines of any slice may be acquired at the isocenter of the magnet. The total FOV required for data collection in SMS imaging is minimized. All slices are acquired along the same spatial trajectory relative to the scanner, and the same phase-encoding trajectory is applied during acquisition. The acquisition trajectories of different slices are incrementally shifted in time. The optimum spatial trajectory through the scanner, which is typically placed around the isocenter of the magnet, is automatically applied to the acquisition of all slices. This reduces artifacts from z-dependent effects, such as distortions from nonlinear gradient fields. Additionally, SMS avoids discontinuities between slices along the scanner's axis and allows for continuous display and "real-time" control of currently acquired images on the user interface (Fig. 4.1a, b).

SMS was implemented as a moving-table scan from head to toe in order to assess potential metastatic

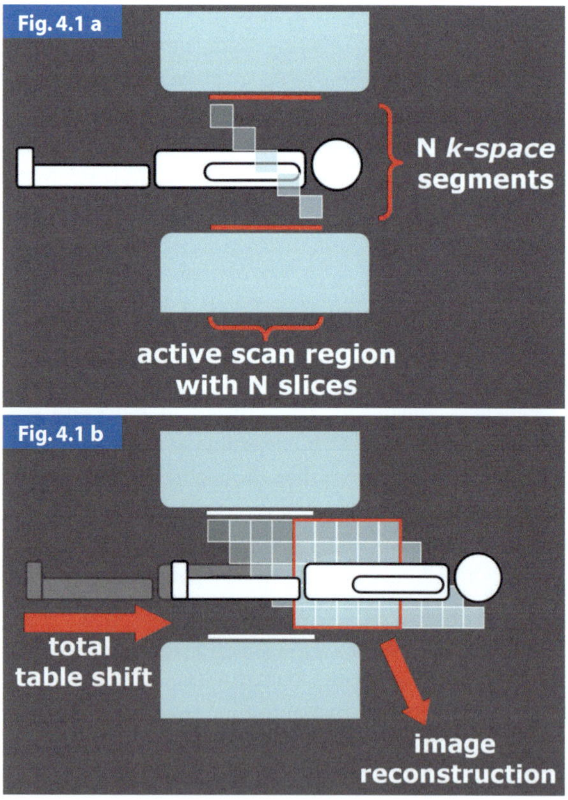

Fig. 4.1 Illustration of SMS continuously moving-table MRI. (**a**) Exemplary k-space trajectory demonstrates acquisition strategy in SMS. (**b**) Continuous table movement allows for seamless acquisition with SMS

spread from rectal cancer as an adjunct to local staging by applying high-resolution pelvic MRI. The major benefit of this new technology is seamless imaging within minutes of acquiring two different MR contrasts. The procedure is also applicable to dedicated tumor staging. Patient repositioning and stepwise examination for whole body coverage are not needed. For SMS moving-table MRI, we currently combine a standard axial T1-weighted fat-saturated contrast-enhanced fast low-angle shot (FLASH) two-dimensional sequence with an axial turbo inversion recovery magnitude (TIRM) sequence. Images are acquired with a table speed of 10 mm/s and 4 mm/s, respectively. The sequence parameters are summarized in Table 4.2. The SMS-FLASH sequence is started 30 s after an intravenous injection of 20 ml Gd-BOPTA. Patients are instructed to hold their breath at the start of the measurement and are told to resume breathing 25 s later while the acquisition is completed. The whole liver can be imaged artifact-free with continuous table movement at a speed of 10 mm/s. Similar to a standard abdominal helical CT, imaging takes place in a portal dominant phase to detect liver metastases from colorectal origin. The free-breathing SMS-TIRM sequence is acquired to get an overview of the lungs, abdomen, and pelvis for pulmonary metastases, nodal disease, and bone marrow infiltration. Within a total acquisition time of 7 min, imaging from the neck to pelvis is feasible. Of note, the examination time of the Freiburg rectal cancer "one-stop-shop" imaging protocol does not exceed 25 min.

Table 4.2 Sequence parameters of Sliding Multislice-MRI

	SMS-FLASH-2D	SMS-TIRM
TR (ms)	102	3,656
TE (ms)	2	101
TI (ms)		150
Slice thickness (mm)	5	6
Matrix	320 × 224	320 × 200
Pixel bandwidth	300 Hz/pixel	445 Hz/pixel
Flip angle	70°	60°
Slices/package	17	8
Measurements	5	16
Pixel size	1.4 × 1.1 × 5.0	1.6 × 1.1 × 6.0
Parallel imaging	Generalized autocalibrating partially parallel acquisition, factor 2	

MRI, magnetic resonance imaging

Our data confirm that the image quality provided by SMS moving-table MRI is comparable to that of a conventional stationary imaging protocol. The reproach associated with inferior lesion characterization using SMS technique instead of standard MRI will be dispelled in the near future with the implementation of additional image contrasts and continual technical optimization. SMS is a cutting-edge technology for rectal cancer work-up using CMT-MRI and has the potential to dramatically improve patient diagnosis and treatment (Baumann et al. 2008, 2009; Schäfer and Langer 2007; Schäfer et al. 2007). To provide an insight into current SMS technique for rectal cancer staging, a case-based demonstration CD-ROM is provided with this book.

4.2.2.2 Diffusion-Weighted Imaging

- In general, DWI explores the random motion of water molecules in the body. The motion of water molecules in the extra- and intracellular spaces and intravascular space contributes to the net water displacement measured by DWI. The technique provides qualitative and quantitative information reflecting tissue cellularity and cell membrane integrity (Koh et al. 2007). Two major problems that arise with whole-body DWI are the presence of motion and susceptibility effects. The introduction of parallel imaging, respiratory gating, and cardiac triggering have helped to improve image quality using echo planar imaging (EPI) for DWI. Currently used imaging strategies for DWI in the body consist of breath-hold single-shot DWI, free-breathing multiple-averaging DWI, and free-breathing multiple-averaging multistation DWI, also called diffusion-weighted whole-body imaging with background body signal suppression (Koh et al. 2007).

- The following section focuses on free-breathing multiple averaging EPI-based DWI as applied in the pelvis. Multiple averaging in DWI allows one to choose a range of *b*-values and thin slices, thus producing images with a high signal-to-noise ratio. In addition, postprocessing methods, such as multiplanar reconstruction and maximum intensity projection, are possible. Another interesting feature is the ability to combine functional and anatomical images by performing image fusion. Moreover, multiple *b*-values enable the apparent diffusion coefficient (ADC) calculation of a target lesion. The ADC is calculated by fitting a decaying exponential function to the signal intensity (SI) on the *y*-axis against the *b*-values on the *x*-axis: $S_i = S_0\, x^{e-b \times D}$, in which S_i is the SI of a given pixel; S_0 is the SI of a given pixel without diffusion sensitization; *e* is the mathematical constant, the base of the natural logarithm; *b* is the attenuation coefficient (mm^2/s); and *D* is the diffusion rate constant for the given pixel (s/mm^2). The slope of the resulting line fitted through plots represents the ADC (Koh and Collins 2007). Tissues with restricted diffusion, such as tumors composed of densely packed cells, exhibit low ADC values.

Free-breathing multiple-averaging DWI allows for both qualitative and quantitative analysis and may therefore be well suited as an adjunct to local rectal cancer staging. DWI is increasingly applied for oncologic staging because it has the capability to detect and characterize tumors. Moreover, DWI provides assessment of treatment response, which renders the technique highly useful for monitoring neoadjuvant radiochemotherapy for advanced rectal carcinomas. Rectal cancer may exhibit either restricted or increased diffusion, depending on its cellular architecture. To put it simply, in tumors with high cellular density, the motion of the water molecules and consequently diffusion are restricted. Loss of cell membrane integrity or decrease in cell density resulting from necrosis increases diffusion. Other sources of increased diffusion are intratumoral edema and cystic tumor components (Kwee et al. 2008).

One of the most intriguing findings associated with the use of DWI in patients with cancer has been that ADC measurements appear to be predictive of tumor response to chemotherapy and radiation treatment. Studies in rectal cancer have shown that cellular tumor with low-baseline pretreatment ADC values respond better to chemotherapy or radiation treatment than tumors that exhibit high-pretreatment ADC values (DeVries et al. 2003; Dzik-Jurasz et al. 2002). One possible explanation is that tumors with high pretreatment ADC values are likely to be more necrotic than those with low values (Koh and Collins 2007). Necrotic tumors are frequently hypoxic, acidodic, and poorly perfused, leading to reduced sensitivity to chemotherapy and radiation treatment. Additionally, it has been observed that an early increase in the ADC after commencing treatment was predictive of better treatment outcome (Theilmann et al. 2004). DWI for rectal cancer staging is typically performed using a range of *b*-values (e.g., 0, 50, 100, 250, 500, 750, 1,000 s/mm^2). A larger *b*-value indicates a greater degree of signal attenuation from water molecules. The relative contribution of T2 SI (known as the T2 shine-through effect) is a potential source of error in image interpretation and can be mistaken for restricted diffusion. With the calculation of the ADC, the effects of T2 shine-through can be overcome.

4.3 MRI for Primary Staging of Rectal Cancer

4.3.1 Introduction

To improve patient selection for individually tailored therapy, a reliable imaging modality capable of differentiating early-stage tumors from advanced tumors is warranted. MRI meets this requirement by accurately defining tumors with a favorable prognosis, regardless of their distance from the anal verge. Additionally, MRI allows for visualization of the entire tumor, its anatomic disposition in any plane extramurally, and its relationship to the circumferential resection margin (CRM) (Brown et al. 2004).

4.3.2 T Staging

Significant progress in the management of locally advanced rectal cancer has been achieved during the last decade. Advacnces include the use of preoperative chemoradiation therapy (Sauer et al. 2004), the widespread implementation of total mesorectal excision (TME) surgery (Martling et al. 2000), and autonomic nerve preservation (Enker et al. 1995). Significant improvement in local control, toxicity profile, and sphincter preservation have been achieved in patients with locally advanced rectal cancer who were treated with preoperative chemoradiation therapy (Sauer et al. 2004). According to the National Institutes of Health consensus conference (1990), adjuvant postoperative combined modality treatment is recommended for all pT3 and/or N+ rectal cancers. However, data now suggest that these criteria may be too broad (Merchant et al. 1999; Picon et al. 2003; Willett et al. 1999). Gunderson et al. (2004) reported a retrospective analysis of pooled data demonstrating similar 5-year overall survival for patients with pT3N0 rectal cancer treated with surgery and chemotherapy alone versus those patients treated only with chemoradiation, further suggesting that trimodality therapy may be excessive for some patients in the T3N0 subset. In contrast, Guillem et al. (2008) demonstrated that 22% of patients with T3N0 rectal cancer that was clinically staged by either EUS or MRI prior to chemoradiation therapy have pathologically involved nodes. Because preoperative chemoradiation may not only reduce the total number of lymph nodes but also sterilize nodes, the true rate of unidentified pathologically involved nodes is likely to be higher. Therefore, preoperative chemoradiation therapy should remain the standard of care for patients with MRI-staged T3 rectal cancers.

These considerations represent an enormous challenge for radiologists because there is a growing need for an accurate imaging tool to help identify patients who are at risk for local recurrence. On the basis of different risk categories, patients should be treated with different regimens of surgery, radiation therapy, and chemotherapy. The assessment of local tumor spread includes determination of the depth of tumor growth in the rectal wall, the CRM at TME, and the depth of tumor invasion in surrounding pelvic structures, as well as the nodal status (Beets-Tan and Beets 2004). In this respect, Brown et al. (2004) reported advantages of thin-slice, T2-weighted, high-resolution MRI over both digital-rectal examination and EUS for preoperative staging of rectal cancer. Important MRI criteria relevant for the vast majority of rectal adenocarcinomas are summarized in accordance with the findings of Brown et al. (2003a) as follows:

- *Stage T1*: low signal in the submucosal layer, replacement of the submucosal layer by abnormal signal not extending into the muscle coat
- *Stage T2*: intermediate SI within muscularis propria
- *Stage T3*: broad-based bulge or nodular projection or intermediate SI projecting beyond outer muscle coat
- *Stage T4*: extension of abnormal signal into adjacent organ, extension of tumor signal through the peritoneal reflection

Obviously, the majority of rectal adenocarcinomas exhibit higher SI than the proper muscle layer but lower SI than the submucosa using T2-weighted fast spin-echo sequences. However, linitis plastica carcinomas tend to display SI as low as that of the proper muscle layer, and mucinous adenocarcinomas show an SI that is higher than that of the submucosa in the region of the mucin lakes (Akasu et al. 2005).

The depth of tumor invasion is known to be an important progno with nodal disease stic factor in rectal carcinoma (Hermanek et al. 1995; Park et al. 1999). The present pT3 category includes carcinomas invading through the muscularis propria into subserosa or into nonperitonealized pericolic or perirectal tissues. The prognostic nonhomogeneity of these pT3 rectal cancer patients has been recognized in several studies (Cawthorn et al. 1990; Krook et al. 1991; Willett et al. 1999). In the Erlangen Registry of Colorectal Carcinomas (ERCRC) series, patients with rectal cancer invading beyond the border of the muscularis propria (5 mm or less [pT3*a*]) had a more favorable prognosis than those with invasion greater than 5 mm (pT3*b*) when considering local recurrence and cancer-related survival. The local recurrence rate was 10% for pT3a and 26% for pT3b. Statistically significant differences in cancer-related 5-year survival rates were found between pT3a and pT3b (85% vs 54%). The subdivision, using a cutoff point of 5 mm in the pT3 category, is important both for predicting survival and for selecting patients eligible for adjuvant treatment. For lymph node-negative patients, the indication for adjuvant therapy is strongly dependent on the pT category. Adjuvant treatment is generally accepted for pT3 and pT4 patients. The analysis of the ERCRC data also demonstrated that some lymph node-negative pT3 patients had results similar to pT2 patients. For node-negative pT3 patients with less than or equal to 5 mm of invasion beyond the muscularis propria (pT3a) and for node-negative pT2 patients, the local recurrence rates were 10% and 9%, with 5-year survival rates of 91% and 94%, respectively (Merkel et al. 2001).

Even if a high-spatial resolution is applied with the new generation of phased-array coils, the accuracy of T staging is not as high as anticipated (ranging from 65% to 86%) or as reproducible as expected, with considerable interobserver variability (Beets-Tan et al. 2001; Blomqvist et al. 1997, 2000; Gagliardi et al. 2002). MRI appears to be poor at consistently distinguishing T1 from T2 tumors and sessile or polypoid adenomas from stage-T1 adenocarcinomas. Most staging failures with MRI occur in the differentiation of stage-T2 and borderline stage-T3 cancers, particularly with overstaging. Overstaging is often caused by reactive changes in the connective tissue around the tumor, including inflammatory cell aggregation, desmoplastic changes, and hypervascularity (Akasu et al. 2005; Beets-Tan et al. 2001; Brown et al. 1999; Vogl et al. 1997). Underestimation is mostly attributable to microscopic invasion that is fundamentally undetectable on MRI (Akasu et al. 2005). Differentiating between minimal T3 infiltration and T2 lesions is probably of little consequence for patient treatment, as patients with minimal T3 infiltration into perirectal fat are at low risk of surgical failure from CRM involvement (Cawthorn et al. 1990; Chung et al. 1983).

4.3.3 N Staging

Nodal involvement is a strong independent predictor of survival and local recurrence in rectal cancer (Quirke and Dixon 1988). The depth of extramural spread and the presence of extramural venous invasion are strongly associated with nodal disease (Saclarides et al. 1994a; Zenni et al. 1998). In addition, patients with stage N2 disease have a significantly higher risk of local recurrence compared with those with N0 or N1 disease (Moran et al. 1992). Definitive nodal staging in rectal cancer is not achieved without histopathologic evaluation of the resected specimen. Preoperative assessment of lymph node status in patients with rectal cancer is therefore critical. First, the number of involved nodes has an influence on the prognosis of the patients (Wolmark et al. 1986; Tang et al. 1995). Second, the presence of tumor-containing lymph nodes near the mesorectal fascia increases the risk of local relapse (Adam et al. 1994). Those that remain unresected may be responsible for local recurrence (Moreira et al. 1994). Evaluation of surgical specimens indicates that rectal cancer most commonly spreads to the lymph nodes located in the mesorectal fat, irrespective of whether the tumor arises from the upper or lower third of the rectum.

Lateral tumor spread to pelvic sidewall nodes is a subject of some controversy. It has been suggested that pelvic sidewall nodal dissemination occurs in 10% to 25% of patients with rectal cancer (Hojo et al. 1982; Morikawa et al. 1994). Lateral spread has been reported more frequently in patients with low rectal cancers (Hocht et al. 2002, 2004). Involved nodes in the pelvic sidewall increase the risk of systemic dissemination (Ueno et al. 2001b). Not surprisingly, the 5-year survival in patients with pelvic sidewall lymph node metastasis is low (25–42%) (Ueno et al. 2001b; Takahashi et al. 2000; Hida et al. 1997a). Unlike mesorectal nodes, pelvic sidewall nodes are not routinely removed during TME surgery and extended lymphadenectomy may be required to achieve clearance of the tumor (Billingham 1994; Suzuki et al. 1995). The use of preoperative neoadjuvant therapy may be influenced by the presence of tumor-containing nodes close to the potential resection plane. The ability to accurately determine node-negative status prior to surgery could result in less aggressive treatment and preoperative therapy for some patients (Brown et al. 2003a).

Hida showed that intramural spread of rectal cancer occurred in 10.6% of cases that extended 1 cm distal to the tumor. Likewise, distal mesorectal nodal metastases were identified in 20.2% of cases that were located up to 4 cm below the distal tumor margin. Retrograde lymphatic flow may trigger nodal dissemination below the distal tumor margin in patients with advanced disease (Koh et al. 2005). The likelihood of metastases was also found to increase with the T stage of the tumor, occurring in up to 50% of patients with stage-T4 disease (Hida et al. 1997b).

The ability to consistently define a safe plane for distal mesorectal transection is desirable. It may ensure complete tumor and nodal clearance at surgery, thus reducing the risk of local pelvic recurrence (Koh et al. 2005). Pathologic studies have shown that the majority of nodes associated with rectal cancer—both malignant and benign—are found within the mesorectum and, to a lesser degree, along the superior rectal artery (Dworak 1991; Steup et al. 2002). Koh et al. (2005) demonstrated that the majority of mesorectal nodes associated with rectal cancer were found at the level of the primary tumor. Mesorectal nodes are seen well on MRI with the use of a small FOV, high-spatial resolution, thin-slice, T2-weighted sequence technique oriented orthogonal to the long axis of the rectum. These images allow for clear identification of nodes within the mesorectal fat. Using T2-weighted MRI, normal mesorectal nodes display low, intermediate, or high SI. For assessment of pelvic sidewall lymph nodes, an additional T2-weighted sequence in the coronal plane can be helpful. Only approximately 65% of mesorectal nodes found by histopathology can be identified on in vivo MRI. However, despite nonvisualization of a substantial proportion of small mesorectal nodes, the incidence of malignancy in these nodes is low (Koh et al. 2006).

Currently, the imaging criteria used for prediction of nodal metastasis vary widely. The maximum diameter of a node has traditionally been used as a major diagnostic criterion in cross-sectional imaging. Some authors regard any visible node in the perirectal fat as metastatic (Okizuka et al. 1996), whereas others employ size criteria with cutoff values for nodal involvement that range from 3 to 10 mm (Vogl et al. 1997; Zerhouni et al. 1996). According to the findings of Matsuoka et al. (2004), a 6-mm longitudinal diameter criterion may serve as a useful parameter for the evaluation of mesorectal lymph node metastasis. However, it is firmly established that size criteria are insufficient to consistently distinguish between malignant and benign lymph nodes in patients with rectal cancer. This is largely because mesorectal nodes, whether benign or malignant, tend to be small. In a study of 424 surgical rectal specimens containing 12,759 nodes, Dworak (1991) found a mean nodal diameter of 3.34 mm and a mean metastasis diameter of 3.84 mm.

Nodal hyperplasia is another common feature that results in benign nodal enlargement. In another pathologic study of 698 lymph nodes (Monig et al. 1999), 53% of nodes containing metastases were < 5 mm in diameter. Thus, the application of a size criterion of 5 mm for the maximum short-axis nodal diameter to discriminate between benign and mailgnant nodes has at best moderate sensitivity and specificity for the detection of nodal metastases (Kim et al. 2000; Hadfield et al. 1997; Matsuoka et al. 2004). Additional MRI criteria, such as border and signal characteristics, have therefore been studied (Kim et al. 2004b; Brown et al. 2003b). Border and signal characteristics of lymph nodes on T2-weighted fast spin-echo sequences have been shown to be useful for prediction of nodal disease. Nodes with mixed SI are likely to contain areas of necrosis or extracellular mucin that correspond to metastatic adenocarcinoma. Areas of mixed SI on MRI images correspond with tumor deposits. Irregular borders may indicate partial or complete nodal replacement with a tumor. Extranodal extension leads to irregularity of the surrounding capsule. When border characteristics and SI were combined, the sensitivity for metastatic nodal detection was reported to increase to 85%, with a high specificity of 98% for detecting nodal metastases in nodes ≥3 mm (Brown et al. 2003b).

Normal or reactive nodes should be characterized by uniform SI and smooth, sharply demarcated borders; the presence of intranodal fat is not a typical feature of mesorectal nodes. As discussed, the prediction of nodal status remains problematic. The results of a meta-analysis suggest that, for identification of nodal disease, EUS, MRI, and CT lack sufficient accuracy for clinical decisionmaking (Lahaye et al. 2005). Ultrasmall superparamagnetic iron oxide (USPIO)-enhanced MRI has been reported to be promising for differentiation between benign and malignant nodes (Will et al. 2006). USPIO consists of low-molecular-weight iron oxide (e.g., coated with dextran) supplied as a powder in a glass vial that may be reconstituted by using 10 ml of normal saline. The recommended USPIO dose is 0.13 ml per kilogram of body weight, which equates to 2.6 mg of iron per kilogram. For infusion, the reconstituted solution is diluted in 100 ml of normal saline. The contrast agent is administered within 45 min by a slow-drip infusion. Administration has to be completed 24 to 36 h before MRI (Koh et al. 2004; Lahaye et al. 2008).

In the literature, two main mechanisms for transportation of nanoparticles to the lymph nodes are described. The major pathway is direct transcapillary passage of the nanoparticles from blood vessels into the medullary sinuses of the node. The other pathway is nonselective endothelial transcytosis across permeable capillaries into the interstitium, from where nanoparticles are transported through the lymphatic system and accumulate in macrophages within the lymph node (Weissleder et al. 1990; Frija et al. 1996). USPIOs cause a decrease in SI within the node, owing to susceptibility artifacts on three-dimensional T2-weighted MRI.

Variation of SI within a node can be explained by the concentration of macrophages in a particular region in the node. A region with a normal concentration of macrophages will produce an area with SI decrease. This means that enlarged inflamed nodes will also show a significant decrease in SI. The involved part of the lymph node is expected to show no SI decrease caused by the replacement of macrophages by tumor cells, creating a region of increased SI within a node—the so-called white region (Lahaye et al. 2008). Four main patterns of nodal enhancement after USPIO administration can be identified (Koh et al. 2004):

- Uniform low-SI
- Central low SI
- Eccentric high SI
- Uniform high SI

The problem occurring with rectal cancer and its associated nodal metastasis is the presence of micrometastase that are ≤1 mm in size and are impossible to detect even with the use of USPIO-enhanced MRI. Nonmalignant nodes usually exhibit uniform low SI or central low SI. Central low SI is a pattern frequently encountered in reactive lymph nodes; it is thought to be related to the distribution of macrophages within the node. When lymph nodes undergo reactive enlargement, there is frequently cortical or paracortical hyperplasia, which results in an increase in size of the lymphoid follicles and the nodal cortical thickness. Because the macrophages remain predominantly within the medullary sinus, the susceptibility effects of USPIO in a reactive lymph node can appear confined to the center of the node, subsequently creating the low SI pattern. Malignant nodes that harbor focal metasases greater than 1 mm in diameter demonstrate uniform or eccentric high SI (Koh et al. 2004). Lymphatic metastases are carried via lymphatic trunks to nodes, where they usually settle within the subcapsular sinus or along the sinusoids within the medulla (Carr 1983). From the intranodal site, the tumor cells proliferate and subsequently replace the node.

In a study conducted by Koh et al. (2004), the rate of matching between nodes seen in vivo and the total number of mesorectal nodes harvested at pathologic analysis was 57%. In another recent study of 28 patients with rectal cancer (Lahaye et al. 2008), MRI detected a total of 362 mesorectal nodes. A total of 333 nodes were found at histopathology. Of those, 27 were malignant and 306 were benign. Of the 333 nodes at histopathology, 236 nodes could be matched with nodes found during MRI, whereas 97 nodes could not. Only 176 nodes were eligible for SI measurements because 60 nodes were too small to be accurately measured.

The estimated percentage of white region within a node seems to be the most practical criterion in the prediction of nodal status with USPIO-enhanced MRI. An estimated area of white region larger than 30% within a node is highly predictive for an involved node, with high sensitivity and specificity. The larger the white region, the more likely the node is malignant. Benign conditions such as focal nodal fibrosis or fatty hilum may also present as white regions because of their lack of macrophages, thus mimicking malignancy. These white regions, however, are usually 30% or less of the total node area. The use of patterns to predict malignant nodes has a major drawback: It involves a certain level of subjectivity and therefore constitutes a potential source of error (Lahaye et al. 2008).

4.3.4 Circumferential Resection Margin

One key source of local recurrence after curative resection of rectal cancer is incomplete removal of the lateral spread of the tumor (Adam et al. 1994; de Haas-Kock et al. 1996). Quirke demonstrated that positive microscopic resection margins result in a local recurrence rate of 83% (Quirke et al. 1986). Attention has also been directed toward the surgical technique itself as a determinant of local recurrence rates (Heald and Ryall 1986). The strong predictive value of CRM has been shown in an number of reports, but the actual critical free distance remains uncertain (Wibe et al. 2002a; Nagtegaal et al. 2002a). Per definition, CRM involvement is predicted when a tumor extends to within 1 mm of the mesorectal fascia on MRI. Histopathology of resected specimens has shown that the frequency of local recurrence greatly decreases when a tumor-free CRM greater than 1 mm can be obtained (Adam et al. 1994; de Haas-Kock et al. 1996; Quirke et al. 1986).

MRI provides detailed and accurate information on CRM status (Brown et al. 2003a). Nevertheless, there is ongoing debate about when to call the CRM positive (Nagtegaal and Quirke 2008). Beets-Tan et al. (2001) found that MRI with a phased-array coil accurately predicted the distance to the mesorectal resection plane. A tumor-free margin of at least 1 mm can be predicted with a high degree of certainty when the measured distance on MRI is at least 5 mm, and a margin of at least 2 mm can be predicted when the MRI distance is at least 6 mm. The MRI prediction of tumor-free margins is currently more reliable than the prediction of the tumor stage. In combination with lymph node status, CRM status provides a better prognostic model than the current tumor-node-metastasis (TNM) system (Nagtegaal et al. 2007; Gosens et al. 2007).

MRI prediction of CRM has some disadvantages. Difficulties in image interpretation can lead to errors when predicting the lateral margins, especially when mesorectal tumor deposits or enlarged lymph nodes are present. Rectal cancer also can provoke desmoplastic reaction, in which fibrous tissue is formed in and around the tumor. MRI cannot reliably distinguish between fibrosis with or without tumor cells (Beets-Tan et al. 2001). In Norway, the indications for preoperative chemoradiotherapy have been extended to include patients in whom the distance from the tumor to mesorectal fascia is ≤ 3 mm, as measured on a good-quality MRI examination (Eriksen et al. 2007). However, the increased cutoff from 1 mm to 5 mm seems to correspond to an unacceptably high false-positive rate and will not enhance accuracy (Brown et al. 2003a). Six distinct types of margin involvement have been described (Quirke et al. 1986; Birbeck et al. 2002):

- Direct tumor spread
- Discontinuous tumor spread
- Lymph node metastases
- Venous invasion
- Lymphatic invasion
- Perineural tumor spread

In approximately 30% of patients, the tumor shows more than one feature of margin involvement. There is an obvious correlation of CRM positivity and TNM stage. Increasing depths of tumor invasion, as well as the presence of tumor deposits and involved lymph nodes, contribute to this correlation (Nagtegaal and Quirke 2008). If the mesorectum is removed as a whole, then few positive margins are present and local recurrence rates are low (Nagtegaal et al. 2002b). In contrast, when the plane of resection is on the muscularis propria, CRM involvement is common and local recurrence rates are high. There are more positive margins in tumors located in the lower rectum (Marr et al. 2005; Wibe et al. 2002b). CRM involvement is even more important in the neoadjuvant setting. In advanced tumors with a positive margin on preoperative imaging, if the margin becomes free after treatment, prognosis is good. In contrast, if the margin remains positive, the prognosis is worse than in cases without neoadjuvant therapy; this is because the remaining tumor consists of a selected population of tumor cells resistant to therapy (Nagtegaal and Quirke 2008). Imaging technology currently allows for fairly accurate determination of two important parameters: the proximity of the cancer to the rectal fascia propria, and the extent by which the cancer has penetrated through the muscularis propria.

The most interesting finding of the Magnetic Resonance Imaging and Rectal Cancer European Equivalence (MERCURY) study is that MRI and histopathologic assessment of tumor spread are equivalent to within 0.5 mm (MERCURY Study Group 2007). Clearly, emphasis has shifted from measurement of tumor extension through the muscularis propria—long believed to correlate with outcome—to the proximity of tumor to the histologic CRM, and hence to the intended CRM on preoperative imaging (Wittekind et al. 2001; Quirke and Dixon 1988). Radiologic prediction of CRM involvement in patients with distal rectal cancers, which often extend below the rectal fascia propria and the mesorectum, is even more difficult. In patients undergoing abdominoperineal resection, the radial resection may be extended outside the levator muscles to allow for wider clearance of the tumor (Marr et al. 2005). The current recommendation in most countries is for the radial excision level to extend to the connective tissue just outside the fascia propria. In a subset analysis of the Dutch trial in which all patients were intended to have TME, the excised mesorectum was judged to be incomplete in 43% of cases (Nagtegaal et al. 2002b).

4.3.5 Negative Prognostic Factors in Rectal Cancer

The prognosis of rectal cancer strongly depends on a number of factors that have traditionally been assessed by histopathologic examination. These factors include the depth of tumor invasion into and beyond the bowel wall (Harrison et al. 1994; Willett et al. 1999), the number of lymph nodes involved with the tumor (Wolmark 1986; Tang 1995), extramural venous invasion (Talbot et al. 1980), involvement of the CRM (Adam 1994), and the presence of ulceration of the peritoneum by tumor (Shepherd et al. 1995). Accurate preoperative assessment of these prognostic factors is a fundamental prerequisite for selecting patients for neoadjuvant therapy and planning surgical approaches to optimize complete excision (Barrett 1998).

4.3.5.1 Perineural Invasion

Several reports have shown that perineural invasion (PNI) is an important prognostic factor in colorectal cancer (CRC) (Guerra et al. 1998; Horn et al. 1991; Knudsen et al. 1983; Krasna et al. 1988; Shirouzu et al. 1993; Ueno et al. 2001a). PNI was defined as the presence of cancer cells in the perineurium in Auerbach's plexus in a prospective study conducted by Fujita and coworkers (Fujita et al. 2007). They found that PNI was a significant prognostic factor in pT3 and pT4 CRC. The incidence of PNI in pT3 and pT4 CRC was 26% in this study. The reported incidence of PNI differs among studies and ranges from 14% to 50% (Knudsen et al. 1983; Ueno et al. 2001a). To date, only a few studies have examined the relationship between PNI and the prognosis of patients with colon cancer (Wied et al. 1985; Takahashi et al. 1997; Burdy et al. 2001). These studies clearly demonstrated that PNI is associated with tumor recurrence and poor survival.

4.3.5.2 Extramural Vascular Invasion

Histologic extramural vascular invasion has long been recognized as an independent predictor of local and distant recurrence and poorer overall survival (Bokey et al. 1997; Harrison et al. 1994; Horn et al. 1991). It is defined as the presence of malignant cells within blood vessels beyond the muscularis propria (Talbot et al. 1980) and is reported to occur in as many as 52% of cases of CRC (Horn et al. 1991). It is possible to detect extramural vascular invasion with MRI (Brown et al. 2003a). Depth of tumor invasion can indicate the potential for extramural vascular invasion. By definition, histologically defined extramural vascular invasion has to be associated with tumors that are at least stage T3. Assessment of MRI for features suggestive of extramural vascular invasion include the following four components:

- Pattern of tumor margin
- Location of tumor relative to majot vessels
- Caliber of vessel
- Vessel border

The tumor margin may appear nodular or smooth. Tumor invasion into the small noncharacterizable veins that radiate outward from the bowel wall gives rise to a nodular border. This finding can be differentiated from desmoplasia, which normally appears as fine stranding of low SI. Whenever a tumor is seen close to a vessel, the possibility of extramural venous invasion should be considered. The presence of tumor SI within a vascular structure is highly suggestive of extramural vascular invasion. As a tumor invades along the lumen, the vessel expands. The tumor may eventually expand through and beyond the vessel wall, disrupting the border, which can be described either as irregular or nodular (Smith et al. 2008a).

4.3.5.3 Mucinous Adenocarcinoma of the Rectum

Mucinous adenocarcinoma of the colon and rectum accounts for 5% to 15% of all primary CRC (Symonds and Vickery 1976; Nozoe et al. 2000). CRC can progress through two pathways of genomic instability: microsatellite instability (MSI) and chromosomal instability (CIN) (Lengauer et al. 1997). CRCs with MSI often present a mucinous carcinoma phenotype (Kim et al. 1994). Kazama et al. (2005) demonstrated that MSI was significantly more frequent and CIN was significantly less frequent in mucinous adenocarcinomas than in well differentiated carcinomas matched for T classification and tumor location. Mucinous adenocarcinoma is one of the subtypes of CRC showing a mucinous pattern on histopathologic examination with extracellular mucin produced by secreting acini (Symonds and Vickery 1976; Hanski 1995). The amount of mucin required to warrant a diagnosis of mucinous carcinoma, as set by the World Health Organization (WHO), is ≥50% of the mucin pool occupying the tumor mass (Hanski 1995). This finding is distinct from signet-ring cell adenocarcinoma, a rare variant in which mucin remains inside the cell (Nissan et al. 1999).

According to the literature, mucinous carcinoma affects younger patients, is more frequent in the proximal portion of the colon, and tends to present at a more advanced stage (Odone et al. 1982; Umpleby et al. 1985). Conflicting results are found in the literature regarding the relationship between mucinous adenocarcinoma and survival. The majority of published series suggest that mucinous adenocarcinoma is associated with a poor outcome (Minsky et al. 1987; Symonds and Vickery 1976). Negri et al. (2005) reported that mucinous CRC is less responsive to 5-FU-based chemotherapy than nonmucinous adenocarcinomas. The mechanism of this resistance is unknown.

Mucinous tumors are associated with a higher proportion of nodal metastases and peritoneal metastases, whereas the most common site of metastasis for patients with nonmucinous histology is the liver. Additionally, mucinous carcinomas of the rectum are associated with a higher rate of local recurrence than nonmucinous carcinomas (Secco et al. 1994). They are also poor candidates for local excision even if confined to the muscularis propria (Masaki et al. 2001). Therefore, preoperative identification of mucinous adenocarcinoma is extremely useful for treatment planning. However, it is sometimes difficult to locate the mucin or estimate its content with small amounts of a biopsy specimen (Younes et al. 1993). Mucinous carcinomas of the rectum tend to show more extensive invasion at the time of presentation (Sasaki et al. 1987). The production of mucus under pressure allows the cancer to separate tissue planes in the bowel wall and thus to more frequently gain access to the peritoneal cavity. In addition, the fluid produced by these tumors is absorbed by lymphatics, which support tumor spread into the regional lymph nodes (Sugarbaker 2001).

Mucinous rectal carcinomas may present as a perirectal cystic mass because of their ablilty to easily penetrate the outside rectal wall. Therefore, knowledge of the imaging features of these tumors is important for radiologists. In a study by Kim et al. (1999), all mucinous carcinomas with mucin pools that were >50% of the tumor showed hyperintense areas on T2-weighted MRI that correlated with the mucin pool in the tumor. Interpretation errors of high-SI areas that mimic mucinous carcinoma can occur in nonmucinous rectal cancers such as intratumoral congestion, abscess, and necrosis in the adjacent rectal wall (Kim et al. 2003). To overcome these limitations, the additional use of gadolinium-enhanced sequences may improve the differentiation of mucin pool from edema, necrosis, or abscess. In one report, the tumor mucin pool showed contrast enhancement (Hussain et al. 1999).

4.3.5.4 Primary Signet-Ring Cell Carcinoma of the Rectum

Primary colorectal signet-ring cell carcinoma is a rare malignancy. More than 96% of signet-ring cell carcinomas begin in the stomach; the others originate from the colon and rectum, gallbladder, pancreas, urinary bladder, and breast (Tung et al. 1996). In a population-based review Kang et al. (2005) reported an incidence rate of 0.6% for colorectal signet-ring cell carcinoma. The diagnosis of primary colorectal signet-ring cell carcinoma is based on the histologic examination of the specimen with exclusion of a gastric primary tumor (Sim et al. 2008). An aggressive clinical course and a poor prognosis are typically associated with signet-ring cell tumors (Secco et al. 1994). There is high incidence of peritoneal metastasis and a relatively low incidence of hepatic metastases, a characteristic feature that distinguishes colorectal signet-ring cell carcinoma from non-signet-ring cell CRC. Secco et al. (1994) reported a 5-year survival rate of primary colorectal signet-ring cell cancer of 0% coupled with a recurrence rate of 100%. It is important to identify peritoneal dissemination at the time of initial diagnosis, as these patients are unlikely to benefit from surgery if symptoms are minimal (Sim et al. 2008).

The histologic appearance of the tumor is characterized by cells with abundant intracytoplasmic mucin, which pushes the nucleus to the periphery. The tumor cells may be arranged individually or in loose clusters, and may spread diffusely through the bowel wall. Mucin lakes also may be present (Almagro 1983). It has been suggested that when a signet-ring cell carcinoma is encountered on colon biopsy, the diagnosis of a colorectal primary is supported by the presence of CK7(−)/CK20(+) immunostaining pattern in the neoplastic cells, whereas gastric primary is diagnosed if the cells have a CK7(+)/CK20(−) staining pattern (Goldstein et al. 2000). Signet-ring cell carcinomas extensively permeate the bowel wall. Yoo et al. (1994) reported the case of a 12-year-old boy, who is believed to be the youngest patient with primary signet-ring cell carcinoma of the rectum. The patient died 4 months after initial diagnosis.

Laufman and Saphir (1951) defined the pathologic criteria for primary signet-ring cell carcinoma of the colon as the presence of signet-ring cells, formation of immature or abortive glands, and the occurrence of anaplastic cells with monocytoid features. This tumor type spreads extensively beneath the mucosal layer and is accompanied by a marked stromal desmoplastic reaction, resulting in a linitis plastica-type appearance. The term linitis plastica has been more commonly used for designating the macroscopic characteristics of rigidity, fibrosis, and diffuse wall thickening (Chowdhury et al. 1975; Vernon et al. 1981). Mucosal ulceration is superficial and some areas of mucosa are preserved, unlike the usual finding in nonsignet-ring cell CRC, which forms deep and extensive ulcerations. The radiographic appearance of signet-ring cell cancer is not sufficient for diagnosis and often mimics inflammatory bowel disease (Rao et al. 1982). Many cases are deemed unresectable because of extensive intraperitoneal seeding and chemoradiation therapy is only of limited benefit (Rao et al. 1982).

4.3.5.5 Small Cell Neuroendocrine Carcinoma of the Rectum

Gastroenteropancreatic neuroendocrine tumors (GEP-NET) are composed of cells with a neuroendocrine phenotype. Well-differentiated tumors, well-differentiated carcinomas, poorly differentiated carcinomas, functioning tumors, and nonfunctioning tumors are commonly seen with GEP-NET (Klöppel et al. 2007). Markers of the neuroendocrine phenotype such as synaptophysin; chromogranins A, B, and C; HISL-19; neuron-specific enolase (NSE); the protein convertases PC2 and PC3; the lymphoreticular epitope Leu-7; and the neural cell adhesion molecule or CD56 reveal the neuroendocrine differentiation of GEP-NETs (Llyod 2003). In the gastrointestinal tract and pancreas, 15 neuroendocrine cell types, which all produce different hormones but express the general neuroendocrine marker synaptophysin, can be distinguished as the sources of GEP-NETs (Klöppel et al. 2007). All GEP-NETs are potentially malignant but differ in their capacity to metastasize. The WHO (Solcia 2000) classification identified three tumor categories, irrespective of their site of origin:

1. Well-differentiated endocrine tumors with benign or uncertain behavior at the time of diagnosis
2. Well-differentiated endocrine tumors with low-grade malignant behavior
3. Poorly differentiated endocrine carcinomas with high-grade malignant behavior

The incidence of all NETs of the gut has been estimated to be 2.0 in 100,000 for men and 2.4 in 100,000 for women (Hemminki and Li 2001). Whereas colon NETs are rare, NETs of the rectum account for 20% of the gastrointestinal NETs (Klöppel et al. 2007). Well-differentiated NETs (carcinoids) are more frequent in the rectum than the colon, whereas poorly differentiated neuroendocrine carcinomas are more common in the colon. Well-differentiated rectal tumors appear during endoscopy as small (<1 cm), movable submucosal tumors. The poorly differentiated neuroendocrine carcinomas of the colon are usually of larger size (>2 cm). Prognostically, well-differentiated NETs of the rectum that are >2 cm in size and have already invaded the muscularis propria are likely to have metastasized to the regional lymph nodes and elsewhere. Well-differentiated NETs of the rectum that are <1 cm in size have a very low risk of metastasis. Poorly differentiated tumors exhibit a high rate of metastasis at the time of diagnosis (Brenner et al. 2004).

Small cell neuroendocrine carcinoma (NEC) of the colon and rectum has been documented under the terms of small cell undifferentiated carcinoma, NEC, and stem cell carcinoma (Vilor et al. 1995). This tumor is a rare aggressive neoplasm that is biologically similar to bronchogenic small cell carcinoma. It has been reported to occur frequently with distant metastases and carries a poor prognosis, even if diagnosed at an early stage (Saclarides et al. 1994b; Gaffey et al. 1990). Okuyama et al. (1999) reported that the NEC component in one patient was characterized by a proliferation of nests of relatively uniform, small-sized carcinoma cells with hyperchromatic nuclei and scanty cytoplasm with delicate fibrovascular stroma, which could be classified as small cell carcinoma according to the WHO classifications (Jass and Sobin 1993). Neuron-specific enolase (NSE) is strongly and uniformly expressed (Vilor et al. 1995; Saclarides et al. 1994b).

NEC is characterized by Grimelius staining, which exhibits fine endocrine granules in the cytoplasm of the cancer cells. Colorectal NEC accounts for less than 0.1% of all malignancies at this anatomical site (Vilor et al. 1995). In the literature, most patients present with metastatic disease in the liver, lymph nodes, bone, lung, or peritoneum, with the liver being the most common site of involvement (Gaffey et al. 1990). Hung (1989) reported a mean survival of approximately 6 months, with only 10% of patients surviving longer than 1 year. The histologic findings revealed that these tumors were frequently associated with adenomatous polyps, and small foci were found scattered in the adenoma (Gaffey 1990).

4.4 MRI After Neoadjuvant Chemoradiation Therapy

The goal of neoadjuvant therapy is to downstage and downsize the tumor to improve resectability and obtain better local control (Sauer et al. 2004; Reerink et al. 2003). Neoadjuvant chemoradiation therapy is often used in patients with extramural spread of rectal cancer in whom the CRM may be at risk of involvement at surgery. Such patients have locally advanced disease, an extramural tumor abutting the levator muscle, or a tumor that lies too close to the anal canal for which sphincter-preserving surgery is being considered (Allen et al. 2007). Preoperative chemoradiation therapy is known to be associated with less acute toxicity, greater tumor response/sensitivity, and higher rates of sphincter-saving procedures when compared with postoperative course (Minsky et al. 1992; Busse et al. 1998).

Tumor downstaging may lead to complete clinical response or complete pathologic response (pT0N0M0). These situations may be observed in 10% to 30% of patients treated by neoadjuvant chemoradiation and may be referred as stage 0 disease (Grann et al. 1997; Habr-Gama et al. 1998; Hiotis et al. 2002; Janjan et al. 1999; Luna-Perez et al. 2001; Medich et al. 2001). A multimodal approach is often the preferred treatment strategy for distal rectal cancer (Guillem et al. 2003; Habr-Gama et al. 1998; Luna-Perez et al. 2001). Radical surgery with TME may result in significantly low recurrence rates only in selected patients (Simunovic et al. 2003). Thus, adjuvant therapy has an important role in the management of rectal cancer despite TME surgery (Colquhoun et al. 2003). Ideally, complete pathologic response is warranted for every patient with distal rectal cancer treated by preoperative chemoradiation.

Local recurrence in patients treated by neoadjuvant therapy has been associated with the grade of primary tumor response. Habr-Gama et al. (2004) reported local recurrence-free follow-up period of 48 months for patients with pT0N0M0. However, preoperative chemoradiation therapy may not prevent control of distant recurrence. A proportion of patients may develop distant metastasis during the course of neoadjuvant therapy, even in the presence of complete pathologic response of the primary tumor. Medich et al. (2001) reported a rate of 20% for patients initially without metastatic disease and treated by preoperative chemoradiation therapy with stage IV disease at operation (pT0N0M1).

MRI has repeatedly been shown to be the most accurate modality for the prediction of mesorectal fascia tumor invasion and could be an important tool in selecting patients for different types of neoadjuvant treatment regimens according to the risk of local recurrence (Beets-Tan et al. 2001; Burton et al. 2006; Lahaye et al. 2005). Vliegen et al. (2008) evaluated the performance of postchemoradiation MRI for the prediction of mesorectal fascia tumor invasion. They found the assessment of diffuse fibrotic tissue in the initial tumor area, which is a feature seen in more than 50% of all patients, to be the main difficulty of postchemoradiation MRI in the evaluation of mesorectal fascia tumor invasion. Residual tumor within these fibrotic areas is often confined to small tumor nests that are beyond the depiction level of MRI (Dworak et al. 1997; Beets-Tan et al. 2000).

Despite the problems of MRI in the interpretation of postradiotherapy fibrosis, some potentially useful specific morphologic patterns can be identified. The presence of diffuse iso- or hyperintense tissue infiltration of the mesorectal fascia on MRI is associated with tumor invasion at histologic examination in 90% of the quadrants in which this pattern is seen (Vliegen et al. 2008). The technique can be performed with reasonable accuracy for documenting decrease in tumor size. In contrast, nodal downstaging is present in most patients after preoperative chemoradiation therapy, even if the tumor has not decreased in size or stage. After chemoradiation therapy, Allen et al. (2007) found that 63% of the tumors shrank sufficiently to constitute a partial response to treatment. Tumor downstaging occurred in only 17% of cases. Nodal downstaging occurred in 68% of the patients. In the study, a combination of size criteria and morphologic features was used to evaluate nodal metastasis (Brown et al. 2003b). A node was considered enlarged if the length was greater than 5 mm (mesorectal), 7 mm (internal iliac), 10 mm (external iliac), or 9 mm (common iliac) (Grubnic et al. 2002).

Identification of nodal disease in patients with rectal cancer remains problematic and represents a major challenge. Reliable differentiation between reactive and metastatic nodes is not always possible because there is a high incidence of microscopic metastasis in normal-looking nodes (Andreola et al. 1996), and enlarged but reactive mesorectal nodes can be present. MRI was only moderately accurate in predicting tumor stage in patients with rectal cancer who had undergone long-course preoperative chemoradiation therapy (Allen et al. 2007). Mucinous tumors tended to retain high SI after chemoradiation therapy in both primary tumors and nodes and did not seem to shrink. These tumors did not seem to respond well to chemoradiation therapy; they had persistent areas of high SI and CRM involvement was found frequently. This finding proved to be a source of error; in many of these cases, histologic evaluation showed no active tumor but only inactive mucin lakes.

Allen et al. (2007) found four additional mucinous tumors after chemoradiation therapy compared to pretreatment MRI. This morphologic change was found in a similar proportion in a previous pathologic study (Nagtegaal et al. 2004). Tumors showing mucinous differentiation only after chemoradiation were responsive to treatment. Another pitfall included discrimination of active tumor and posttreatment fibrosis, particularly when differentiating stage T2 and T3 carcinomas. This phenomenon occurred even though the observers based the MRI diagnosis of T3 lesions on the method described by Brown et al. (1999). This method of classification and other criteria are based on observations of patients receiving short-course chemoradiation therapy (Brown et al. 2005). Short-course radiation therapy 1 week prior to surgery resulted in no discernible histopathologic evidence of a radiation therapy effect on the tumor. In particular, there was no evidence of florid inflammation or fibrosis (Brown et al. 1999).

After a long course of chemoradiation therapy, a reliable differentiation of active tumor from posttreatment fibrosis is impossible, as demonstrated in the study by Kuo et al. (2005) with an overall tumor staging accuracy of 47%. CRM tumor regression was frequently found, and the distance between tumor and CRM was accurately predicted to within a few millimeters. Chen et al. (2005) reported an overall accuracy for T stage after neoadjuvant therapy of 52% of patients using phased-array pelvic MRI, whereas overstaging occurred in 38% and understaging in 10% of patients, respectively. For N stage, accurate staging was noted in 68% of patients, whereas 24% were overstaged and 8% were understaged.

From a clinical point of view, overstaging is much more acceptable than understaging. Understaging may lead to incomplete tumor resection and an unacceptably high risk of local tumor recurrence (Govindarajan et al. 2006; Lehnert et al. 2002; Luna-Perez et al. 2005). Peschaud et al. (2005) evaluated the accuracy of MRI in predicting CRM involvement in patients receiving long- or short-course chemoradiation therapy. Involvement was indicated if the measurable distance of the tumor on MRI was <2 mm from the CRM. CRM involvement in patients who had received long-course chemoradiation was predicted in 70% of cases, but most of the tumors were midrectal. The rate of CRM prediction of low rectal tumors was as low as 22%.

4.5 MRI for the Detection of Recurrent Rectal Cancer

4.5.1 Introduction

CRC is the third leading cancer type in the United States in both males and females, with an estimated number of 148,810 new cases annually. CRC was responsible for approximately 49,960 deaths in 2008 (Jemal et al. 2008). Eighty percent of patients with CRC present with local disease amenable to surgery with curative intent (Jessup et al. 1997). Unfortunately, around 40% of these patients will develop recurrent cancer, mainly within the first 3 years after treatment (Abir et al. 2006; Arriola et al. 2006; Desch et al. 2005; Kraemer et al. 2001). About 1 of every 5 patients will go on to develop liver metastases, and 1 of every 12 patients will develop lung metastases (Kievit 2002). Pelvic recurrence remains a significant problem with rectal cancer, occurring in 3% to 47% of patients (Abulafi and Williams 1994; Sagar and Pemberton 1996; Titu et al. 2006). Relapse after initial surgery of CRC is responsible not only for significant morbidity and mortality, but also for impaired quality of life (Beets-Tan and Beets 2004; Camilleri-Brennan and Steele 2001; Miller 1998).

MRI has the potential to directly visualize local and distant relapse of CRC. Unlike other malignancies, both local recurrence and metastatic spread from CRC can be addressed by curative-intent surgery. However, only between 20% and 30% of patients with local relapse detected during follow-up have tumors that are deemed resectable at the time of diagnosis (Goldberg et al. 1998).

Aggressive surgical approaches for CRC recurrence confined to a single organ are associated with a 5-year survival rate of up to 30% in selected patient populations (Abir et al. 2006; Arriola et al. 2006; Huguier et al. 2001; Titu et al. 2006). Thus, early diagnosis of local recurrence and small volume metastases are two of the primary goals of surveillance strategies; salvage surgery has a higher chance of success in the asymptomatic patient with limited disease (Arriola et al. 2006; Huguier et al. 2001). Consequently, surveillance should enhance the proportion of resectable cases to increase survival.

In rectal cancer, the majority of local recurrences originate from the tumor bed, which emphasizes the importance of direct visualization of the perirectal tissues as part of postoperative follow-up (Titu et al. 2006). In addition to carcinoembryonic antigen (CEA) monitoring and endoscopy, CT, MRI, and positron emission tomography (PET) are used as diagnostic imaging modalities for the detection of local and distant relapse of CRC. The role of diagnostic imaging for routine follow-up of CRC patients remains controversial because no single strategy for postoperative surveillance has been unequivocally shown to improve survival or cure rate (Guillem et al. 2005; Giordano et al. 2006; Longo and Johnson 2002).

A number of single-center clinical trials have examined the usefulness of various surveillance strategies. Only two (Pietra et al. 1998; Secco et al. 2002) of the currently existing six randomized studies (Kjeldsen et al. 1997; Makela et al. 1995; Ohlsson et al. 1995; Pietra et al. 1998; Schoemaker et al. 1998; Secco et al. 2002) demonstrated significant improvements in survival for those patients receiving intensive surveillance; however, the definition of intensive varied widely between those trials (Arriola et al. 2006). The findings were corroborated by three high-quality meta-analyses (Figueredo et al. 2003; Jeffery et al. 2002; Renehan et al. 2002), which suggests a survival benefit correlated with intensive follow-up. Additionally, patients with more intensive surveillance had earlier documentation of recurrences, although the number of recurrences was comparable with those patients receiving less intensive follow-up. Patients with more intensive postoperative surveillance, including thoracic and abdominal imaging studies, were more likely to have surgery for metastatic or recurrent disease (Figueredo et al. 2003; Jeffery et al. 2002; Renehan et al. 2002).

4.5.2 Risk-Adapted Surveillance

To advance the idea of risk-adapted follow-up, Secco et al. (2002) randomly assigned patients with two different risk profiles to intensive and minimal follow-up. Patients were preoperatively judged at high risk for recurrence if they had adenocarcinoma of the low rectum treated by low anterior resection, a preoperative CEA value of ≥7.5 ng/ml, Dukes C stage, poorly differentiated carcinoma (G3), and mucinous adenocarcinoma or signet ring cells. Patients who did not meet these criteria were considered to be at low risk. The results of this trial clearly showed that prospective stratification of patients with CRC in subgroups at higher and lower risk of recurrence according to established prognostic factors would be rational and clinically reliable. Patients classified as being at high risk developed recurrence 2.5 times more frequent than patients at low risk. Only patients at high risk who were randomly assigned to the minimal follow-up group had a shorter median disease-free interval compared with high-risk patients who underwent intensive surveillance. The proposed risk-adapted follow-up strategy allowed for a significantly higher number of curative-intent surgical procedures and helped to reduce costs.

4.5.3 Imaging for Recurrent Colorectal Cancer

Local recurrence is defined as clinical, radiologic, and/or pathologic determination of rectal cancer recurrence in the prior pelvic treatment field (Guillem et al. 2005). According to Abulafi and Williams (1994), local relapse can be further divided into extraluminal recurrence (in which tumor regrowth occurs in and around the tumor bed, including the pericolic fat, the adjoining mesentery, and the lymph nodes) and intramural recurrence (in which the tumor regrowth involves the region of the bowel anastomosis). Distant recurrence is defined as clinical, radiologic, and/or pathologic determination of rectal cancer recurrence at any other site—mainly the liver, lungs and retroperitoneum (Guillem et al. 2005). In one of the largest single-institution analyses of long-term oncologic outcome, a total of 297 patients with locally advanced rectal cancer were observed. Of these, 67 patients (23%) had either local or distant relapse, with a 10-year overall survival rate of 58% (Guillem et al. 2005).

In general, diagnostic imaging for postoperative surveillance of rectal cancer should have the potential to differentiate between scar and extraluminal recurrence, as well as to detect anastomotic recurrence. To guide salvage surgery, an anatomically correct description of the location and extent of relapse is essential. Additionally, staging for metastatic spread should be possible within one examination, rendering a multimodal approach unnecessary (Schaefer and Schlemmer 2006). In this respect, one diagnostic challenge for all imaging strategies for detecting recurrence consists of the alteration of the pelvic anatomy associated with previous surgery and chemoradiation therapy.

4.5.3.1 Assessment of Local Relapse of Colorectal Cancer

Despite the increasing number of reports on the accuracy of diagnostic imaging for preoperative workup of patients with rectal cancer patients, data reflecting the role of state-of-the-art imaging for local relapse of CRC are scarce. In the opinion of the authors, MRI is currently the best-suited imaging modality for the detection of pelvic recurrence of CRC. Its excellent soft-tissue resolution provides detailed anatomic information (Markus et al. 1997; Stoker et al. 2000). Compared to other imaging modalities, the distinction of recurrent cancer within a presacral scar seems to be more accurate. This finding is based on differences in SI between tumor and fibrosis using T2-weighted sequences or contrast-enhanced imaging techniques (Dicle et al. 1999).

Despite these advantages over other imaging tests, a recent study (Titu et al. 2006) concluded that the use of MRI as part of routine pelvic surveillance after curative resection of CRC is not justified. Instead, MRI should be reserved for selective imaging of patients with clinical, colonoscopic, and/or biochemical suspicion of recurrent disease. The study examined 226 patients who underwent curative surgery for CRC. An intensive follow-up program included clinical examination, CEA measurements, colonoscopy, and MRI at 3- to 6-month intervals. The separate contribution of these diagnostic tests to the final diagnosis was assessed. The median clinical follow-up was 42 months, with a median MRI surveillance period of 21 months and a median number of 3 MRI scans per patient. Local recurrence was detected in 30 of 226 patients (13%). The median interval between initial surgery and recurrence was 15 months. MRI detected 26 (87%) of the 30 local recurrences and missed 3 of the 4 anastomotic recurrences. In summary, the sensitivity, specificity, positive predictive value, and negative predictive value were 87, 86, 48, and 98%, respectively. MRI was the only positive diagnostic test in four (13%) patients with pelvic recurrence located in the perirectal tissue. Only two of these patients were determined to have resectable disease. Resection of local relapse was possible in six (20%) patients. MRI correctly diagnosed four of these six cases. The median surival time in the surgically treated group was 13 months. In contrast, the median survival time of the unresectable patient group was 9 months. In light of these results, the authors strongly question the use of MRI in the routine postoperative follow-up of CRC patients. A total of 576 examinations were performed in the 226 patients in order to detect 4 (<2%) cases with local recurrence missed by other tests.

Twenty-five patients were enrolled in a study by Blomqvist et al. (1996) who received CT, MRI, and CEA scintigraphy for the detection of recurrent rectal cancer. As a result of the study, MRI was the most effective imaging modality with an accuracy of 87.5% compared to CT, which correctly diagnosed recurrent cancer in 76%. In a comparative study, Pema et al. (1994) analyzed the value of CT and MRI in diagnosing recurrent rectal cancer. Eighteen patients were included in this study. MRI was the superior imaging method with a sensitivity of 91%, a specificity of 100%, and an overall accuracy of 95%.

4.5.3.2 Assessment of Distant Relapse of Colorectal Cancer

The liver is one of the main targets of metastatic spread of CRC (Bhattacharjya et al. 2004). Early detection of limited disease is of particular importance for patient management and outcome. A meta-analysis conducted by Kinkel et al. (2002) compared ultrasound (US), CT, MRI, and PET for hepatic metastases from cancers of the gastrointestinal tract. In cases with a specificity greater than 85%, the mean weighted sensitivity for the detection of liver metastases was 55% for US, 72% for CT, 76% for MRI, and 90% for PET. Bipat (2005) also performed a meta-analysis to obtain the estimates of sensitivity of CT, MRI, and PET for the detection of colorectal liver metastases. Sensitivity estimates on a per-patient basis for nonhelical CT, helical CT, 1.5-T MRI, and FDG-PET were 60.2, 64.7, 75.8, and 94.6%, respectively. On a per-lesion basis, sensitivity estimates for nonhelical CT, helical CT, 1.0-T MRI, 1.5-T MRI, and FDG-PET were 52.3, 63.8, 66.1, 64.4, and 75.9%, respectively. For lesions of 1 cm or larger, superparamagnetic iron oxide-enhanced MRI has turned out to be the most accurate modality.

Parallel acquisition technique, multiple phased-array surface coils, and receiver channels (e.g., total imaging matrix) opened the door for whole-body MRI with highly resolved spin echo and/or gradient echo sequences in acceptable imaging time. Thus, tumor staging is now possible. Compared with CT or PET/CT, total-body MRI seems to be more sensitive for brain, liver, and bone metastases, although it still offers lower sensitivity for lung metastases. However, detectability is strongly related to lesion size and number of sequences performed. In the meantime, comparable sensitivities for nodules greater than 4 mm in size were found (Schaefer and Schlemmer 2006).

Schmidt (2005) compared whole-body MRI with PET/CT in a study including 41 patients with malignant disease. PET/CT detected 7 of 7 tumors (sensitivity 100%, specificity 100%), whereas whole-body MRI diagnosed 6 of the 7 tumors (sensitivity 86%, specificity, 100%). A total of 60 metastatic lymph nodes were diagnosed with a sensitivity of 98% for PET/CT and 80% for whole-body MRI. PET/CT found more lymph nodes of all size groups and was superior to whole-body MRI in small-sized nodes. Using PET/CT, distant metastases were detected with a sensitivity and a specificity of 82%. Whole-body MRI had a diagnostic sensitivity of 96% and a specificity of 82%. Regarding TNM, stage reliable assessment was possible with each modality (diagnostic accuracy of PET/CT 96% and of whole-body MRI 91%).

4.5.3.3 Future Perspectives

For pre- and postoperative workup of patients with rectal cancer, pelvic MRI is routinely combined with abdominal and thoracic CT. Although MRI of the upper abdomen is an alternative to CT, the combination with high-resolution pelvic MRI during one examination is time consuming and normally requires patient repositioning. When workflow and cost effectiveness are considered, an integrated one-stop examination for both local staging and screening for distant metastases is a possibility. In this regard, the implementation of moving-table MRI represents a possible alternative to traditional multimodality approaches. Because of its high image quality and relatively short acquisition times, it appears reasonable to combine SMS with pelvic MRI for follow-up of patients with rectal cancer (Baumann et al. 2008; Fautz and Kannengiesser 2006; Schäfer and Langer 2007; Sommer et al. 2008, see also Section 4.2.2 and enclosed CD-ROM).

4.6 Integrative Decisions in Rectal Cancer

The management of rectal cancer patients should be coordinated by an MDT composed of specialist surgeons, oncologists, radiologists, histopathologists, and specialist nurses. The participation of all members of the MDT in the discussion of staging and other characteristics before any therapeutic intervention is crucial. According to Cervantes et al. (2007), the important activities of the MDT include the following:

- Reviewing all new or recently diagnosed cases prior to therapeutic decision making
- Sharing all data concerning diagnosis and staging of new patients, especially MRI features
- Discussing and deciding the therapeutic approach for all newly diagnosed patients
- Reviewing the pathology report of all operated patients, including TNM stage, CRM status, and quality of the surgical specimen
- Selecting patients for adjuvant therapy
- Reviewing and discussing all local and systemic relapses

The MDT should implement an agreed-upon treatment strategy based on accepted guidelines with the aim of standardizing and improving outcomes (Burton et al. 2006). In the past, the main outcome measures of rectal cancer treatment were local recurrence rate, development of distant metastases, and overall survival. More recently, CRM has been identified as an indicator of surgical quality, and there is now good evidence to relate CRM status to improved outcomes (Birbeck et al. 2002; Nagtegaal et al. 2002a). The presence of a positive CRM has been shown to correlate with an increasing incidence of local recurrence, systemic failure, and poor survival (Hall et al. 1998; Delany et al. 2002; Nagtegaal et al. 2002a).

In addition to CRM status, increasing depth of spread has also been identified as a poor prognostic factor (Merkel et al. 2001). Other poor prognostic features include N2 nodal disease, T4 disease, and extramural venous invasion (Shepherd et al. 1995). It appears that the positive CRM rate is reducible, but only in the presence of robust MRI staging, preoperative MDT discussion of all staging investigations, specialized surgery, the availability of effective preoperative therapies, and standardized histopathology reporting with comprehensive data collection (Burton et al. 2006). The radiologists' role in the preoperative decision-making process has become crucial; the information provided by specific MRI of the primary tumor guides the team in achieving improved outcomes for patients with rectal cancer. Rectal MRI is highly dependent on specialized MRI radiologists who are familiar with pelvic anatomy in order to plan MRI acquisition and obtain consistently high image quality (Brown 2005).

4.7 Selected Differential Diagnoses Mimicking Rectal Cancer

4.7.1 Anal Cancer

Squamous cell carcinoma of the anus is rare and accounts for only 1.5% of cases of gastrointestinal tract cancer in the United States (Ryan et al. 2000). A TNM staging system for anal cancer has been developed by the American Joint Committee on Cancer and the International Union Against Cancer (UICC 1995) (Table 4.3). Because few tumors are surgically removed, the system is based on clinical factors and places particular emphasis on tumor size, which is known to be an important prognostic indicator (Uronis and Bendell 2007). From 50% to 60% of patients present with T1 or T2 lesions, for which the 5-year survival rate is between 80% and 90%. A smaller percentage of patients present with T4 lesions, which have a 5-year survival rate <50%. The incidence of nodal metastasis can range from 20% to 60% for T4 lesions (Salmon et al. 1986).

Table 4.3 TNM classification for anal cancer (Uronis and Bendell 2007)

Primary tumor (T)	
TX	Primary tumor cannot be assessed
T0	No evidence of primary tumor
Tis	Carcinoma in situ
T1	Tumor ≤ 2 cm in greatest dimension
T2	Tumor > 2 cm but not ≥5 cm in greatest dimension
T3	Tumor > 5 cm in greatest dimension
T4	Tumor of any size invades adjacent organ(s), e.g., vagina, urethra, bladder (involvement of the sphincter muscle[s] alone is not classified as T4)
Regional lymph nodes (N)	
NX	Regional lymph nodes cannot be assessed
N0	No regional lymph node metastases
N1	Metastasis in perirectal lymph node(s)
N2	Metastasis in unilateral internal iliac and/or inguinal lymph nodes
N3	Metastasis in perirectal and inguinal lymph nodes and/or bilateral internal iliac and/or inguinal lymph nodes
Distant metastasis (M)	
MX	Distant metastasis cannot be assessed
M0	No distant metastasis
M1	Distant metastasis

Adapted from the AJCC Cancer Staging Manual, 5th edition (1997) published by Lippincott-Raven Publishers, Philadelphia, PA
TNM, tumor- node metastasis

The standard treatment for anal cancer is concurrent chemotherapy and radiotherapy (Chauveinc et al. 2003). The effects of chemoradiation on anal cancer can be present for weeks after completion of treatment. Treatment response is best assessed at least 6 to 8 weeks after completion. Metastatic disease develops in 10% to 17% of patients treated with chemoradiation therapy (Bartelink et al. 1997). The most common site of distant metastasis is the liver. A discrimination of low-lying rectal cancer and anal cancer seems to be impossible in many cases, relying on MRI only. For this reason, biopsy with histopathologic evaluation is the decisive factor in diagnosis.

4.7.2 Cancer Arising from Anorectal Fistula

Adenocarcinoma associated with a fistula-in-ano is rare (Hama et al. 2006; Ky et al. 1998; Patrinou et al. 2001). The incidence of fistula-related carcinoma is approximately 0.7% (Ky et al. 1998). Perianal fistulae are a common manifestation of Crohn's disease (Lockhart-Mummery 1975). The average duration of Crohn's disease before diagnosis of fistula-associated carcinoma is 15.5 years (Connell et al. 1994). The malignancies arising in this setting are usually squamous cell carcinomas (thought to arise from the squamous epithelium of the fistula tract) or mucinous adenocarcinomas (thought to arise from anal glands) (Smith et al. 2008b; Ky et al. 1998). The cause of fistula-related cancer is not clearly understood. Traube et al. (1980) suggested that cancer arises as a result of chronic stimulation of mucosal regeneration. This theory may not adequately explain the development of adenocarcinoma.

Smith et al. (2008b) documented pathologically that mucinous adenoarcinoma can arise in a fistula tract in association with adenomatous mucosa. The colonic epithelialization of the fistula tract may have a dysplastic potential that gives rise to subsequent mucinous adenocarcinoma. In contrast, Wong et al. (2002) suggested that these adenocarcinomas without associated intestinal involvement arise from the anal glands. Another interesting theory is that deposition of malignant cells in the granulation tissue of a fistula comes from a proximal gastrointestinal cancer. It is therefore advisable to evaluate the entire gastrointestinal tract before assuming that the carcinoma is primary to the fistula (Gaertner et al. 2008).

Mucinous adenocarcinoma in a long-standing fistula-in-ano is known to be a slow growing, locally aggressive neoplasm with a low-grade histologic appearance that is rarely metastatic. Tumor spread is usually lymphatic, and the inguinal lymph nodes are the most frequent site of metastasis (Lee et al. 1981b). Treatment can be curative if the diagnosis is made early (Lee et al. 1981b). The standard treatment option for these patients has been surgical. Abdominoperineal resection is the most frequently employed operation (Abel et al. 1993). Neoadjuvant therapy may be another chance to improve the outcome of patients with anal adenocarcinoma. Tarazi and Nelson (1994) reported a good response rate for patients with anal adenocarcinoma treated under a Nigro protocol. Gaertner et al. (2008) also found that cancer along the fistula tract was never clearly obvious. The most consistent finding was mucinous material in the fistula tract. Other characteristics that should raise suspicion include chronic anorectal disease (>10 years), Crohn's disease, the presence of a mass, and distorted anatomy. Frequently, several of these five features are present. Patients with mucinous adenocarcinoma complicating a chronic anorectal fistula usually do not present with complaints such as diarrhea or obstruction (Getz et al. 1981).

Carcinoma arising in chronic, complex fistulas—especially in patients with underlying Crohn's disease—can be very difficult to diagnose. Biopsy of the external openings of the fistula is often not conclusive because the biopsied tissue is superficial and may only reveal an inflammatory reaction, especially when scarring and fibrosis are present (Heidenreich et al. 1966). Therefore, EUS and MRI are used to establish the diagnosis.

4.7.3 Gastrointestinal Stromal Tumor of the Rectum

Gastrointestinal stromal tumor (GIST) was first described in 1983 by Mazur and Clark as a "nonepithelial tumor group consisting of spindle cells and epitheloid cells" (Mazur and Clark 1983). In the past, these tumors were mistaken for smooth muscle tumors, such as leiomyosarcomas, which they resemble on light microscopy (Sandrasegaran et al. 2005). GIST develops in the gastrointestinal tract and the mesentery, from the esophagus to the rectum. This tumor entity expresses CD117 (*c-kit* proto-oncogene), which can be detected with immunohistochemistry. CD117 is the most important GIST marker (Fletcher et al. 2002).

Approximately 20% of GISTs are malignant. However, the malignant potential of GIST is not always predictable using conventional prognostic factors. High cellularity, prominent nuclear pleomorphism, and intratumoral necrosis are indicative of a poor prognosis (Pidhorecky et al. 2007). Rectal GIST accounts for 0.1% of all tumors that originate in the rectum (Conlon et al. 1995). Complete surgical resection remains the most definitive treatment for localized GIST (DeMatteo et al. 2000). However, there is a substantial recurrence rate of up to 90% following surgery (Sandrasegaran et al. 2005).

- The prognostic factors of GIST include invasion to adjacent organs; formation of metastasis; range of resection; and pathologic findings such as size, hemorrhage, necrosis, cell density, nuclear aplasia, proliferation pattern (Baik et al. 2007). A major cause of death after curative resection of GISTs is distant metastasis, not local recurrence (Lewis et al. 1998). Metastatic disease is most commonly found in the liver followed by the mesentery. Liver and mesenteric masses respond to imatinib therapy by rapidly showing cystic change (Sandrasegaran et al. 2005). Rectal GIST tends to show homogeneous contrast enhancement on cross-sectional imaging studies. A crescent-shaped necrosis, the Torricelli-Bernouilli sign, has been reported to be a typical imaging feature of large GISTs (Rioux and Mailloux 1997). An intraluminal component is more common in gastric and rectal GISTs.

4.7.4 Tumors of the Retrorectal Space

Retrorectal masses are uncommon lesions. Although the vast majority of these lesions are benign, a substantial number have malignant potential and therefore require aggressive surgical management (Hobson et al. 2005). The retrorectal space is commonly known as the presacral space. It is defined anteriorly by the fascia propria of the rectum and posteriorly by the presacral fascia overlying the sacrum. Laterally, it is delimited by the lateral stalks of the rectum, the uterus, and the iliac vessels. The retrorectal space extends superiorly to the peritoneal reflection of the rectum and inferiorly to the Waldeyer's fascia, which is located between 3 and 5 cm proximal to the anorectal junction (Hobson et al. 2005).

Retrorectal masses can generally be divided into five categories: congenital, inflammatory, neurogenic, osseous, and miscellaneous (Uhlig and Johnson 1975). Congenital lesions are by far the most common tumor type, accounting for between 55% and 70% of all retrorectal tumors (Stewart et al. 1986). These lesions consist primarily of teratomas, developmental cysts, chordomas, anterior meningoceles, rectal duplications, and adrenal rest tumors. Inflammatory lesions are less common than the congenital lesions and include foreign body granulomas and abscesses (Freier et al. 1971). Neurogenic etiologies account for 10% of retrorectal lesions including neurofibromas, neurolemmomas, ependymomas, ganglioneuromas, and neurofibrosarcomas (Stewart et al. 1986). Osseous lesions can also arise in the retrorectal space, comprising approximately 5 to 10% of all retrorectal tumors. These lesions mainly consist of osteomas, sarcomas, sacral bone cysts, and giant cell tumors (Uhlig and Johnson 1975). The miscellaneous group of retrorectal tumors accounts for between 10 and 25% of all masses in the retrorectal space. This category includes metastatic disease secondary to rectal cancer, sarcomas, malignant fibrous histiocytomas, and lymphangiomas (Uhlig and Johnson 1975; Stewart et al. 1986).

Because of its inherently superior soft-tissue resolution, MRI is increasingly used for the characterization of retrorectal masses. MRI is particularly helpful in delineating soft-tissue planes and evaluating the presence or absence of bony invasion and nerve involvement. Such information is vital for surgical planning. When examining a retrorectal lesion, the mass should only be biopsied if the lesion appears to be unresectable and a tissue diagnosis is required to guide adjuvant therapy (Hobson et al. 2005). Studies indicate that tumor seeding can occur through unaffected tissue planes (Jao et al. 1985). As stated above, approximately 9 to 45% of retrorectal masses are malignant. Local control is difficult to achieve for malignant lesions, as evidenced by a study from the Memorial Sloan-Kettering Cancer Center, which demonstrated a 48% recurrence rate for patients with malignant retrorectal lesions and a poor 5-year overall survival of only 17% (Cody et al. 1981).

4.7.4.1 Tailgut Cyst with Malignant Transformation

Tailgut cysts are rare lesions that are believed to originate in the presacral space in young adults. Between 75 and 90% of the reported cases occur in females (Andea and Klimstra 2005). It is hypothesized that regression failure of the embryologic tailgut results in the formation of a tailgut cyst (Hjermstad and Helwig 1988). About 50% of the cases are discovered incidentally; the other cases are discovered in patients who present with various symptoms related to the retrorectal location, such as rectal fullness, constipation, discomfort while sitting, rectal bleeding, or infections (Levert et al. 1996).

Grossly, taligut cysts have a unilocular or a multilocular cystic appearance (Kim et al. 1997), range in size from 1 to 15 cm, and show a clear to thick mucoid or opaque greenish content. Microscopically, the cysts are lined by a variety of epithelia, including stratified squamous, columnar, cuboidal, ciliated columnar, mucinous, gastric, and transitional (Hjermstad and Hellwig 1988). Rarely, malignant transformation of the tailgut cyst has been reported, in which adenocarcinoma, mucinous adenocarcinoma, neuroendocrine tumors, and sarcoma arise within the cyst (Andea and Klimstra 2005). Differential diagnoses of tailgut cysts include sacrococcygeal teratomas, epidermoid and dermoid cysts, rectal duplication cysts, and anal gland cysts (Tampi et al. 2007).

On MRI, most tailgut cysts display low SI on T1-weighted images and high SI on T2-weighted images. However, they will sometimes show high signal on T1-weighted images because of the presence of mucinous material, high protein content, or hemorrhage within the cyst (Kim et al. 1997; Lim et al. 1998; Moulopoulos et al. 1999). In cases of malignant transformation of a tailgut cyst, irregular wall thickening or a polypoid mass with intermediate signal on both T1- and T2-weighted images and enhancement after intravenous administration of gadolinium have been reported (Yang et al. 2005).

4.7.5 Anorectal Giant Condyloma Acuminatum: Buschke-Loewenstein Tumor

Giant condyloma acuminatum is a variant of venereal warts, with similar etiology and histologic features; however, it can be distinguished by its large size and local infiltration of adjacent structures (Balthazar et al. 1984). It was first described by Buschke and Loewenstein as a large, slowly growing, cauliflower-like tumor, involving mainly the genitourinary tract and often presenting with necrosis, secondary infections, hemorrhage, and fistulizations (Alexander and Kaminsky 1979). The biologic potential of condyloma acuminatum to undergo mailgnant transformation is well recognized (Lee et al. 1981a). Until now, only a few patients with malignant perianal and anorectal condyloma have been reported (Lee et al. 1981a).

It is believed that the giant condyloma represents an intermediate state in the development of carcinoma (Lee et al. 1981a). This is because some of the tumors show a complex histologic pattern, with large areas of benign condyloma intermixed with areas of epithelial dysplasia, verrucous carcinoma, and well-differentiated squamous cell carcinoma. On cross-sectional imaging, especially pelvic MRI, the primary tumor and the extent of perineal, anorectal and perirectal involvement can be precisely determined. However, discriminating between different histologic types of soft-tissue infiltration is almost impossible. The associated inflammatory and fibrotic induration, as well as the type of benign and malignant tumor infiltration, have generally similar imaging characteristics. In these cases, the detection of extensive lymphadenopathy or distant metastases may help to clarify the malignant nature of the anorectal lesion (Balthazar et al. 1984).

References

Abel ME, Chiu YS, Russel TR et al (1993) Adenocarcinoma of the anal glands: results of a survey. Dis Colon Rectum 36:383–387

Abir F, Alva S, Longo WE et al (2006) The postoperative surveillance of patients with colon cancer and rectal cancer. Am J Surg 192:100–108

Abulafi AM, Williams NS (1994) Local recurrence of colorectal cancer: the problem, mechanisms, management and adjuvant therapy. Br J Surg 81:7–19

Adam IJ, Mohamdee MO, Martin IG et al (1994) Role of circumferential margin involvement in the local recurrence of rectal cancer. Lancet 344:707–711

Akasu T, Iinuma G, Fujita T et al (2005) Thin-section MRI with a phased-array coil for preoperative evaluation of pelvic anatomy and tumor extent in patients with rectal cancer. AJR Am J Roentgenol 184:531–538

Alexander RM, Kaminsky DB (1979) Giant conyloma acuminatum (Buschke-Loewenstein tumor) of the anus. Case report and review of the literature. Dis Colon Rectum 22:561–565

Allen SD, Padhani AR, Dzik-Jurasz AS et al (2007) Rectal carcinoma: MRI with histologic correlation before and after chemoradiation therapy. AJR Am J Roentgenol 188:442–451

Almagro UA (1983) Primary signet-ring carcinoma of the colon. Cancer 52:1453–1457

Andea AA, Klimstra DS (2005) Adenocarcinoma arising in a tailgut cyst with prominent meningothelial proliferation and thyroid tissue: case report and review of the literature. Virchows Arch 446:316–321

Andreola S, Leo E, Belli F et al (1996) Manual dissection of adenocarcinoma of the lower third of the rectum specimens for detection of lymph node metastases smaller than 5 mm. Cancer 77:607–612

Arriola E, Navarro M, Pares D et al (2006) Imaging techniques contribute to increased surgical rescue of relapse in the follow-up of colorectal cancer. Dis Colon Rectum 49:478–484

Baik SH, Kim NK, Lee CH et al (2007) Gastrointestinal stromal tumor of the rectum: an analysis of seven cases. Surg Today 37:455–459

Balthazar EJ, Streiter M, Megibow AJ (1984) Anorectal giant condyloma acuminatum (Buschke-Loewenstein tumor): CT and radiographic manifestations. Radiology 150:651–653

Barkhausen J, Quick HH, Lauenstein T (2001) Whole-body MR imaging in 30 seconds with real-time true FISP and a continuously rolling table platform: feasibility study. Radiology 220:252–256

Barrett MW (1998) Chemoradiation for rectal cancer: current methods. Semin Surg Oncol 15:114–119

Bartelink H, Roelofsen F, Eschwege F et al (1997) Concomitant radiotherapy and chemotherapy is superior to radiotherapy alone in the treatment of locally advanced anal cancer: results of a phase III randomized trial of the European organization for research and treatment of cancer radiotherapy and gastrointestinal cooperative groups. J Clin Oncol 15:2040–2049

Baumann T, Ludwig U, Pache G et al (2008) Detection of pulmonary nodules with move-during-scan magnetic resonance imaging using a free-breathing turbo inversion recovery magnitude sequence. Invest Radiol 43:359–367

Baumann T, Ludwig U, Pache G et al (2009) Continuously moving table MRI with sliding multislice for rectal cancer staging: image quality and lesion detection. Eur J Radiol [ahead of print]

Beets-Tan RG, Beets GL (2004) Rectal cancer: review with emphasis on MR imaging. Radiology 232:335–346

Beets-Tan RG, Beets GL, Borstlap AC et al (2000) Preoperative assessment of local tumor extent in advanced rectal cancer: CT or high resolution MRI. Abdom Imaging 25:533–541

Beets-Tan RG, Beets GL, Vliegen RF et al (2001) Accuracy of magnetic resonance imaging in prediction of tumor-free resection margin in rectal cancer surgery. Lancet 357:497–504

Bhattacharjya S, Bhattacharjya T, Baber S et al (2004) Prospective study of contrast-enhanced computed tomography, computed tomography during arterioportography, and magnetic resonance imaging for staging of colorectal liver metastases for liver resection. Br J Surg 91:1361–1369

Billingham RP (1994) Extended lymphadenectomy for rectal cancer: cure vs quality of life. Int Surg 79:11–22

Bipat S, van Leeuwen MS, Comans EFI et al (2005) Colorectal liver metastases: CT, MR imaging, and PET for diagnosis – meta-analysis. Radiology 237:123–131

Birbeck KF, Macklin CP, Tiffin NJ et al (2002) Rates of circumferential resection margin involvement vary between surgeons and predict outcomes in rectal cancer surgery. Ann Surg 235:449–457

Blomqvist L, Holm T, Goranson H et al (1996) MR imaging, CT and CEA scintigraphy in diagnosis of local recurrence of rectal cancer. Acta Radiol 37:779–784

Blomqvist L, Holm T, Rubio C et al (1997) Rectal tumours: MR imaging with and/or phased-array coils, and histopathological staging on giant sections – a comparative study. Acta Radiol 38:437–444

Blomqvist L, Machado M, Rubio C et al (2000) Rectal tumor staging: MR imaging using pelvic phased-array and endorectal coils vs endoscopic ultrasonography. Eur Radiol 10:653–660

Bokey EL, Chapuis PH, Dent OF et al (1997) Factors affecting survival after excision of the rectum for cancer: a multivariate analysis. Dis Colon Rectum 40:3–10

Börnert P, Aldefeld B (2008) Principles of whole-body continuously-moving-table MRI. J Magn Reson Imaging 28:1–12

Brenner B, Tang LH, Klimstra DS et al (2004) Small-cell carcinomas of the gastrointestinal tract: a review. J Clin Oncol 22:2730–2739

Brown G (2005) Thin section MRI in multidisciplinary preoperative decision making for patients with rectal cancer. Br J Radiol 78:117–127

Brown G, Davies S, Williams GT et al (2004) Effectiveness of preoperative staging in rectal cancer: digital rectal examination, endoluminal ultrasound or magnetic resonance imaging? Br J Cancer 91:23–29

Brown G, Radcliffe AG, Newcombe RG et al (2003a) Preoperative assessment of prognostic factors in rectal cancer using high-resolution magnetic resonance imaging. Br J Surg 90:355–364

Brown G, Richards CJ, Bourne MW et al (2003b) Morphologic predictors of lymph node status in rectal cancer with use of high-spatial-resolution MR imaging with histopathologic comparison. Radiology 227:371–377

Brown G, Richards CJ, Newcombe RG et al (1999) Rectal carcinoma: thin-section MR imaging for staging in 28 patients. Radiology 211:215–222

Burdy G, Panis Y, Alves A et al (2001) Identifying patients with T3-T4 node-negative colon cancer at high risk of recurrence. Dis Colon Rectum 44:1682–1688

Burton S, Brown G, Daniels I et al (2006) MRI directed multidisciplinary team preoperative treatment strategy: the way to eliminate positive circumferential margins? Br J Cancer 94:351–357

Busse PM, Ng A, Recht A (1998) Induction therapy for rectal carcinoma. Semin Surg Oncol 15:120–125

Camilleri-Brennan J, Steele RJ (2001) The impact of recurrent rectal cancer on the quality of life. Eur J Surg Oncol 27:349–353

Carr I (1983) Lymphatic metastasis. Cancer Metastasis Rev 2:307–317

Cawthorn SJ, Parums DV, Gibbs NM et al (1990) Extent of mesorectal spread and involvement of lateral resection margin as prognostic factors after surgery of rectal cancer. Lancet 335:1055–1059

Cervantes A, Rodriguez-Braun E, Navarro S et al (2007) Integrative decisions in rectal cancer. Ann Oncol 18:127–131

Chauveinc L, Buthaut X, Falcou MC et al (2003) Anal cancer treatment: practical limitations of routine prescription of concurrent chemotherapy and radiotherapy. Br J Cancer 89:2057–2061

Chen CC, Lee RC, Lin JK et al (2005) How accurate is magnetic resonance imaging in restaging rectal cancer in patients receiving preoperative combined chemoradiotherapy? Dis Colon Rectum 48:722–728

Chung CK, Stryker JA, Demuth WE (1983) Patterns of failure following surgery alone for colorectal carcinoma. J Surg Oncol 22:65–70

Cody HS 3rd, Marcove RC, Quan SH (1981) Malignant retrorectal tumors: 28 years' experience at Memorial Sloan-Kettering Cancer Center. Dis Colon Rectum 24:501–506

Colquhoun P, Wexner SD, Cohen A (2003) Adjuvant therapy is valuable in the treatment of rectal cancer despite total mesorectal excision. J Surg Oncol 83:135–139

Conlon KC, Casper ES, Brennan MF (1995) Primary gastrointestinal sarcomas: analysis of prognostic variables. Ann Surg Oncol 2:26–31

Connell WR, Sheffield JP, Kamm MA et al (1994) Lower gastrointestinal malignancy in Crohn's disease. Gut 35:347–352

de Haas-Kock DF, Baeten CG, Jager JJ et al (1996) Prognostic significance of radial margins of clearance in rectal cancer. Br J Surg 83:781–785

Delany CP, Lavery IC, Brenner A et al (2002) Preoperative radiotherapy improves survival for patients undergoing total mesorectal excision for stage T3 low rectal cancers. Ann Surg 236:203–207

DeMatteo RP, Lewis JJ, Leung D et al (2000) Two hundred gastrointestinal tumors: recurrence patterns and prognostic factors for survival. Ann Surg 231:51–58

Desch CE, Benson AB, Somerfield MR et al (2005) Colorectal cancer surveillance: 2005 update of an American Society of Clinical Oncology practice guideline. J Clin Oncol 23: 8512–8519

DeVries AF, Kremser C, Hein PA et al (2003) Tumor microcirculation and diffusion predict therapy outcome for primary rectal carcinoma. Int J Radiat Oncol Biol Phys 56: 958–965

Dicle O, Obuz F, Cakmakci H (1999) Differentiation of recurrent rectal cancer and scarring with dynamic MR imaging. Br J Radiol 72:1155–1159

Dixon WT, Brummer ME, Malko JA (1988) Acquisition order and motional artifact reduction in spin warp images. Magn Reson Med 6:74–83

Dworak O (1991) Morphology of lymph nodes in the resected rectum of patients with rectal carcinoma. Pathol Res Pract 187:1020–1024

Dworak O, Keilholz L, Hoffmann A (1997) Pathological features of rectal cancer after preoperative radiochemotherapy. Int J Colorectal Dis 12:19–23

Dzik-Jurasz A, Domenig C, George M et al (2002) Diffusion MRI for prediction of response of rectal cancer to chemoradiation. Lancet 360:307–308

Enker WE, Thaler HT, Cranor ML et al (1995) Total mesorectal excision in the operative treatment of carcinoma of the rectum. J Am Coll Surg 181:335–346

Eriksen MT, Wibe A, Haffner J et al (2007) Prognostic groups in 1,676 patients with T3 rectal cancer treated without preoperative radiotherapy. Dis Colon Rectum 50:1–11

Fain SB, Browning FJ, Polzin JA et al (2004) Floating table isoropic projection (FLIPR) acquisition: a time-resolved 3D method for extended field-of-view MRI during continuous table motion. Magn Reson Med 52:1093–1102

Fautz HP, Honal M, Saueressig U et al (2007) Artifact reduction in moving-table acquisitions using parallel imaging and multiple averages. Magn Reson Med 57:226–232

Fautz HP, Kannengiesser SAR (2006) Sliding Multislice (SMS): a technique for minimum FOV usage in axial continuously moving-table acquisitions. Magn Reson Med 55:363–370

Figueredo A, Rumble RB, Maroun J et al (2003) Follow-up of patients with curatively resected colorectal cancer: a practice guideline. BMC Cancer 3:26

Fletcher CD, Berman JJ, Corless C et al (2002) Diagnosis of gastrointestinal stromal tumors: a consensus approach. Hum Pathol 33:459–465

Freier DT, Stanley JC, Thomson NW (1971) Retrorectal tumors in adults. Surg Gynecol Obstet 132:681–686

Frija G, Clement O, Le Guen O et al (1996) Experimental investigation of the delivery pathway of ultrasmall superparamagnetic iron oxide to lymph nodes. Acta Radiol 3:299–300

Fujita S, Nakanisi Y, Taniguchi H et al (2007) Cancer invasion to Auerbach's plexus is an important prognostic factor in patients with pT3-pT4 colorectal cancer. Dis Colon Rectum 50:1860–1866

Gaertner WB, Hagerman GF, Finne CO et al (2008) Fistula-associated anal adenocarcinoma: good results with aggressive therapy. Dis Colon Rectum 51:1061–1067

Gaffey MJ, Mills SE, Lack EE (1990) Neuroendocrine carcinoma of the colon and rectum – a clinicopathologic, ultrastructural and immunohistochemical study of 24 cases. Am J Surg Pathol 14:1010–1023

Gagliardi G, Bayar S, Smith R et al (2002) Preoperative staging of rectal cancer using magnetic resonance imaging with external phased-array coils. Arch Surg 137:437–444

Getz SB Jr, Ough YD, Patterson RB et al (1981) Mucinous adenocarcinoma developing in chronic anal fistula: report of two cases and review of the literature. Dis Colon Rectum 24:562–566

Giordano P, Efron J, Vernava AM et al (2006) Strategies of follow-up for colorectal cancer: a survey of the American Society of Colon and Rectal Surgeons. Tech Coloproctol 10:199–207

Goh JS, Goh JP, Wansaicheong GK (2002). Methylcellulose as a rectal cotrast agent for MR imaging of rectal carcinoma. AJR Am J Roentgenol 178:1145–1146

Goldberg RM, Fleming TR, Tangen CM et al (1998) Surgery for recurrent colon cancer: strategies for identifying resectable recurrence and success rates after resection. Eastern cooperative oncology group, the North central cancer treatment group, and the Southwest oncology group. Ann Intern Med 129:27–35

Goldstein NS, Long A, Kuan SF et al (2000) Colon signet ring cell adenocarcinoma: immunohistochemical characterization and comparison with gastric and typical colon adenocarcinoma. Appl Immunohistochem Mol Morphol8: 183–188

Gosens MJ, Van Krieken JH, Marijnen CA et al (2007) Improvement of staging by combining tumor and treatment parameters: the value of prognostication in rectal cancer. Clin Gastroenterol Hepatol 5:997–1003

Govindarajan A, Coburn N, Kiss A et al (2006) Population based assessment of the surgical management of locally advanced rectal cancer. J Natl Cancer Inst 98:1474–1481

Grann A, Minsky BD, Cohen AM et al (1997) Preliminary results of preoperative 5-fluorouracil, low-dose leucovorin, and concurrent radiation therapy for clinically resectable T3 rectal cancer. Dis Colon Rectum 40:512–522

Griswold MA, Jakob PM, Heidemann RM et al (2002) Generalized autocalibrating partially parallel acquisitions (GRAPPA). Magn Reson Med 47:1202–1210

Grubnic S, Vinniecombe SJ, Norman AR et al (2002) MR evaluation of normal retroperitoneal and pelvic lymph nodes. Clin Radiol 57:193–200

Guerra A, Borda F, Javier Jimenez F et al (1998) Multivariate analysis of prognostic factors in resected colorectal cancer: a new prognostic index. Eur J Gastroenterol Hepatol 10:51–58

Guillem JG, Chessin DB, Cohen AM et al (2005) Long-term oncologic outcome following preoperative combined modality therapy and total mesorectal excision of locally advanced rectal cancer. Ann Surg 241:829–838

Guillem JG, Diaz-Gonzalez JA, Minsky BD et al (2008) cT3N0 rectal cancer: potential overtreatment with preoperative chemoradiotherapy is warranted. 26:368–373

Guillem JG, Moore HG, Paty PB et al (2003) Adequacy of distal resection margin following preoperative combined modality therapy for rectal cancer. Ann Surg Oncol 10:824

Gunderson LL, Sargent DJ, Tepper JE et al (2004) Impact of T and N stage and treatment on survival and relapse in adjuvant rectal cancer: a pooled analysis. J Clin Oncol 22:1785–1796

Habr-Gama A, de Souza PM, Ribeiro U et al (1998) Low rectal cancer: impact of radiation and chemotherapy on surgical treatment. Dis Colon Rectum 41:1087–1096

Habr-Gama A, Perez RO, Nadalin W et al (2004) Operative versus nonoperative treatment for stage 0 distal rectal cancer following chemoradiation therapy. Ann Surg 240:711–718

Hadfield MB, Nicholson AA, MacDonald AW et al (1997) Preoperative staging of rectal carcinoma by magnetic resonance imaging with a pelvic phased-array coil. Br J Surg 84:529–531

Hall NR, Finan PJ, al-Jaberi T et al (1998) Circumferential margin involvement after mesorectal excision of rectal cancer with curative intent. Predictor of survival but not local recurrence? Dis Colon Rectum 41:979–983

Hama Y, Makita K, Yamana T et al (2006) Mucinous adenocarcinoma arising from fistula in ano: MRI findings. AJR Am J Roentgenol 187:517–521

Hanski C (1995) Is mucinous carcinoma of the colorectum a distinct genetic entity? Br J Cancer 72:1350–1356

Harrison JC, Dean PJ, el-Zeky F et al (1994) From Dukes through Jass: pathological prognostic indicators in rectal cancer. Hum Pathol 25:498–505

Heald RJ, Ryall RD (1986) Recurrence and survival after total mesorectal excision for rectal cancer. Lancet 1:1479–1482

Heidenreich A, Collarini HA, Paladino AM et al (1966) Cancer in anal fistulas: report of two cases. Dis Colon Rectum 9:371–376

Hemminki K, Li X (2001) Incidence trends and risk factors of carcinoid tumors. A nationwide epidemiologic study from Sweden. Cancer 92:2204–2210

Hermanek P, Gospodarowicz MK, Hutter RVP, Sobin LH (eds) (1995) Prognostic factors in cancer. Springer, Berlin

Hida J, Yasutomi M, Fujimoto K et al (1997a) Does lateral lymph node dissection improve survival in rectal cancer? Examination of node metastases by the clearing method. J Am Coll Surg 184:475–480

Hida J, Yasutomi M, Maruyama T et al (1997b) Lymph node metastases detected in the mesorectum distal to carcinoma of the rectum by the clearing method: justification of total mesorectal excision. J Am Coll Surg 184:584–588

Hiotis SP, Weber SM, Cohen AM et al (2002) Assessing the predictive value of clinical complete response to neoadjuvant therapy for rectal cancer: an analysis of 448 patients. J Am Coll Surg 194:131–135

Hjermstad BM, Helwig EB (1988) Tailgut cysts. Report of 53 cases. Am J Clin Pathol 89:139–147

Hobson KG, Ghaemmaghami V, Roe JP et al (2005) Tumors of the retrorectal space. Dis Colon Rectum 48:1964–1974

Hocht S, Mann B, Germer CT et al (2004) Pelvic sidewall involvement in recurrent rectal cancer. Int J Colorectal Dis 19:108–113

Hocht S, Wiegel T, Hammad R et al (2002) Pelvic sites of recurrence in rectal cancer. Lancet 360:879–880

Hojo K, Koyama Y, Moriya A et al (1982) Lymphatic spread and its prognostic value in patients with rectal cancer. Am J Surg 144:350–354

Horn A, Dahl O, Morild I (1991) Venous and neural invasion as predictors of recuurence in rectal adenocarcinoma. Dis Colon Rectum 34:798–804

Huguier M, Houry S, Barrier A (2001) Local recurrence of cancer of the rectum. Am J Surg 182:437–439

Hung SSJ (1989) Small cell carcinoma of the colon – a case report and literature review. J Clin Gastroenterol 11:335–339

Hussain SM, Outwater EK, Siegelman ES (1999) Mucinous versus non-mucinous rectal carcinomas: differentiation with MR imaging. Radiology 213:79–85

Janjan NA, Khoo VS, Abbruzzese J et al (1999) Tumor downstaging and sphincter preservation with preoperative chemoradiation in locally advanced rectal cancer: the M. D. Anderson Cancer Center experience. Int J Radiat Oncol Biol Phys 44:1027–1038

Jao SW, Beart RW Jr, Spencer RJ et al (1985) Retrorectal tumors. Mayo Clinic experience, 1960–1979. Dis Colon Rectum 28:644–652

Jass JR, Sobin LH (1993) World Health Organization, International Histological Classification of Tumours, 2nd edn. Springer, Berlin

Jeffery GM, Hickey BE, Hider P (2002) Follow-up strategies for patients treated for non-metastatic colorectal cancer. (Cochrane Database System Review) Oxford United Kingdom, Cochrane Library, CD002200

Jemal A, Siegel R, Ward E et al (2008) Cancer statistics, 2008. CA Cancer J Clin 58:71–96

Jessup JM, Menk HR, Fremgen A et al (1997) Diagnosing colorectal carcinoma: clinical and molecular approaches. CA Cancer J Clin 47:70–92

Johnson KM, Leavitt GD, Kayser HW (1997) Total-body MR imaging in as little as 18 seconds. Radiology 202:252–256

Kang H, O'Connell JB, Maggard MA et al. (2005) A 10-year outcomes evaluation of mucinous and signet-ring cell carcinoma of the colon and rectum. Dis Colon Rectum 48:1161-1168

Kazama Y, Watanabe T, Kanazawa T et al (2005) Mucinous carcinoma of the colon and rectum show higher rates of microsatellite instability and lower rates of chromosomal instability. Cancer 103:2023–2029

Kievit J (2002) Follow-up of patients with colorectal cancer: numbers needed to test and treat. Eur J Cancer 38: 986–999

Kim H, Jen J, Vogelstein B et al (1994) Clinical and pathological characteristics of sporadic colorectal carcinomas with DNA errors in microsatellite sequences. Am J Pathol 145: 148–156

Kim JH, Beets GL, Kim MJ et al (2004a) High-resolution MR imaging for nodal staging in rectal cancer: are there any criteria in addition to the size? Eur J Radiol 52:78–83

Kim MJ, Huh YM, Park YN et al (1999) Colorectal mucinous carcinoma: findings on MRI. J Comput Assist Tomogr 23:291–296

Kim MJ, Kim WH, Kim NK et al (1997) Tailgut cyst: multilocular cystic appearance on MRI. J Comput Assist Tomogr 21:731–732

Kim MJ, Lim JS, Oh YT et al (2004b) Preoperative MRI of rectal cancer with and without rectal water filling: an intraindividual comparison. AJR Am J Roentgenol 182:1469–1476

Kim MJ, Park JS, Park SI et al (2003) Accuray in differentiation of mucinous and nonmucinous rectal carcinoma on MR imaging. J Comput Assist Tomogr 27:48–55

Kim NK, Kim MJ, Park JK et al (2000) Preoperative staging of rectal cancer with MRI: accuracy and clinical usefulness. Ann Surg Oncol 7:732–737

Kim SH, Lee JM, Lee MW et al (2008) Sonography transmission gel as endorectal contrast agent for tumor visualization in rectal cancer. AJR Am J Roentgenol 191:186–189

Kinkel K, Lu Y, Both M et al (2002) Detection of hepatic metastases from cancers of the gastrointestinal tract by using noninvasive imaging methods (US, CT, MR imaging, PET): a meta-analysis. Radiology 224:748–756

Kjeldsen BJ, Kronborg O, Fenger C et al (1997) A prospective randomized study of follow-up after radical surgery of colorectal cancer. Br J Surg 84:666–669

Klöppel G, Rindi G, Anlauf M et al (2007) Site-specific biology and pathology of gastroenteropancreatic neuroendocrine tumors. Virchows Arch 451:29–38

Knudsen JB, Nilsson T, Sprechler M et al (1983) Venous and nerve invasion as prognostic factors in postoperative survival of patients with resectable cancer of the rectum. Dis Colon Rectum 26:613–617

Koh DM, Brown G, Husband JE (2006) Nodal staging in rectal cancer. Abdom Imaging 31:652–659

Koh DM, Brown G, Temple L et al (2004) Rectal cancer: mesorectal lymph nodes at MR imaging with USPIO versus histopathologic findings – initial observations. Radiology 231:91–99

Koh DM, Brown G, Temple L et al (2005) Distribution of mesorectal lymph nodes in rectal cancer: in vivo MR imaging compared with histopathological examiantion. Initial observations. Eur Radiol 15:1650–1657

Koh DM, Collins DJ (2007) Diffusion-weighted MRI in the body: applications and challenges in oncology. AJR Am J Roentgenol 188:1622–1635

Koh DM, Takahara T, Imai Y et al (2007) Practical aspects of assessing tumors using clinical diffusion-weighted imaging in the body. Magn Reson Med Sci 6:211–224

Kraemer M, Wiratkapun S, Seow-Choen F et al (2001) Stratifying risk factors for follow-up: a comparison of recurrent and nonrecurrent colorectal cancer. Dis Colon Rectum 44:815–821

Krasna MJ, Flancbaum L, Cody RP et al (1988) Vascular and neural invasion in colorectal carcinoma. Incidence and prognostic significance. Cancer 61:1018–1023

Krook JE, Moertel CG, Gunderson LL et al (1991) Effective surgical adjuvant therapy for high-risk rectal carcinoma. N Engl J Med 324:709–715

Kruger DG, Riederer SJ, Grimm RC et al (2002) Continuously moving table data acquisition method for long FOV contrast enhanced MRA and whole body MRI. Magn Reson Med 47:224–231

Kuo LJ, Chern MC, Tsou MH et al (2005) Interpretation of magnetic resonance imaging for locally advanced rectal carcinoma after preoperative chemoradiation therapy. Dis Colon Rectum 48:23–28

Kwee TC, Takahara T, Ochiai R et al (2008) Diffusion-weighted whole-body imaging with background body signal suppression (DWIBS): features and potential applications in oncology. Eur Radiol 18:1937–1952

Ky A, Sohn N, Weinstein MA et al (1998) Carcinoma arising in anorectal fistulas of Crohn's disease. Dis Colon Rectum 41:992–996

Lahaye MJ, Engelen SM, Kessels AG et al (2008) USPIO-enhanced MR imaging for nodal staging in patients with primary rectal cancer: predictive criteria. Radiology 246:804–811

Lahaye MJ, Engelen SM, Nelemans PJ et al (2005) Imaging for predicting the risk factors – the circumferential resection margin and nodal disease – of local recurrence in rectal cancer: a meta-analysis. Semin Ultrasound CT MR 26:259–268

Laufman H, Saphir O (1951) Primary linits plastica type of carcinoma of the colon. Arch Surg 62:79–91

Lee SH, McGregor DH, Kuziez MN (1981a) Malignant transformation of perianal condyloma acuminatum. A case report with review of the literature. Dis Colon Rectum 24:462–467

Lee SH, Zucker M, Sato T (1981b) Primary adenocarcinoma of the anal gland with secondary perianal fistula. Hum Pathol 12:1034–1037

Lehnert T, Methner M, Pollok A et al (2002) Multivisceral resection for locally advanced primary colon and rectal cancer: an analysis of prognostic factors in 201 patients. Ann Surg 235:217–225

Leiner T, Nijenhuis RJ, Maki JH (2004) Use of a three-station phased array coil to improve peripheral contrast-enhanced magnetic resonance angiography. J Magn Reson Imaging 20:417–425

Lengauer C, Kinzler KW, Vogelstein B (1997) Genetic instability in colorectal cancers. Nature 386:623–627

Levert LM, Van Rooyen W, Van Den Bergen HA (1996) Cysts of the tailgut. Eur J Surg 162:149–152

Lewis JJ, Leung D, Woodruff JM et al (1998) Retroperitoneal soft-tissue sarcoma: analysis of 500 patients treated and followed at a single institution. Ann Surg 228:355–365

Lim KE, Hsu WC, Wang CR (1998) Tailgut cyst with malignancy: MR imaging findings. AJR Am J Roentgenol 170:1488–1490

Llyod RV (2003) Practical markers used in the diagnosis of neuroendocrine tumors. Endocr Pathol 14:293–301

Lockhart-Mummery HE (1975) Symposium. Crohn's disease: anal lesions. Dis Colon Rectum 18:200–202

Longo WE, Johnson FE (2002) The preoperative assessment and postoperative surveillance of patients with colon and rectal cancer. Surg Clin North Am 82:1091–1108

Ludwig U, Sommer G, Zaitsev M et al (2006) 2D axial moving table acquisitions with dynamic slice adaption. Magn Reson Med 55:423–430

Luna-Perez P, Bustos-Cholico E, Alvarado I et al (2005) Prognostic significance of circumferential margin involvement in rectal adenocarcinoma treated with preoperative chemradiotherapy and low anterior resection. J Surg Oncol 90:20–25

Luna-Perez P, Rodriguez-Ramirez S, Rodriguez-Coria DF et al (2001) Preoperative chemoradiation therapy and anal sphincter preservation with locally advanced rectal adenocarcinoma. World J Surg 25:1006–1011

Maier AG, Kersting-Sommerhoff B, Reeders JW et al (2000) Staging of rectal cancer by double-contrast MR imaging using the rectally administered superparamagnetic iron oxide contrast agent ferristine and i.v. gadodiamide injection: results of a multicenter phase II trial. J Magn Reson Imaging 12:651–660

Makela JT, Laitinen SO, Kairaluoma MI (1995) Five-year follow-up after radical surgery for colorectal cancer: results of a prospective randomized trial. Arch Surg 130:1062–1067

Markus J, Morrissey B, deGara C et al (1997) MRI of recurrent rectosigmoid carcinoma. Abdom Imaging 22:338–342

Marr R, Birbeck K, Garvican J et al (2005) The modern abdominoperineal excision. The next challenge after total mesorectal excision. Ann Surg 242:74–82

Martling AL, Holm T, Rutqvist LE et al (2000) Effect of a surgical training programme on outcome of rectal cancer in the county of Stockholm: Stockholm colorectal cancer study group, basingstoke bowel cancer research project. Lancet 356:93–96

Masaki T, Sugiyama M, Atomi Y et al (2001) The indication of local excision for T2 rectal carcinomas. Am J Surg 181:133–137

Mathur P, Smith JJ, Ramsey C et al (2003) Comparison of CT and MRI in the pre-operative staging of rectal adenocarcinoma and prediction of circumferential margin involvement by MRI. Colorectal Dis 5:396–401

Matsuoka H, Nakamura A, Sugiyama M et al (2004) MRI diagnosis of mesorectal lymph node metastasis in patients with rectal carcinoma. What is the optimal criterion? Anticancer Res 24:4097–4102

Mazur MT, Clark HB (1983) Gastric stromal tumors: reappraisal of histogenesis. Am J Surg Pathol 7:507–519

Medich D, McGinty J, Parda D et al (2001) Preoperative chemoradiotherapy and radical surgery for locally advanced distal rectal adenocarcinoma: pathologic findings and clinical implications. Dis Colon Rectum 44:1123–1128

Merchant NB, Guillem JG, Paty PB et al (1999) T3N0 rectal cancer: results following sharp mesorectal excision and no adjuvant therapy. J Gastrointest Surg 3:642–647

MERCURY Study Group (2007) Extramural depth of tumor invasion at thin-section MR in patients with rectal cancer: results of the MERCURY Study. Radiology 243: 132–139

Merkel S, Mansmann U, Siassi M et al (2001) The prognostic inhomogeneity in pT3 rectal carcinomas. Int J Colorectal Dis 16:298–304

Miller AR (1998) Multidisciplinary management of recurrent colorectal cancer. Surg Oncol 7:209–221

Minsky BD, Cohen AM, Kemeny N et al (1992) Combined modality therapy of rectal cancer: decreased acute toxicity with the preoperative approach. J Clin Oncol 10: 1218–1224

Minsky BD, Mies C, Rich TA et al (1987) Colloid carcinoma of the colon and rectum. Cancer 60:3103–3112

Monig SP, Baldus SE, Zirbes TK et al (1999) Lymph node size and metastatic infiltration in colon cancer. Ann Surg Oncol 6:579–581

Moran MR, James EC, Rothenberger DA et al (1992) Prognostic value of positive lymph nodes in rectal cancer. Dis Colon Rectum 35:579–581

Moreira LF, Hizuta A, Iwagaki H et al (1994) Lateral lymph node dissection for rectal carcinoma below the peritoneal reflection. Br J Surg 81:293–296

Morikawa E, Yasutomi M, Shindou K et al (1994) Distribution of metastatic lymph nodes in colorectal cancer by the modified clearing method. Dis Colon Rectum 37:219–223

Moulopoulos LA, Karvouni E, Kehagias D et al (1999) MR imaging of complex tail-gut cysts. Clin Radiol 54:118–122

Nagtegaal ID, Gaspar C, Marijnen CA et al (2004) Morphological changes in tumor type after radiotherapy are accompanied by changes in gene expression profile but not clinical behaviour. J Pathol 204:183–192

Nagtegaal ID, Gosens M J, Marijnen CA et al (2007) Combinations of tumor and treatment parameters are more discriminative for prognosis than the present TNM system in rectal cancer. J Clin Oncol 25:1647–1650

Nagtegaal ID, Marijnen CA, Kranenbarg EK et al (2002a) Circumferential margin involvement is still an important predictor of local recurrence in rectal carcinoma: not one millimeter but two millimeters is the limit. Am J Surg Pathol 26:350–357

Nagtegaal ID, Quirke P (2008) What is the role for the circumferential margin in the modern treatment of rectal cancer? J Clin Oncol 28:303–312

Nagtegaal ID, van der Velde CJ et al (2002b) Macroscopic evaluation of rectal cancer resection specimen: clinical significance of the pathologist in quality control. J Clin Oncol 20:1729–1734

National Institutes of Health Consensus Conference. (1990) JAMA 246:1444–1450

Negri FV, Wotherspoon A, Cunningham D et al (2005) Mucinous histology predicts for reduced fluorouracil responsiveness and survival in advanced colorectal cancer. Ann Oncol 16:1305–1310

Nissan A, Guillem JG, Paty PB et al (1999) Signet-ring cell carcinoma of the colon and rectum: a matched control study. Dis Colon Rectum 42:1176–1180

Nozoe T, Anai H, Nasu S et al (2000) Clinicopathological characteristics of mucinous carcinoma of the colon and rectum. J Surg Oncol 75:103–107

Odone V, Chang L, Caces J et al (1982) The natural history of colorectal carcinoma in adolescents. Cancer 49:1716–1720

Ohlsson B, Breland U, Ekberg H et al (1995) Follow-up after curative surgery for colorectal carcinoma: randomized comparison with no follow-up. Dis Colon Rectum 38:619–626

Okizuka H, Sugimura K, Yoshizako T et al (1996) Rectal carcinoma: prospective comparison of conventional and gadopentate dimeglumine enhanced fat-suppressed MR imaging. J Magn Reson Imaging 6:465–471

Okuyama T, Korenaga D, Tamura S et al (1999) The effectiveness of chemotherapy with cisplatin and 5-fluorouracil for recurrent small cell neuroendocrine carcinoma of the rectum: report of a case. Jpn J Surg 29:165–169

Panaccione JL, Ross PR, Torres GM et al (1991) Rectal barium in pelvic MR imaging: initial results. J Magn Reson Imaging 1:605–607

Park YJ, Youk EG, Choi HS et al (1999) Experience of 1446 rectal cancer patients in Korea and analysis of prognostic factors. Int J Colorectal Dis 14:101–106

Patrinou V, Petrochilos J, Batistatou A et al (2001) Mucinous adenocarcinoma arising in chronic perianal fistula. J Clin Gastroenterol 33:175–176

Pema PJ, Bennett WF, Bova JG et al (1994) CT vs MRI in diagnosis of recurrent rectosigmoid carcinoma. J Comp Assist Tomogr 18:256–261

Peschaud F, Cuenod CA, Benoist S et al (2005) Accuracy of magnetic resonance imaging in rectal cancer depends on location of the tumor. Dis Colon Rectum 8:1603–1609

Picon AI, Moore HG, Sternberg SS et al (2003) Prognostic significance of depth of gross or microscopic perirectal fat invasion in T3N0M0 rectal cancers following sharp mesorectal excision and no adjuvant therapy. Int J Colorectal Dis 18: 487–492

Pidhorecky I, Cheney RT, Kraybill WG et al (2007) Gastrointestinal stroma tumors: current diagnosis, biologic behaviour, and management. Ann Surg Oncol 7:705–712

Pietra N, Sarli L, Costi R et al (1998) Role of follow-up in management of local recurrences of colorectal cancer: a prospective, randomized study. Dis Colon Rectum 41:1127–1133

Quirke P, Dixon MF (1988) The prediciton of local recurrence in rectal adenocarcinoma by histopathological examination. Int J Colorectal Dis 3:127–131

Quirke P, Durdey P, Dixon MF, et al (1986) Local recurrence of rectal adenocarcinoma due to inadequate surgical resection: histopathological study of lateral tumor spread and surgical excision. Lancet 2:996–999

Rao TR, Hambrick E, Abcarian H et al (1982) Colorectal linits plastica. Dis Colon Rectum 25:239–244

Reerink O, Verschueren R, Szabo B et al (2003) A favourable pathological stage after neo-adjuvant radiochemotherapy in patients with initially irresectable rectal cancer correlates with a favourable prognosis. Eur J Cancer 39:1127–1132

Renehan AG, Egger M, Saunders MP et al (2002) Impact on survival of intensive follow-up after curative resection for colorectal cancer: systematic review and meta-analysis of randomised trials. BMJ 324:1–8

Rioux M, Mailloux C (1997) Crescent-shaped necrosis: a new imaging sign suggestive of stromal tumor of the small bowel. Abdom Imaging 22:376–380

Ryan DP, Compton CC, Mayer RJ (2000) Carcinoma of the anal canal. N Engl J Med 342:792–800

Saclarides TJ, Bhattacharyya AK, Britton-Kuzel C et al (1994a) Predicting lymph node metastases in rectal cancer. Dis Colon Rectum 37:52–57

Saclarides TJ, Szeluga D, Staren ED (1994b) Neuroendocrine carcinoma of the colon and rectum – results of a ten-year experience. Dis Colon Rectum 37:635–642

Sabati M, Lauzon ML, Mahallati H et al (2006) Interactive continuously moving table (iCMT) large field-of-view real-time MRI. Magn Reson Med 55:1202–1209

Sagar PM, Pemberton JH (1996) Surgical management of locally recurrent rectal cancer. Br J Surg 83:293–304

Salmon RJ, Zafrani B, Labib A et al (1986) Prognosis of cloacogenic ans squamous cancers of the anal canal. Dis Colon Rectum 29:336–340

Sandrasegaran K, Rajesh A, Rushing DA et al (2005) Gastrointestinal stromal tumors: CT and MRI findings. Eur Radiol 15:1407–1414

Sasaki O, Atkin WS, Jass JR (1987) Mucinous carcinoma of the rectum. Histopathology 11:259–272

Sauer R, Becker H, Hohenberger W et al (2004) Preoperative versus postoperative chemoradiotherapy for rectal cancer. N Engl J Med 351:1731–1740

Schäfer AO, Baumann T, Pache G (2007) Preoperative staging of rectal cancer. Radiologe 47:635–651

Schäfer O, Langer M (2007) Detection of recurrent rectal cancer with CT, MRI and PET/CT. Eur Radiol 17:2044–2054

Schaefer JF, Schlemmer HP (2006) Total-body MR-imaging in oncology. Eur Radiol 16:2000–2015

Schmidt GP, Baur-Melnyk A, Herzog P et al (2005) High-resolution whole-body magnetic resonance image tumor staging with the use of parallel imaging versus dual-modality positron emission tomography-computed tomography: experience on a 32-channel system. Invest Radiol 40:743–753

Schoemaker D, Black R, Giles L et al (1998) Yearly colonoscopy, liver CT, and chest radiography do not influence 5-year survival of colorectal cancer patients. Gastroenterology 114:7–14

Secco GB, Fardelli R, Campora E et al (1994) Primary mucinous adenocarcinomas and signet-ring cell carcinomas of colon and rectum. Oncology 51:30–34

Secco GB, Fardelli R, Gianquinto D et al (2002) Efficacy and cost of risk-adapted follow-up in patients after colorectal cancer surgery: a prospective, randomized and controlled trial. J Surg Oncol 28:418–423

Shankaranarayanan A, Herfkens R, Hargreaves BM et al (2003) Helical MR: continuously moving table axial imaging with radial acquisitions. Magn Reson Med 50:1053–1060

Shepherd NA, Baxter KJ, Love SB (1995) Influence of local peritoneal involvement on pelvic recurrence and prognosis in rectal cancer. J Clin Pathol 48:849–855

Shirouzu K, Isomoto H, Kakegawa T (1993) Prognostic evaluation of perineural invasion in rectal cancer. Am J Surg 165:233–237

Sim HL, Tan KY, Poon PL et al (2008) Primary signet ring cell carcinoma with peritoneal dissemination and gastric secondaries. World J Gastroenterol 14:2118–2120

Simunovic M, Sexton R, Rempel E et al (2003) Optimal preoperative assessment and surgery for rectal cancer may greatly limit the need for radiotherapy. Br J Surg 90:999–1003

Smith NJ, Shihab O, Arnaout A et al (2008a) MRI for detection of extramural vascular invasion in rectal cancer. AJR Am J Roentgenol 191:1517–1522

Smith R, Hicks D, Tomljanovich PI et al (2008b) Adenocarcinoma arising from chronic perianal Crohn's disease: case report and review of the literature. Am Surg 74:59–61

Sommer G, Fautz HP, Ludwig U et al (2006) Multicontrast sequences with continuous table motion: a novel acquisition technique for extended field of view imaging. Magn Reson Med 55:918–922

Sommer G, Schaefer AO, Baumann T et al (2008) Sliding Multislice MRI for abdominal staging of patients with pelvic malignancies: a pilot study. J Magn Reson Imaging 27:666–672

Steup WH, Moriya Y, van de Velde CJ (2002) Patterns of lymphatic spread in rectal cancer. A topographical analysis on lymph node metastases. Eur J Cancer 38:911–918

Stoker J, Rociu E et al (2000) Imaging of anorectal disease. Br J Surg 87:10–27

Stewart BW, Kleihues P (eds) (2003) World Health Organization World Cancer Report. International Agency for Researh on Cancer, pp 12–21

Stewart RJ, Humphreys WG et al (1986) The presentation and management of presacral tumors. Br J Surg 73:153–155
Sugarbaker PH (2001) Mucinous colorectal carcinoma. J Surg Oncol 77:282–283
Suzuki K, Muoto T, Sawada T (1995) Prevention of local recurrence by extended lymphadenectomy for rectal cancer. Surg Today 25:795–801
Symonds DA, Vickery AL (1976) Mucinous carcinoma of the colon and rectum. Cancer 37:1891–1900
Takahashi T, Ueno M, Azekura K et al (2000) Lateral node dissection and total mesorectal excision for rectal cancer. Dis Colon Rectum 43:59–68
Takahashi Y, Tucker SL, Kitadai Y et al (1997) Vessel counts and expression of vascular endothelial growth factor as prognostic factors in node-negative colon cancer. Arch Surg 132:541–546
Talbot IC, Ritchie S, Leighton MH et al (1980) The clinical significance of invasion of veins by rectal cancer. Br J Surg 67:439–442
Tampi C, Lotwala V, Lakdawala M et al (2007) Retrorectal cyst hamartoma (tailgut cyst) with malignant transformation. Gynecol Oncol 105:266–268
Tang R, Wang JY, Chen JS et al (1995) Survival impact of lymph node metastasis in TNM stage III carcinoma of the colon and rectum. J Am Coll Surg 180:705–712
Tarazi R, Nelson RL (1994) Anal adenocarcinoma: a comprehensive review. Semin Surg Oncol 10: 235–240
Theilmann RJ, Borders R, Trouard TP et al (2004) Changes in water mobility measured by diffusion MRI predict response of metastatic breast cancer to chemotherapy. Neoplasia 6:831–837
Titu LV, Nicholson AA, Hartley JE et al (2006) Routine follow-up by magnetic resonance imaging does not improve detection of resectable local recurrences from colorectal cancer. Ann Surg 243:348–352
Traube J, Simpson S, Riddell RH et al (1980) Crohn's disease and adenocarcinoma of the bowel. Dig Dis Sci 25: 939–944
Tung SY, Wu CS, Chen PC (1996) Primary signet ring cell carcinoma of colorectum: an age- and sex-matched controlled study. Am J Gastroenterol 91:2195–2199
Ueno H, Hase K, Mochizuki H (2001a) Criteria for extramural perineural invasion as a prognostic factor in rectal cancer. Br J Surg 88:994–1000
Ueno H, Mochizuki H, Hashiguchi Y et al (2001b) Prognostic determinants of patients with lateral nodal involvement by rectal cancer. Ann Surg 234:190–197
Uhlig BE, Johnson RL (1975) Presacral tumors and cysts in adults. Dis Colon Rectum 18:581–589
Umpleby HC, Ranson DL, Williamson RC (1985) Peculiarities of mucinous colorectal carcinoma. Br J Surg 72:715–718
Uronis HE, Bendell JC (2007) Anal cancer: an overview. Oncologist 12:524–534
van Lingen CP, Zeebregts CJ, Gerritsen JJ et al (2003) Local recurrence of rectal cancer after total mesorectal excision without preoperative radiotherapy. Int J Gastrointest Cancer 34:129–134
Vernon SE, Unger H, Traitz JJ (1981) Diffusely infiltrating carcinoma of the colon (linitis plastica type). Dis Colon Rectum 24:391–394
Vilor M, Tsutsumi Y, Osamura Y et al (1995) Small cell neuronedocrine carcinoma of the rectum. Pathol Int 45:605–609
Vliegen RF, Beets GL, Lammering G et al (2008) Mesorectal fascia invasion after neoadjuvant chemotherapy and radiation therapy for locally advanced rectal cancer: accuracy of MR imaging for prediction. Radiology 246:454–462
Vliegen RF, Beets GL, von Meyenfeldt MF et al (2005) Rectal cancer: MR imaging in local staging – is gadolinium-based contrast material helpful? Radiology 234:179–188
Vogl TJ, Pegios W, Mack MG et al (1997) Accuracy of staging rectal tumors with contrast-enhanced transrectal MR imaging. AJR Am J Roentgenol 168:1427–1434
Wallengren NO, Holtas S, Andren-Sandberg A et al (2000) Rectal carcinoma: double-contrast MR imaging for preoperative staging. Radiology 215:108–114
Weissleder R, Elizondo G, Wittenberg J et al (1990) Ultrasmall superparamagnetic iron oxide: characterization of a new class of contrast agents for MR imaging. Radiology 175:489–493
Wibe A, Rendedal PR, Svensson E et al (2002a) Prognostic significance of the circumferential resection margin following total mesorectal excision for rectal cancer. Br J Surg 89:327–334
Wibe A, Syse A, Anderson E et al (2002b) Oncological outcomes after total mesorectal excision for cure of cancer of the lower rectum: anterior vs abdominoperineal resection. Dis Colon Rectum 47:48–58
Wied U, Nilsson T, Knudsen JB et al (1985) Postoperative survival of patients with potentially curable cancer of the colon. Dis Colon Rectum 28:333–335
Will O, Purkayastha S, Chan C et al (2006) Diagnostic precision of nanoparticle-enhanced MRI for lymph-node metastases: a meta-analysis. Lancet Oncol 7:52–60
Willett CG, Badizadegan K, Ancukiewicz M et al (1999) Prognostic factors in stage T3N0 rectal cancer: do all patients require postoperative pelvic irradiation and chemotherapy? Dis Colon Rectum 42:167–173
Wittekind C, Henson DE, Hutter RV et al (2001) TNM Supplement. A commentary for uniform use, 2nd edn. Wiley, New York, pp 117–119
Wolmark N, Fisher B, Wieand HS (1986) The prognostic value of the Dukes' C class of colorectal cancer: an analysis of the NSABP clinical trials. Ann Surg 203:115–122
Wong NA, Shirazi T, Hamer-Hodges DW et al (2002) Adenocarcinoma arising within a Crohn's-related anorectal fistula: a forum of anal gland carcinoma? Histopathology 40:302–304
Yang DM, Park CH, Jin W et al (2005) Tailgut cyst: MRI evaluation. AJR Am J Roentgenol 184:1519–1523
Yoo SY, Lee JH, Park KR et al (1994) Primary signet-ring-cell carcinoma of the rectum in a 12-year-old boy. Pediatr Surg Int 9:284–286
Younes M, Katikaneni PR, Lechago J (1993) The value of preoperative mucosal biopsy in the diagnosis of colorectal mucinous adenocarcinoma. Cancer 72:3588–3592
Zenni GC, Abraham K, Harford FJ et al (1998) Characteristics of rectal carcinomas that predict the presence of lymph node metastases: implications for patient selection for local therapy. J Surg Oncol 67:99–103
Zerhouni EA, Rutter C, Hamilton SR et al (1996) CT and MR imaging in the staging of colorectal carcinoma: report of the Radiology Diagnostic Oncology Group II. Radiology 200:443–451

Clinical Atlas

5

Arnd-Oliver Schäfer

5.1 Introduction

The key component in the accurate radiological staging of rectal cancer is experience. Although individual experience cannot be entirely replaced by reading, it is the aim of this chapter to familiarize the reader with the most important features of local disease, typical patterns of metastatic spread, negative prognostic factors that can be revealed by MR images, appearance of the postsurgical anatomy and an array of possible differential diagnoses. To convey the idea of experience, not only are single images being presented for each aspect, but a total of 133 cases have been selected, reviewed, and adapted for this clinical atlas. Often the cases encompass MR images from different time points as well as multislice computed tomography (MSCT) or positron emission tomography (PET) images or histopathological microphotographs to illustrate the course of the disease. Furthermore, ink drawings by the author are provided in individual cases to clarify certain aspects in the sometimes complex MR images. The numerous images are accompanied by detailed legends with additional information on patient history, treatment, clinical and pathologic TNM staging, and follow-up or outcome.

It is the intention of the author to confront the reader with recurring problems in the assessment of the tumor stage, typical pitfalls related to tissue changes initiated by neoadjuvant radiochemotherapy, and unexpected histopathologic results.

Additionally, the CD-ROM that is provided with this book can be seen as an adjunct to the atlas section. It shows the prospects of continuously-moving-table MRI, an examination of the chest and abdomen that can be combined with high-resolution pelvic MRI to serve as a one-stop-shop staging concept for patients with rectal cancer.

A-O. Schäfer
Department of Diagnostic Radiology, Freiburg University Hospital, Hugstetter Strasse 55, 79106 Freiburg, Germany
e-mail: arnd-oliver.schaefer@uniklinik-freiburg.de

A-O. Schäfer, M. Langer, *MRI of Rectal Cancer*,
DOI: 10.1007/978-3-540-72833-7_5, © Springer-Verlag Berlin Heidelberg 2010

5.2 Stage T1 Rectal Cancer

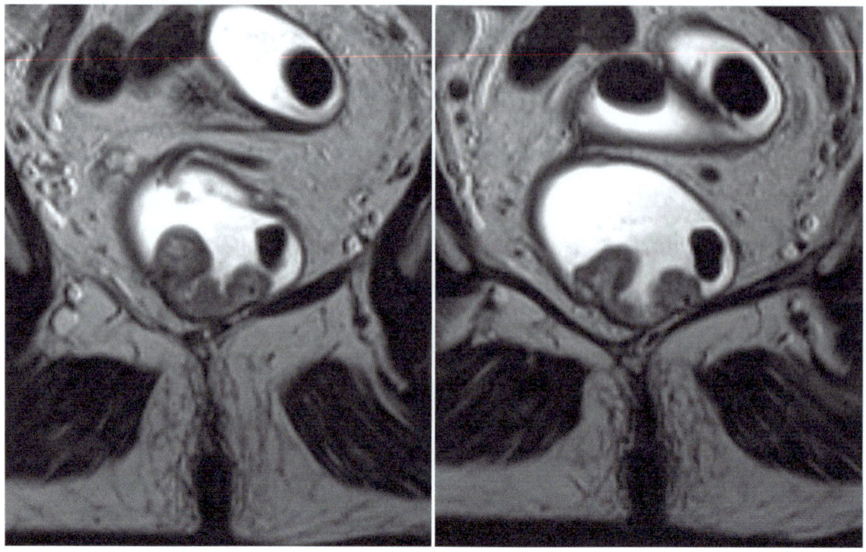

Fig. 5.1 Tubulovillous adenoma of the rectum. The para-coronal T2-TSE images reveal a digitate tumor located in the lower rectum. A differentiation between tubulovillous adenoma and stage T1–2 carcinoma is impossible based solely on MRI.

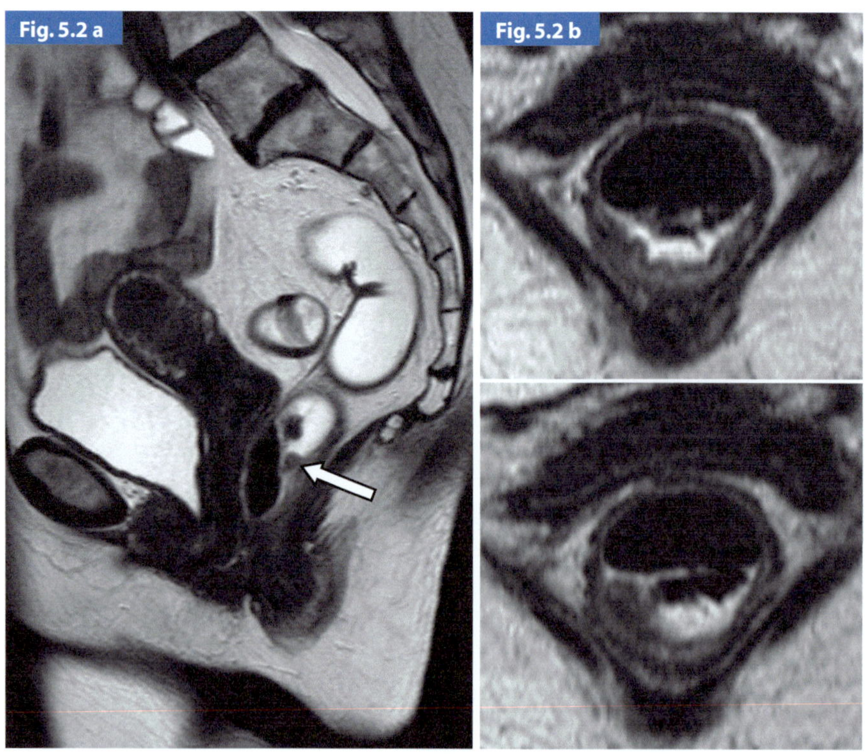

Fig. 5.2 (**a**) Sagittal T2-TSE image reveals a small polyp in the lower rectum (*arrow*). (**b**) Axial T2-TSE images demonstate normal wall architecture. On T2-weighted images, the mucosal layer appears hypointense, the submucosa has an intermediate signal intensity, and the muscle layer exposes the lowest signal intensity of all three wall components. The small tumor, which bioptically contained malignant cells, seems to penetrate the submucosal layer and was clinically staged as cT1N0. Histopathology confirmed the diagnosis and the ultimate stage was defined as pT1N0L1V0Pn0.

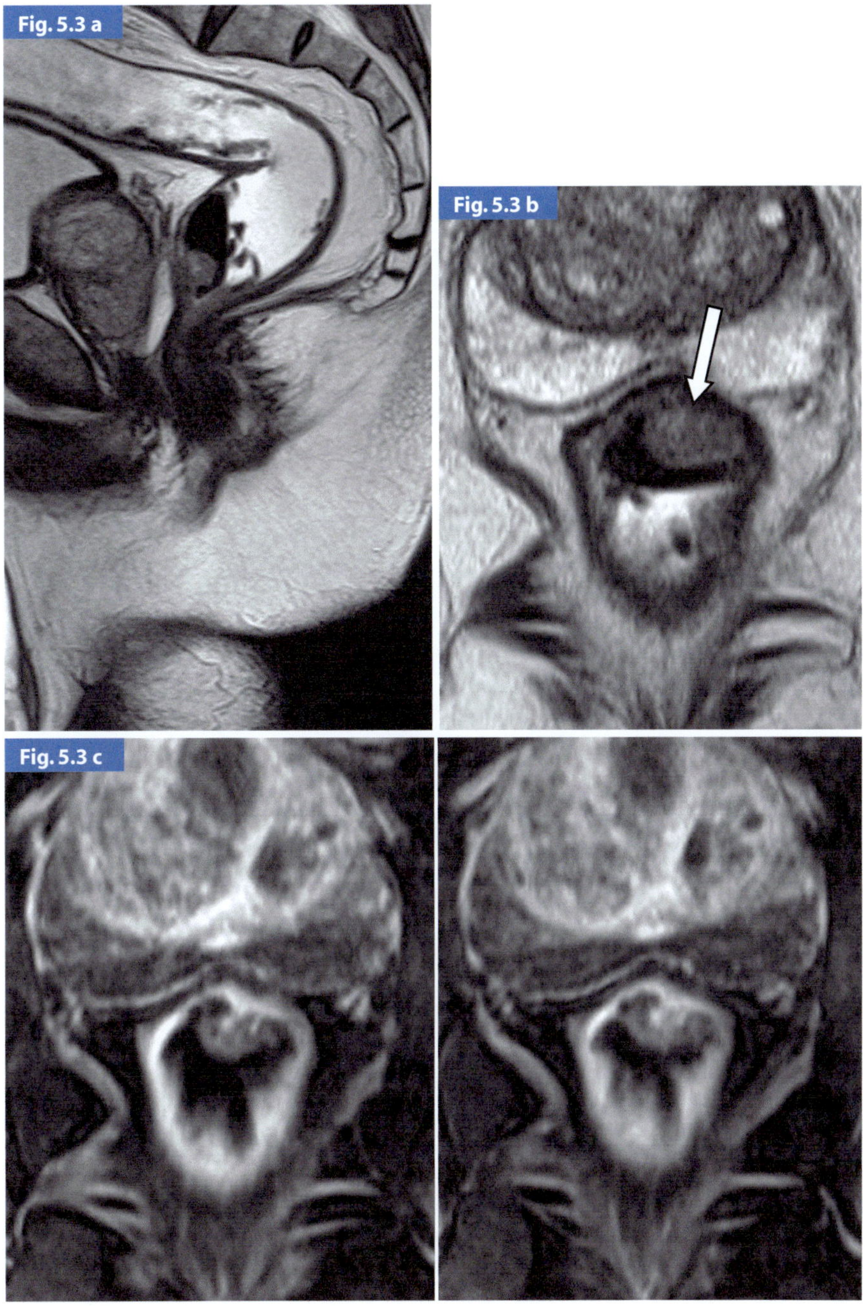

Fig. 5.3 (**a**, **b**) Sagittal and axial T2-TSE images show a small polypoid intermediate signal tumor of the anterior lower rectum. The tumor respects the muscle layer, whereas tumor signal is seen within the submucosa. (**c**) The axial CE-VIBE images support these findings. The contrast enhancement of the tumor is clearly inferior to that of the normal wall layers, which cannot be differentiated on the VIBE sequence. Histopathologic analysis resulted in a stage pT1N0L0V0 rectal cancer derived from a tubulovillous adenoma.

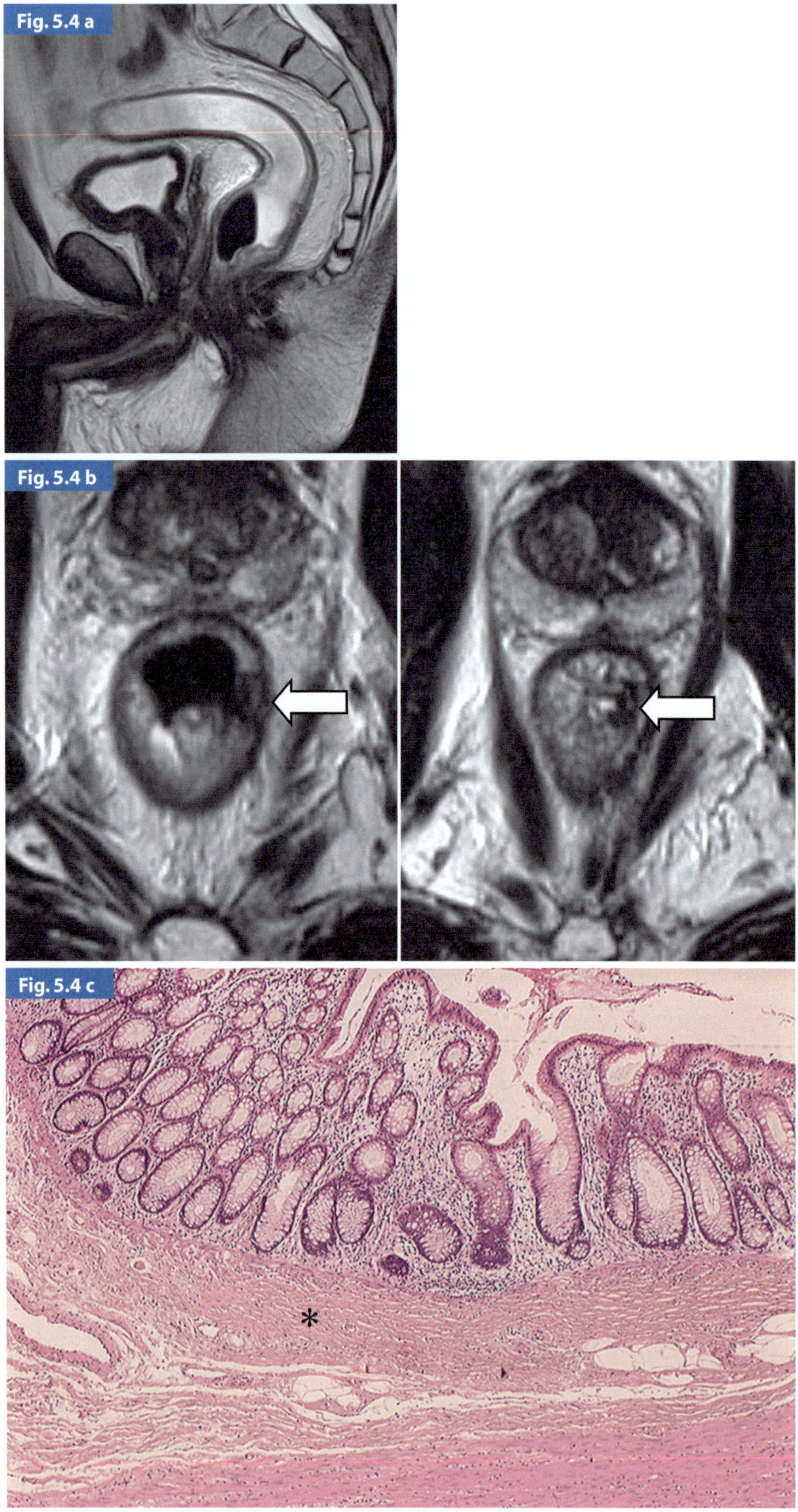

Fig. 5.4 (**a**) Sagittal T2-TSE image obtained after neoadjuvant therapy shows submucosal swelling. (**b**) On the para-axial T2-TSE images, tumor fibrosis is visible as hypointense foci in the lower rectal mucosa and submucosa at 3-o'clock lithotomy position (*arrows*). Problem: Grade of regression after radiochemotherapy. Image characteristics indicate that a grade between T0 and T2 is probable. The histopathologic stage was defined as ypT1N0G2. (**c**) Radiotherapy-associated fibrosis located in the submucosa, shown by the *asterisk* (H&E, ×5).

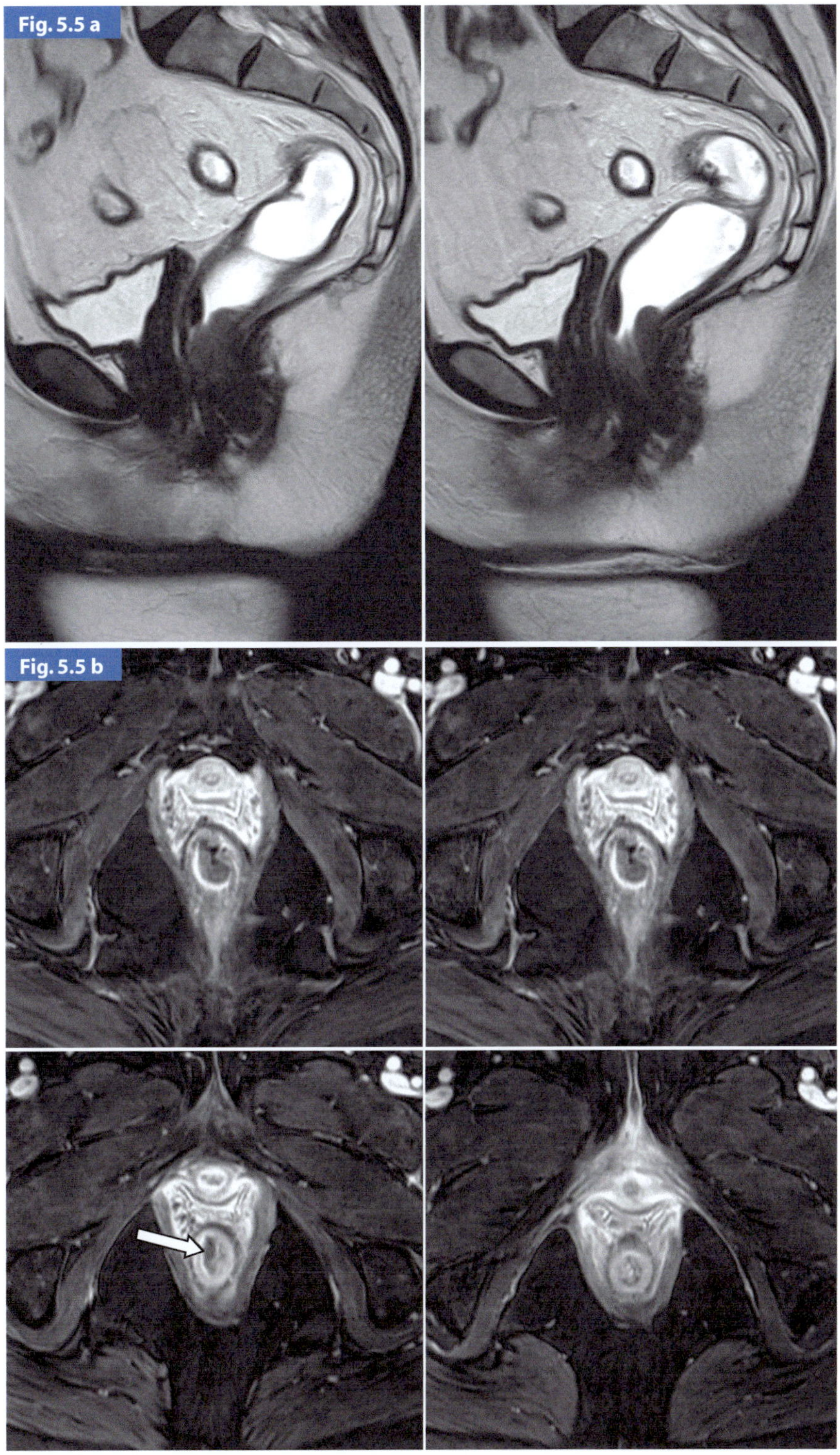

Fig. 5.5 Pretreatment MRI. (**a**) The sagittal T2-TSE images display a tumor mass originating from the anorectal junction. (**b**) The corresponding para-axial CE-VIBE 3D images reveal a hypovascular tumor formation between the 4- and 12-o'clock lithotomy positions limited to the rectal wall. The tumor involves the upper anal channel (*arrow*) and was clinically staged cT3N0. For this reason, neoadjuvant radiochemotherapy was carried out.

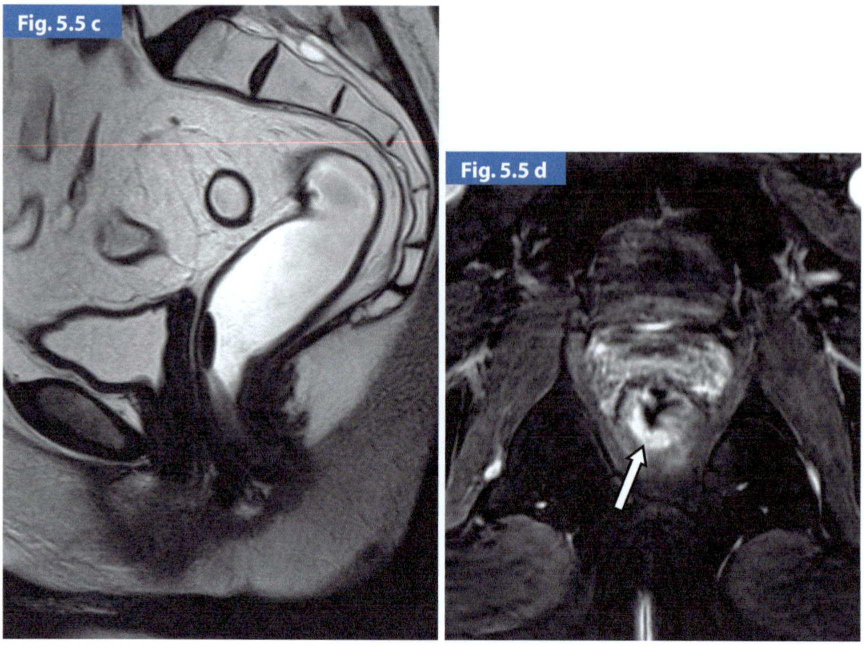

Fig. 5.5 (**c**, **d**) Post-neoadjuvant therapy MRI. (**c**) On the sagittal T2-TSE image, residual thickening of the supraanal rectal wall and anal channel with low signal due to fibrosis can be observed. (**d**) The tumor bed shows intensive enhancement on the representative CE-VIBE 3D image as a result of radiotherapy (*arrow*). The intraoperative histopathologic evaluation of tissue samples indicated microfocal residual tumor within the submucosa of the anorectal junction. Abdominoperineal resection had to be performed. Histopathology of the specimen revealed stage ypT1N0 rectal cancer.

Fig. 5.6 a

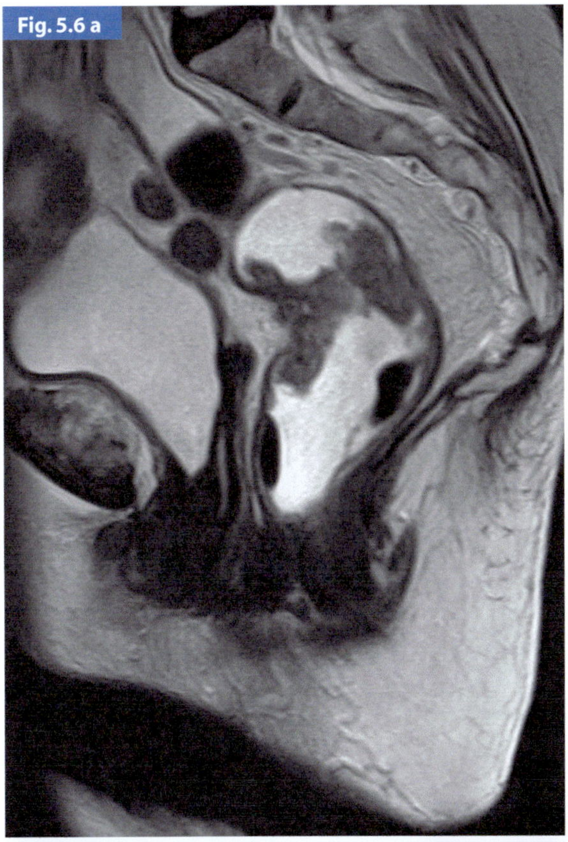

Fig. 5.6 Stage ypT1 rectal cancer. (**a**, **b**) Pretreatment MRI. Sagittal (**a**) and axial (**b**) T2-TSE images of a midrectal cancer show a wall-exceeding tumor (*arrow*) with small surrounding lymph nodes.

Fig. 5.6 b

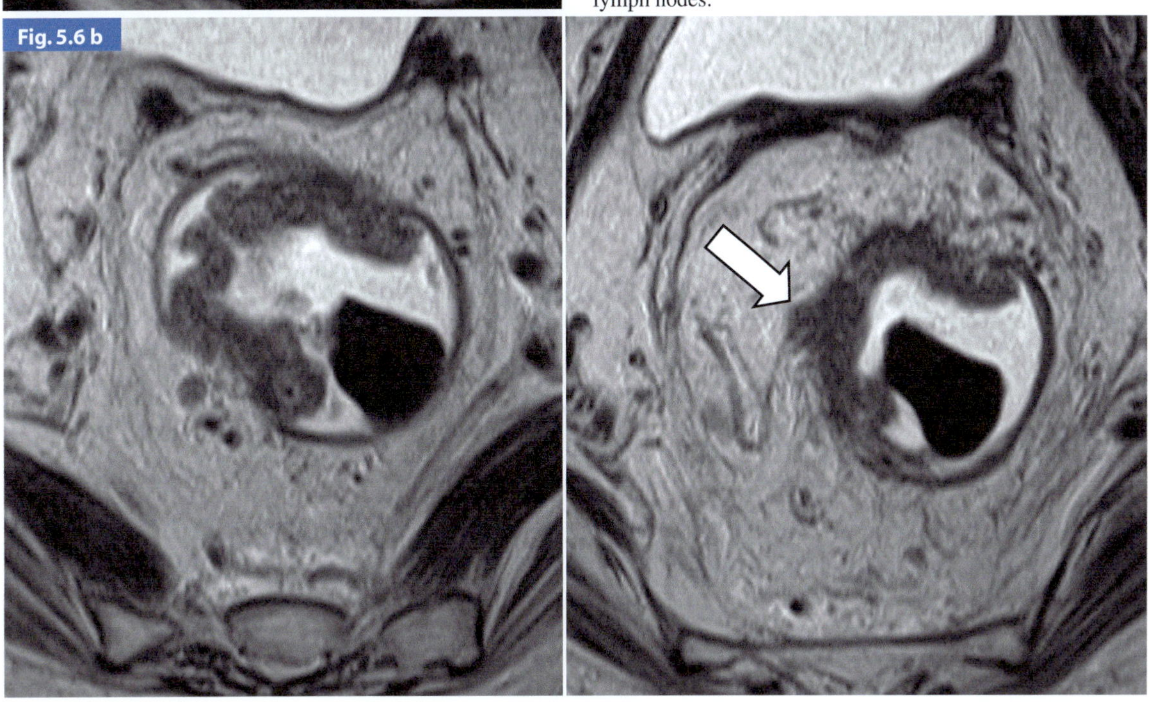

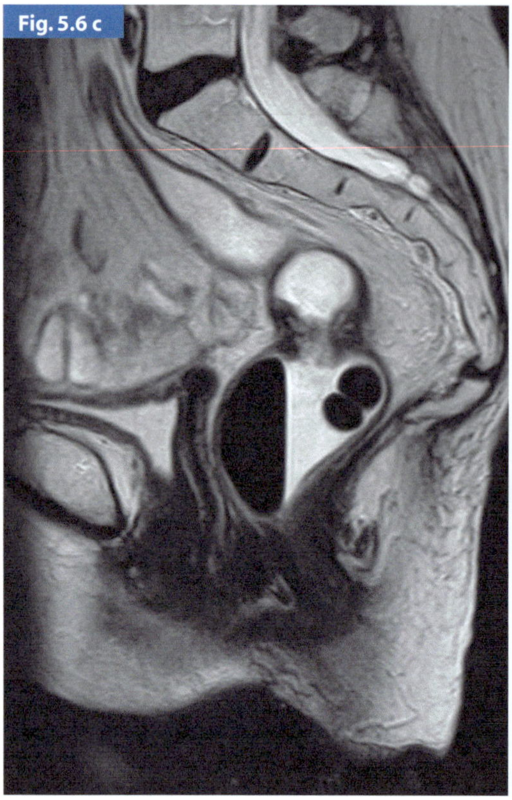

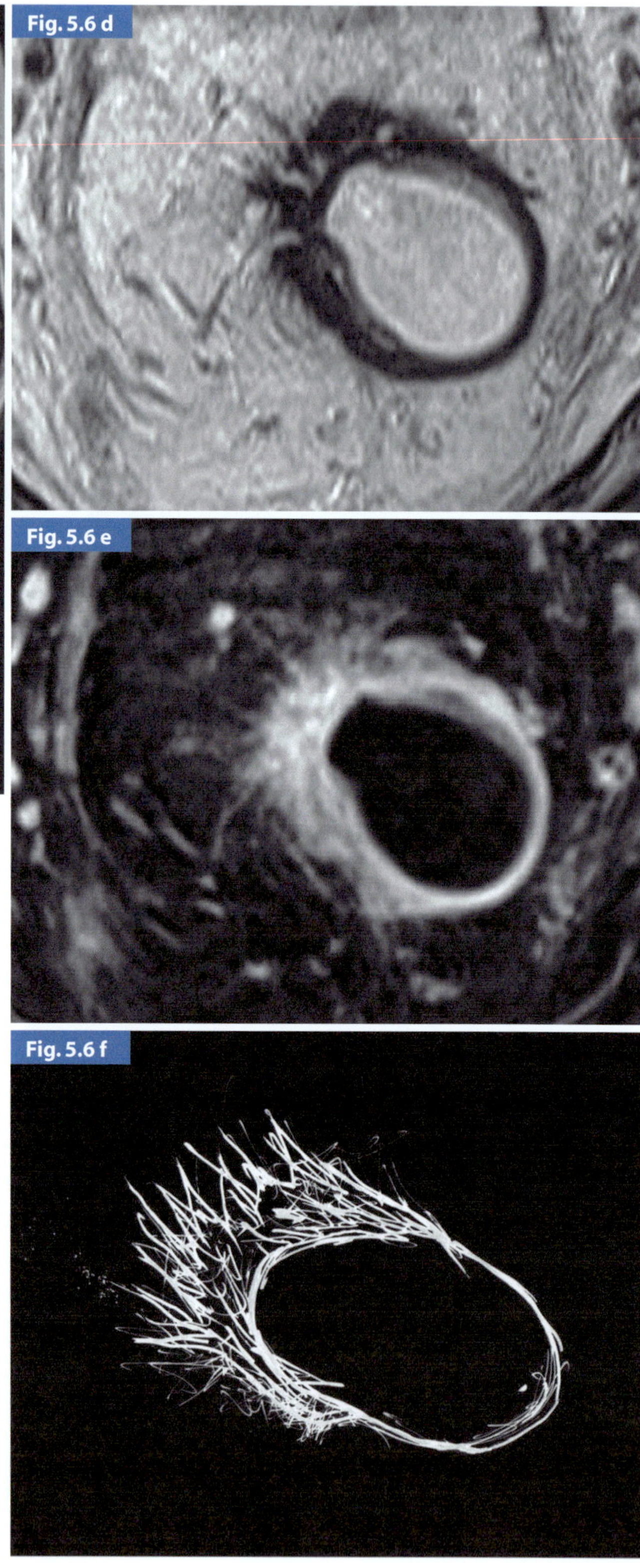

Fig. 5.6 (**c**–**e**) Post-chemoradiation MRI. Sagittal (**c**), axial T2-TSE (**d**), and axial CE-VIBE (**e**) three-dimensional images reveal tumor downsizing. Problem: Marked enhamcement of the tumor bed and the peritumorous tissue coupled with hypervascularization are indicative of inflammation and impede classification of the residual tumor. The definitive stage was ypT1OL0V0Pn0. (**f**) Ink drawing: Peritumorous inflammation.

5.3 Stage T2 Rectal Cancer

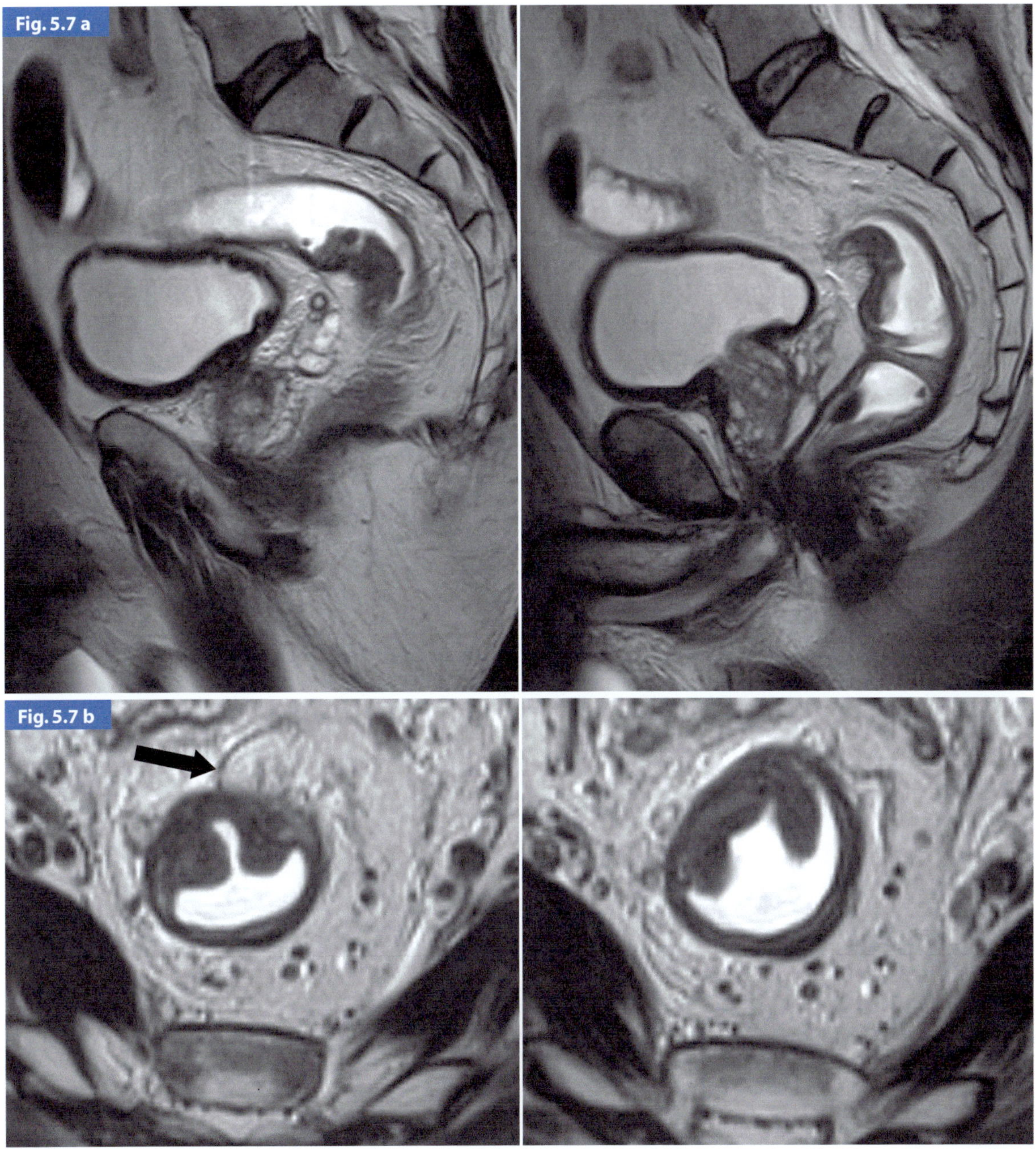

Fig. 5.7 Sagittal (**a**) and para-axial (**b**) T2-TSE images delineate a tumor of the midrectum at the level of the peritoneal reflection (*arrow*). The tumor involves the muscle layer with no signs of mesorectal invasion. Histopathologic examination of the specimen revealed stage pT2N0L0V0Pn0 rectal cancer.

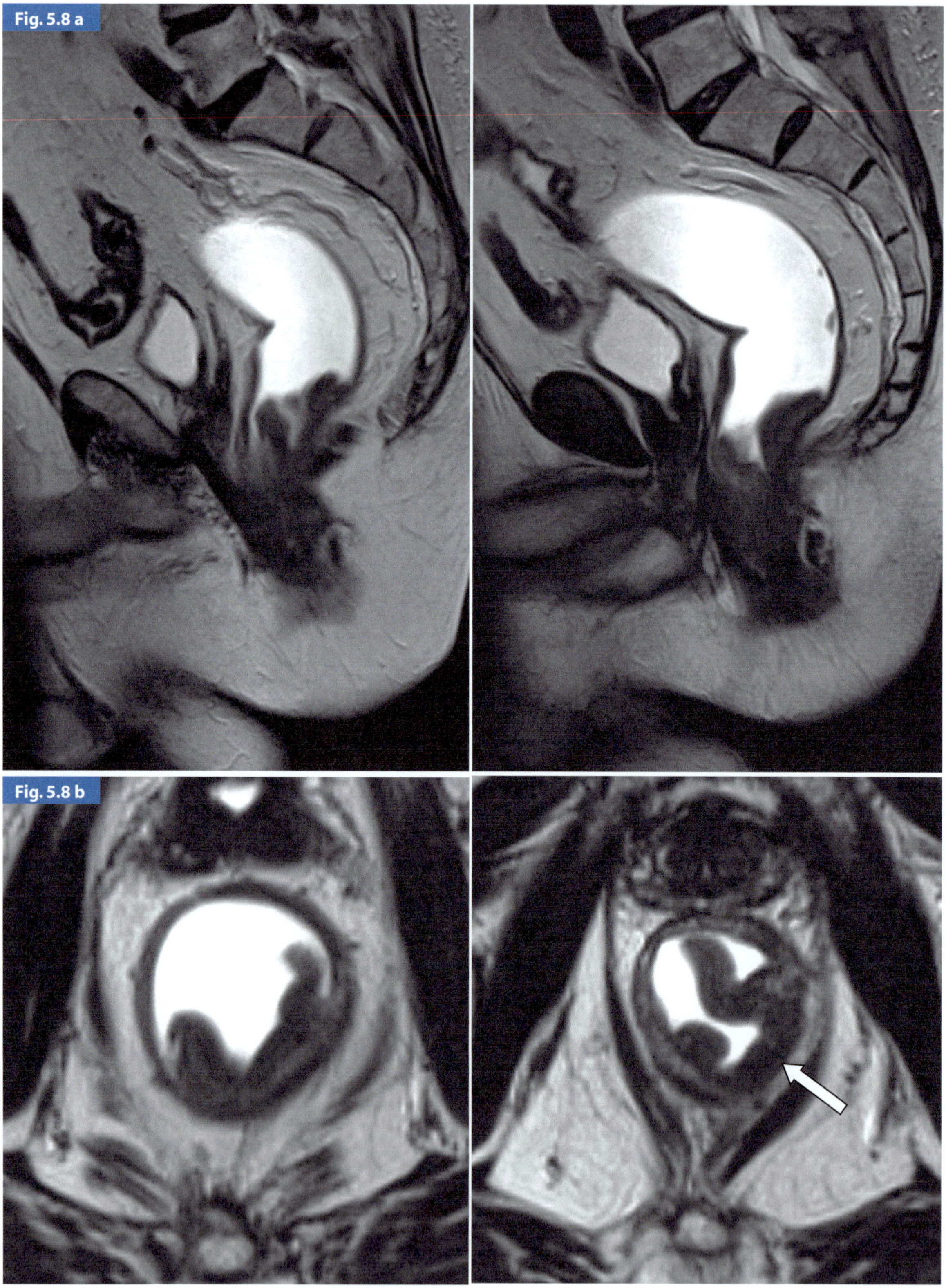

Fig. 5.8 The sagittal (**a**) and corresponding para-axial (**b**) T2-TSE images show supraanal rectal tumor. Status after prostate cancer: The tumor signal reaches the muscularis propria (*arrow*). The findings were confirmed by histopathology revealing pT2N0 G2 rectal cancer.

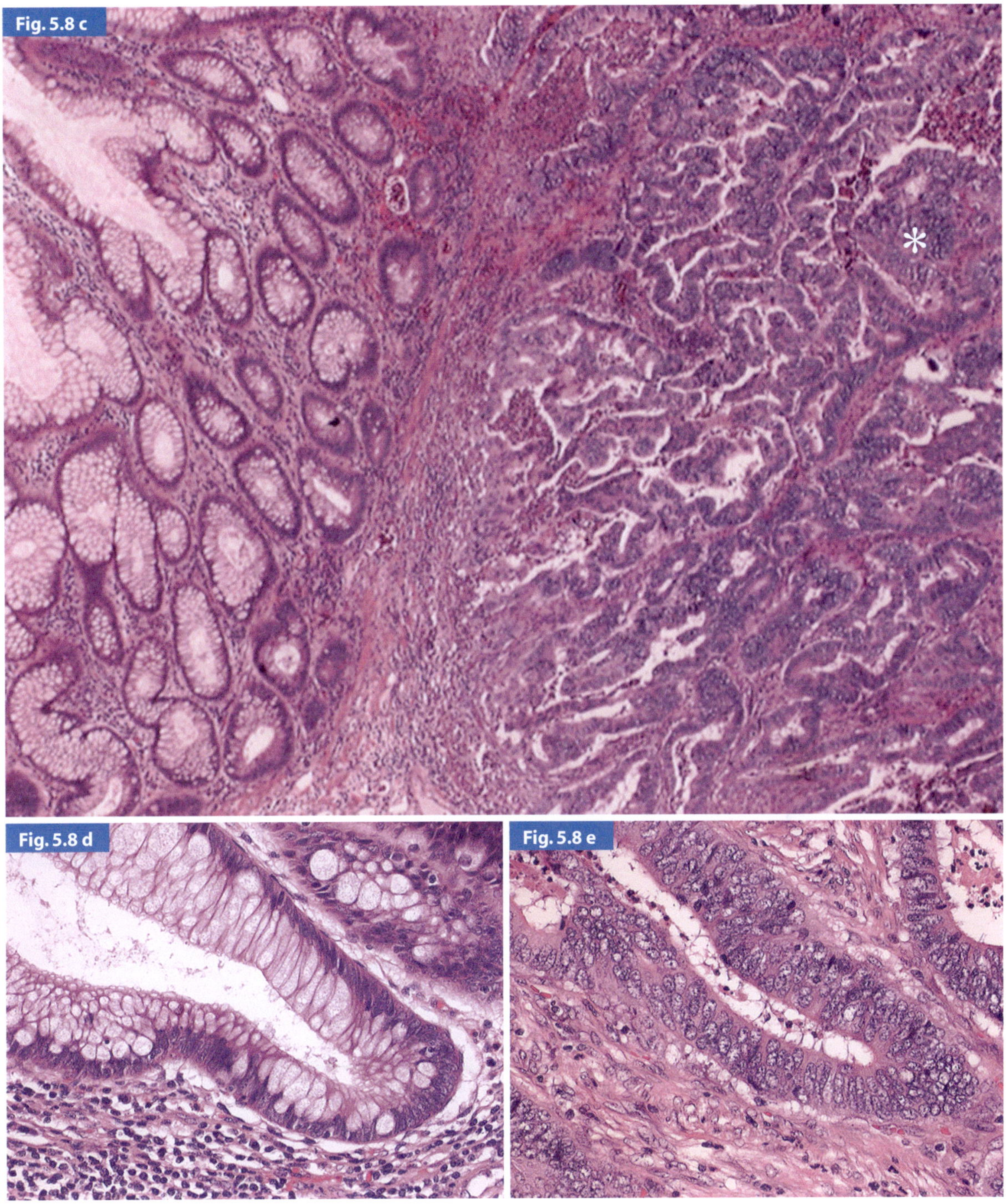

Fig. 5.8 (**c–e**) Comparsion of normal colonic crypt architecture and crypts inflitrated by tumor cells in this patient example, shown by the *asterisk* in (**c**) (H&E, ×5). (**d**) Normal crypt (H&E, ×20). (**e**) Colonization of neighboring crypts by malignant cells (H&E, ×20).

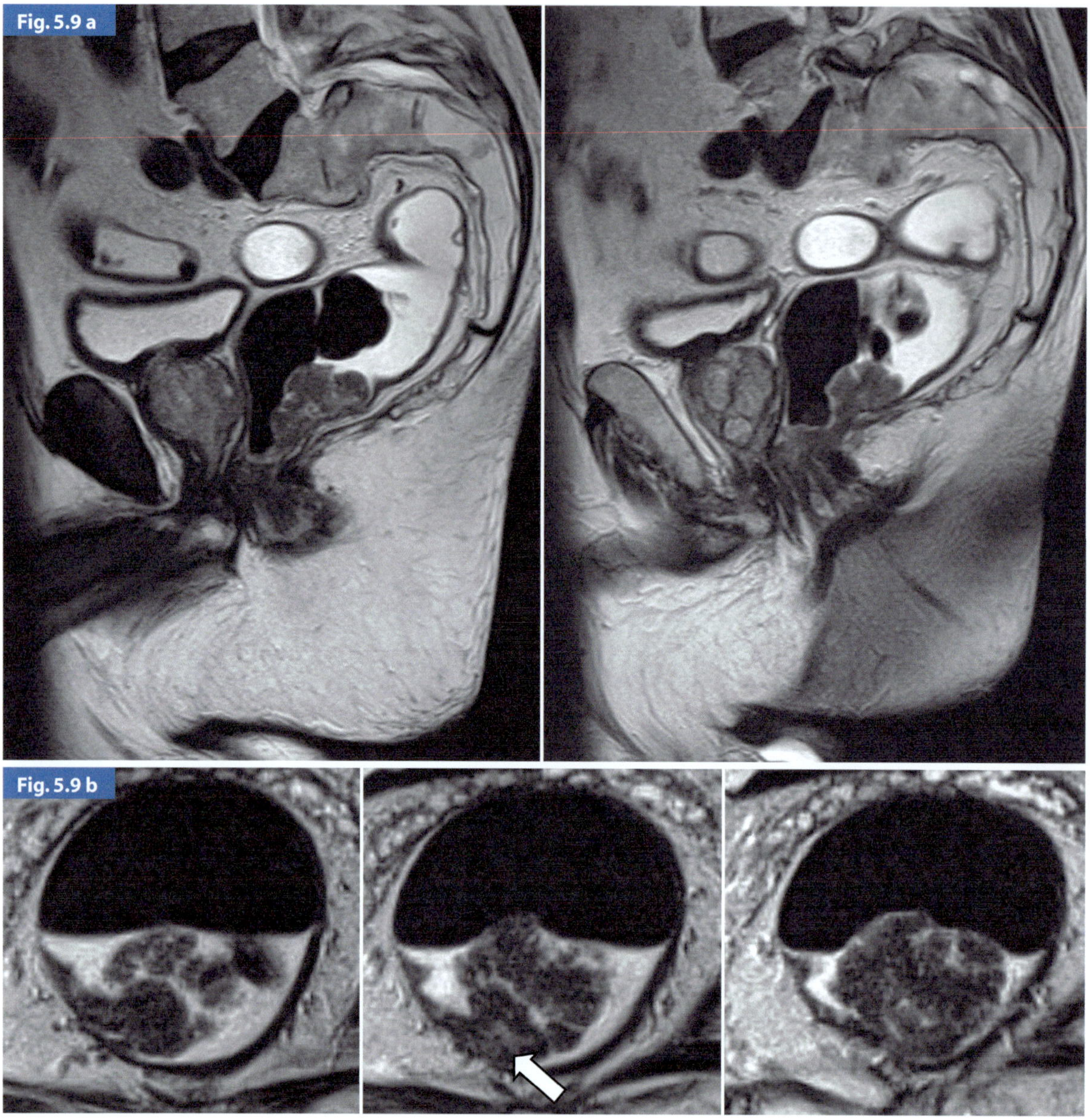

Fig. 5.9 (**a**) Sagittal T2-TSE images show a tubulovillous adenoma of the lower rectum. (**b**) Representative axial T2-TSE images demonstrate the villous and fissured surface of the tumor. At the stalk-basis, conspicuous changes in signal intensity can be observed, which indicate malignant transformation (*arrow*). Concurrently, there are no signs of mesorectal infiltration. Patient history: The patient received transanal endoscopic microsurgery (TEM) of the sessile poly. Histopathology detected malignant transformation of the deep layers of the tubulovillous adenoma, indicating incomplete removal. Additionally, microscopic venous invasion was detected. The final decision to perform abdominoperineal resection was based on these findings. The histopathologic stage was ypT2N0V1Pn1 G2.

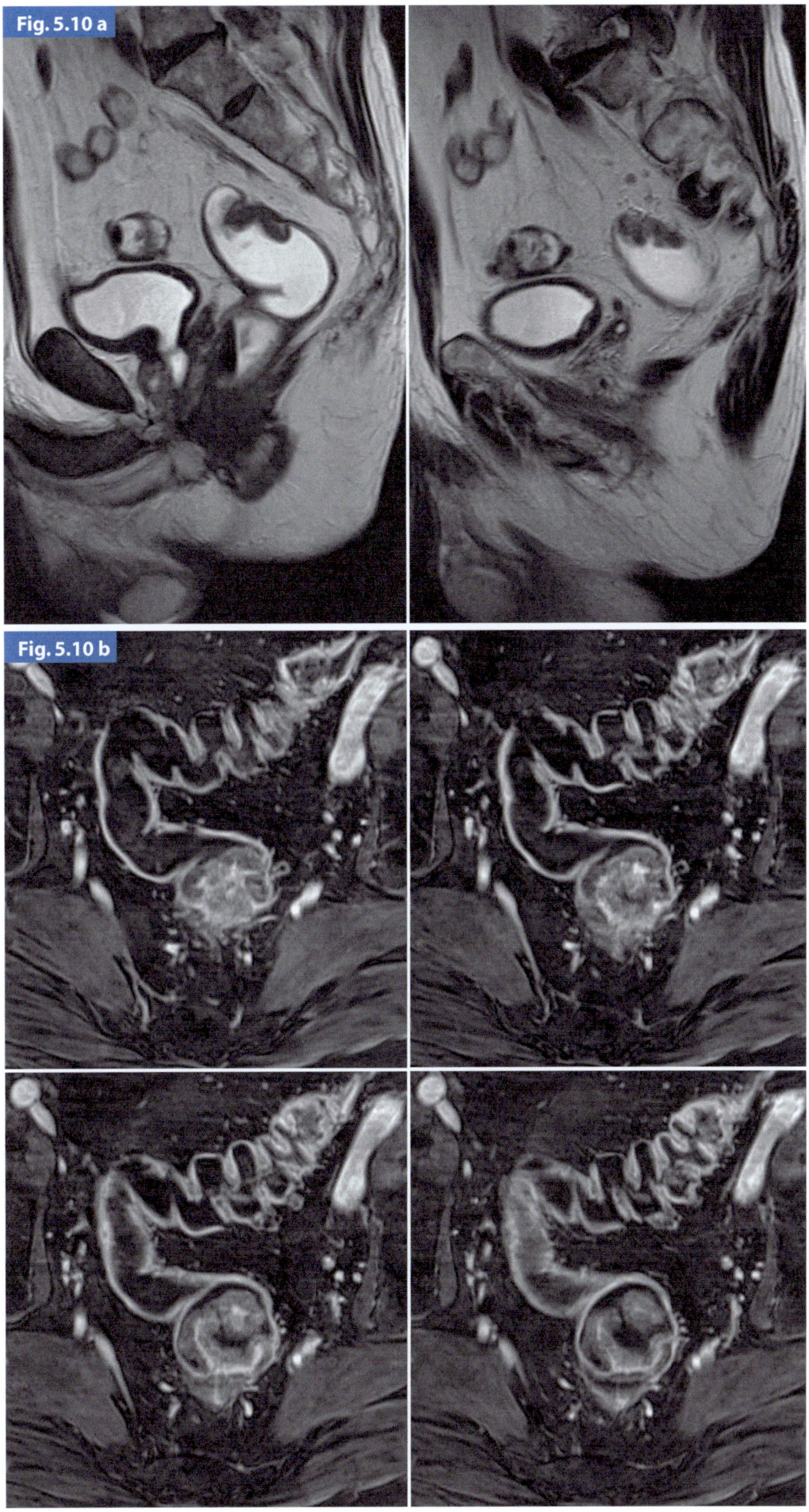

Fig. 5.10 (**a**) On the sagittal T2-TSE images, a bowl-shaped tumor of the upper rectum is evident with adjacent small mesorectal nodes. (**b**) The corresponding CE-VIBE 3D images reflect typical contrast-agent uptake of colonic adenocarcinoma, which is inferior to that of normal bowel wall. The histopathologic stage was pT2N0V0L0Pn0 G2.

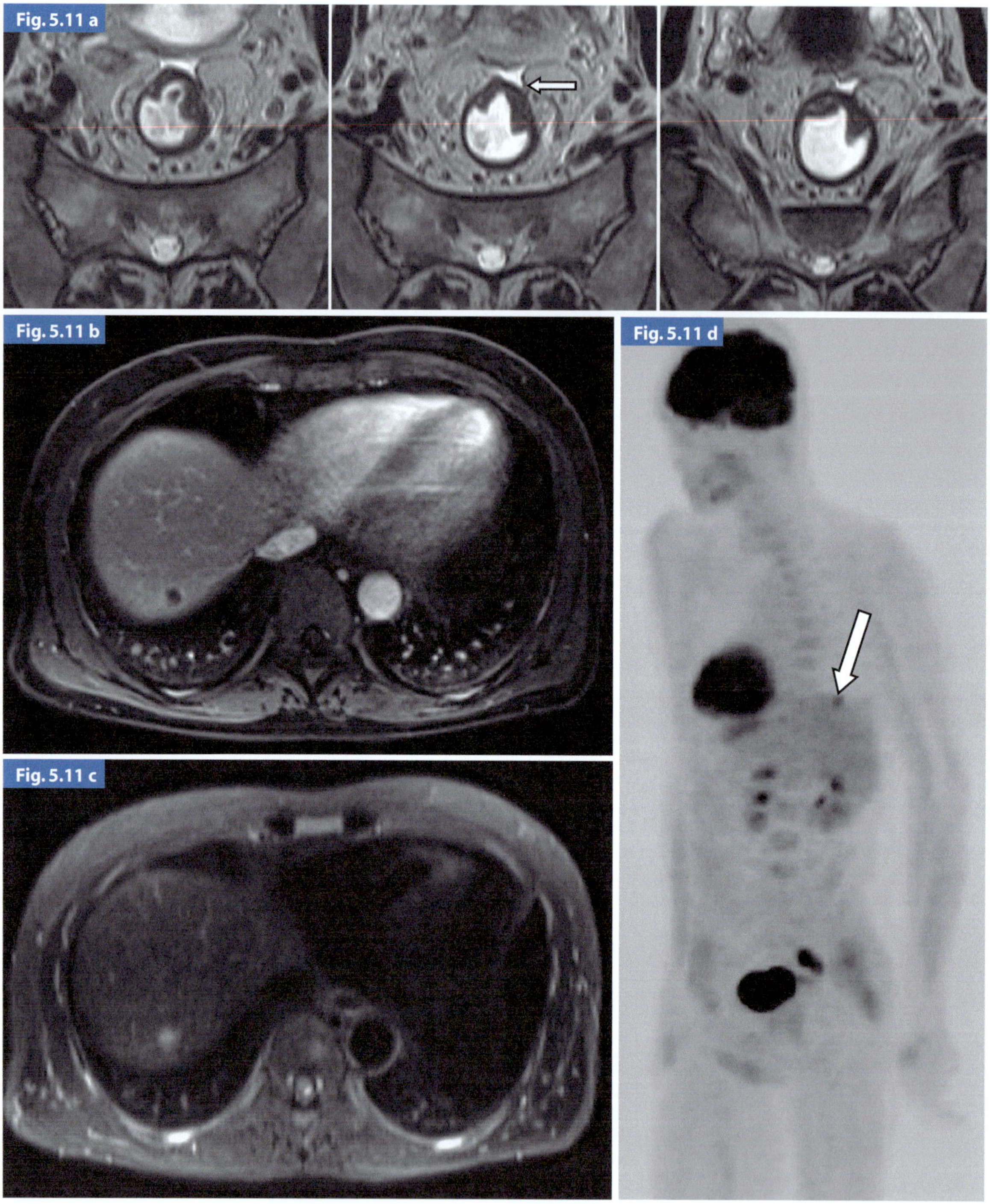

Fig. 5.11 (**a**–**d**) Pretreatment MRI. (**a**) On the axial T2-TSE images, small anterior rectal carcinoma at the level of the peritoneal reflection is distinguishable. The slight thickening of the peritoneal reflection (*arrow*) and small amounts of ascites are indicative of peritoneal infiltration. The tumor was diagnosed at clinical stage T4. (**b**–**d**) SMS staging with breath-hold CE-FLASH 2D (**b**) and free-breathing TIRM (**c**) revealed a small metastasis in the hepatic dome that was confirmed by PET examination (**d**, *arrow*).

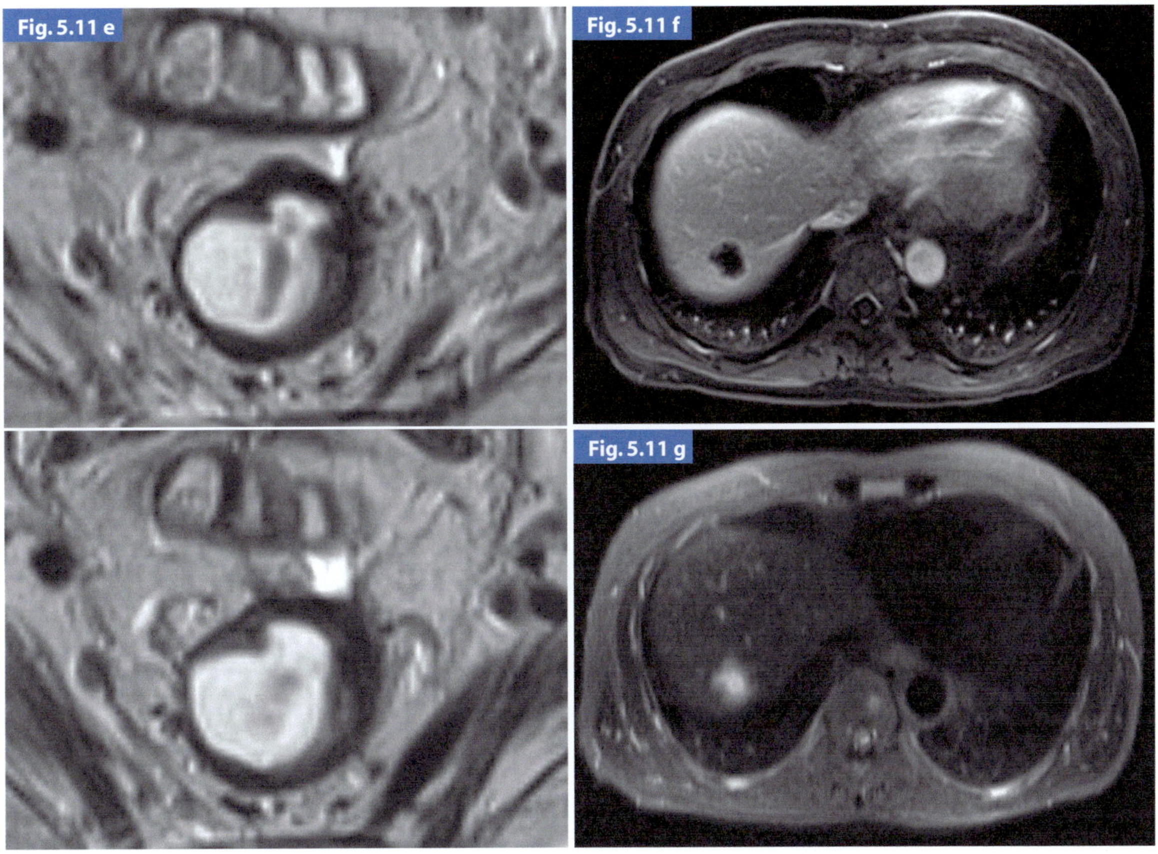

Fig. 5.11 (**e–g**) Post-radiochemotherapy MRI. (**e**) The axial T2-TSE images confirm signal changes of the tumor resulting from fibrosis and a distinct thickening of the peritoneal reflection with few ascites. (**f, g**) Of note, liver metastasis was increasing in size. Despite the small size of the initial tumor, histopathology indicated stage ypT2N0M1L0V0 G2 rectal cancer.

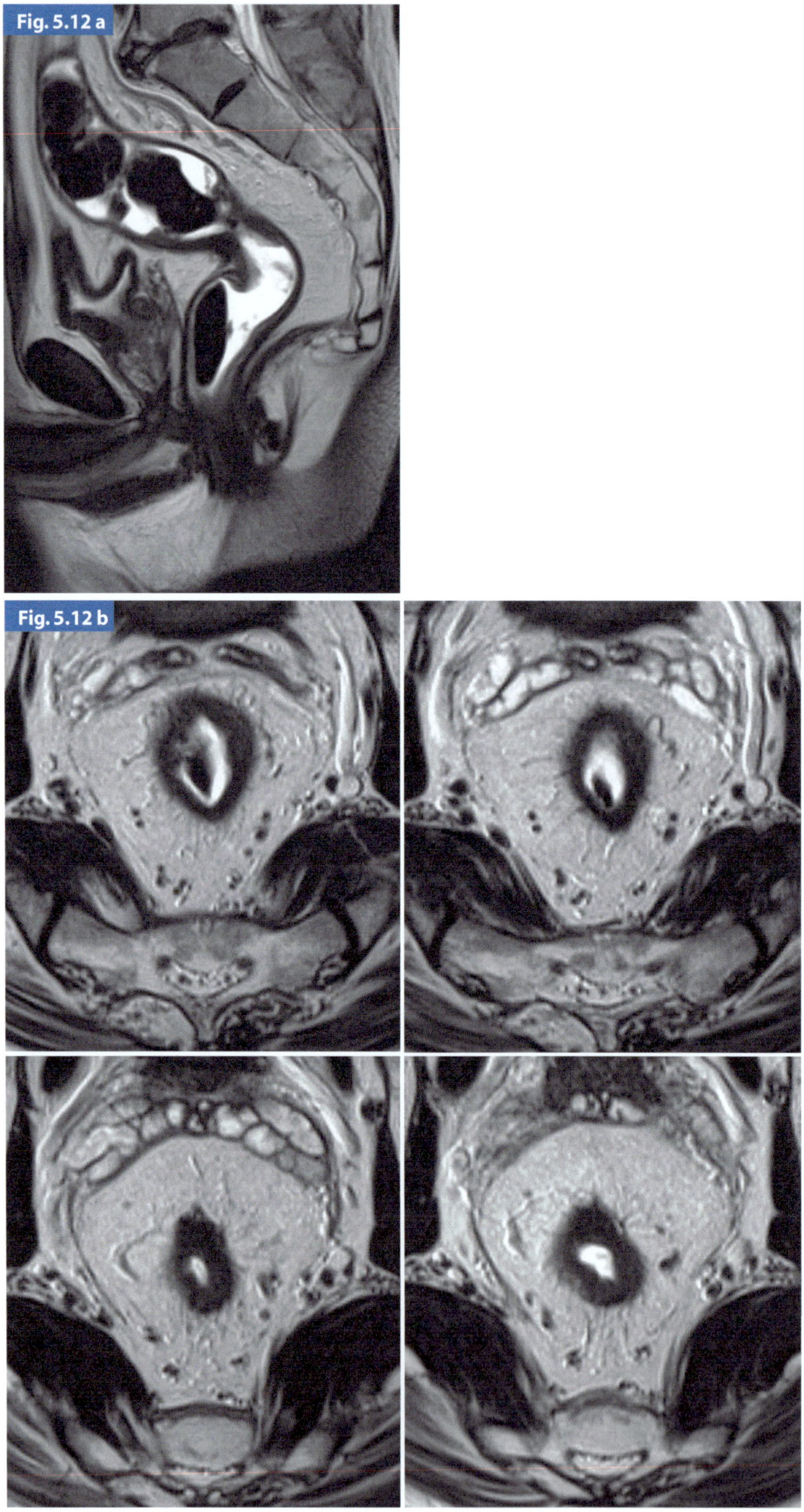

Fig. 5.12 (**a**, **b**) Pretreatment MRI. Sagittal (**a**) and axial (**b**) T2-TSE images show a circular stenosing midrectal cancer. The tumor signal is comparable to that of the normal muscle layer, indicative of linitis plastica carcinoma. The tumor involves all layers of the rectal wall. A differentiation between desmoplastic reaction and mesorectal fat invasion is imposssible because the diffuse, streak-like, hypointense perimuscular tissue changes surrounding the tumor in this example can occur in both situations. Radiologically, the clinical tumor stage was therefore reported as cT3N0.

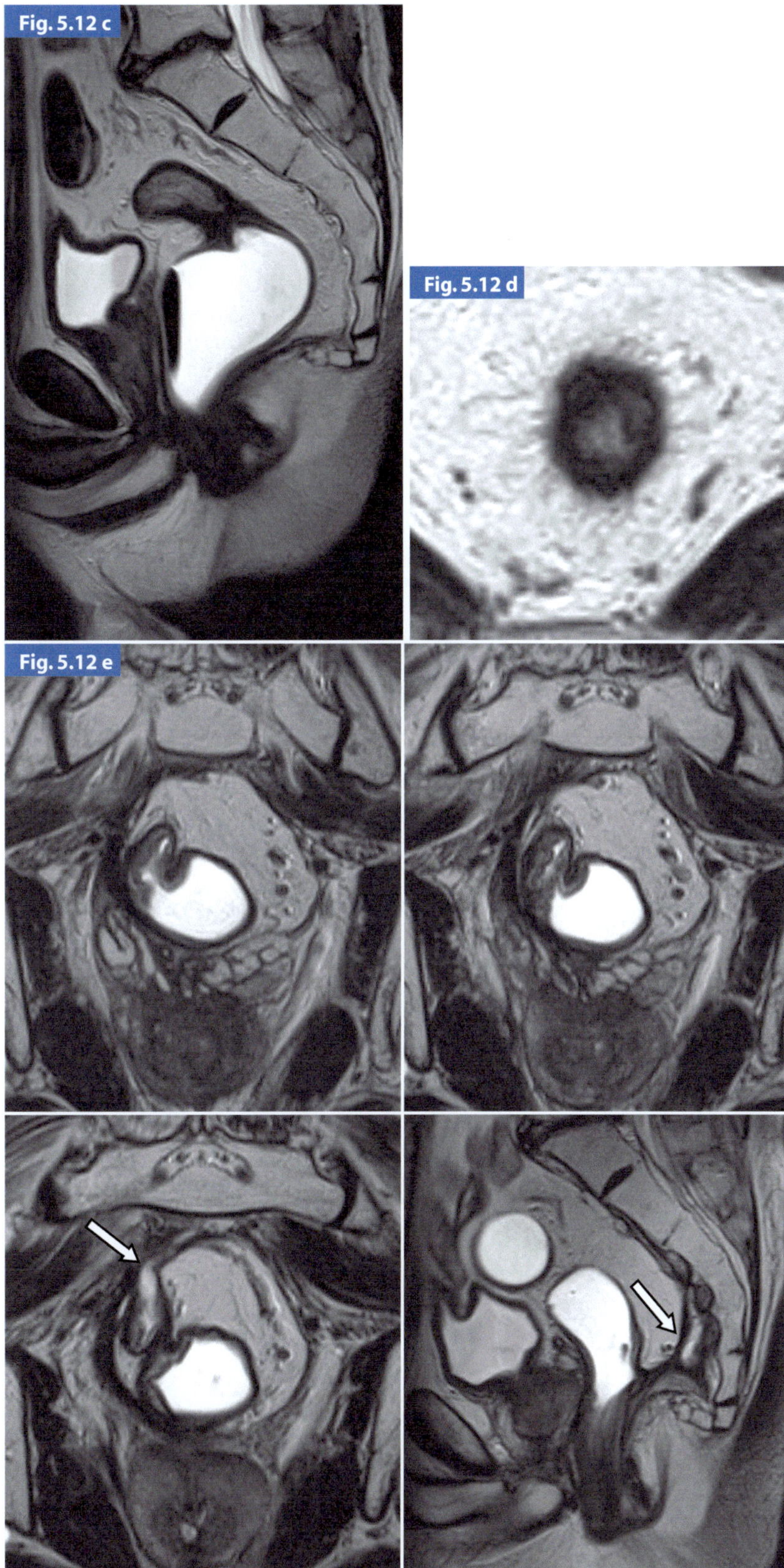

Fig. 5.12 (**c**, **d**) MRI following neoadjuvant radiochemotherapy. On the sagittal (**c**) and para-axial (**d**) T2-TSE images, tumor shrinkage is evident. Zones of increased signal can be seen as suggestive of necrosis. The changes of the perimuscular fat are still present. The final stage was ypT2N0L0V0Pn0R0. During histopathologic work-up, mucinous lakes within the junction of the muscularis propria and perimuscular fat were interpreted as residuals of an initially higher tumor stage prior to treatment. (**e**) Follow-up MRI. Status: 1 year post-anterior resection and colonic J-pouch. Neither luminal nor extraluminal local recurrence is present on the sagittal and para-coronal T2-TSE images. Instead, a fistula arising from the colonic pouch reaches the presacral scar formation, distinguishable as fluid-filled track (*arrows*).

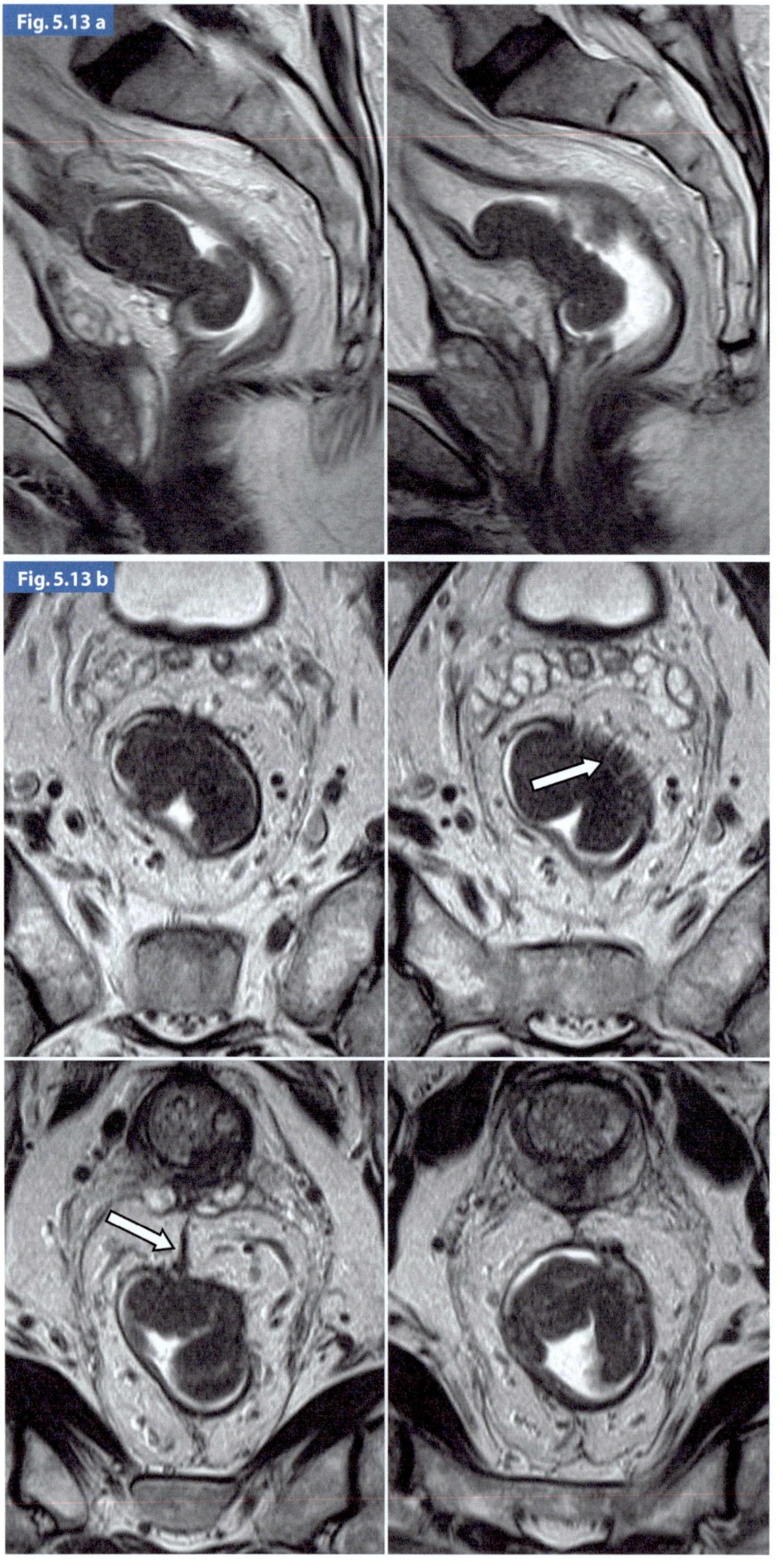

Fig. 5.13 (**a**, **b**) Pretreatment MRI. (**a**) On the sagittal T2-TSE images, a polypoid midrectal tumor is seen. (**b**) The para-axial T2-TSE images show streaky changes of the muscle layer between the 12- and 3-o'clock lithotomy position, which reach the perimuscular fat—indicative of either tumor infiltration or desmoplastic reaction (*arrow*). Additionally, the peritoneal reflection is thickened, indicating possible tumor infiltration (*arrow*).

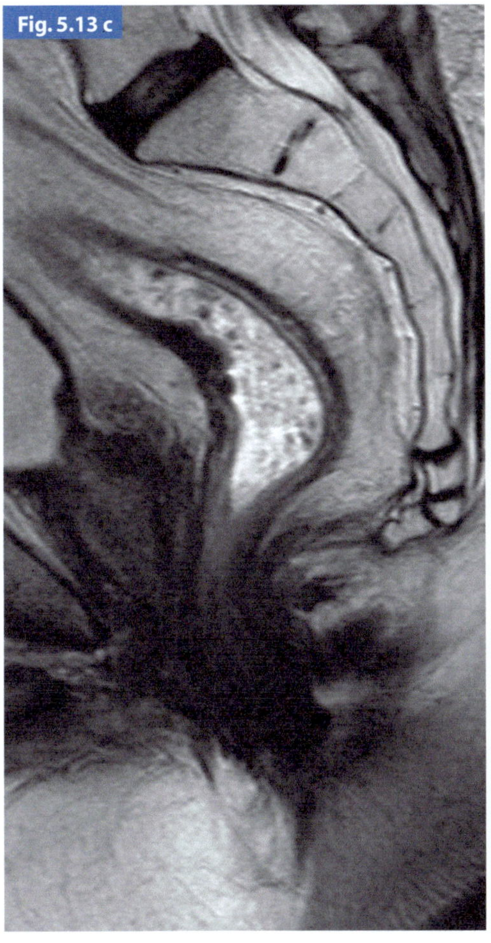

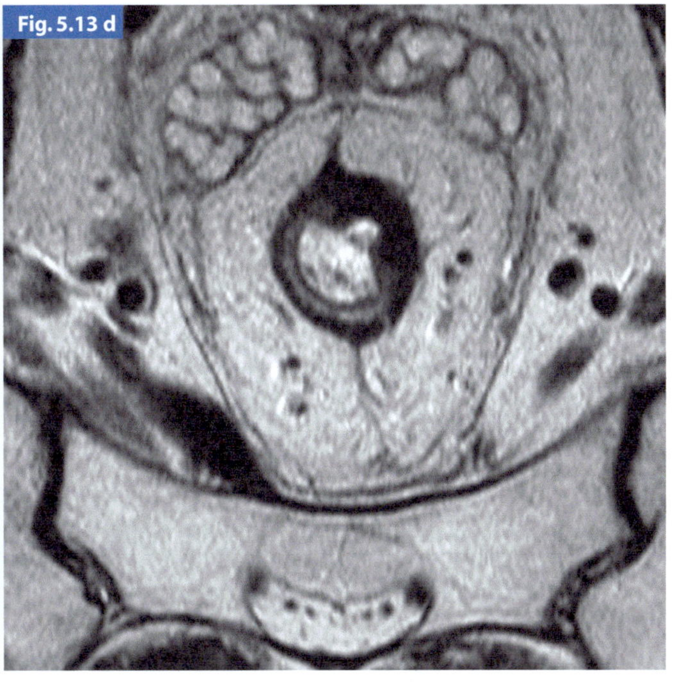

Fig. 5.13 (**c**, **d**) Post-neoadjuvant therapy MRI. Compared with the initial findings, tumor shrinkage and fibrosis can be observed on the sagittal (**c**) and para-axial (**d**) T2-TSE images. The signal drop of the tumor bed involved the entire rectal wall. The signal changes of the adjacent mesorectal fat completely disappeared. The tumor was clinically staged as cT2N0. Deep anterior resection was performed and histopathology diagnosed stage ypT2N0 rectal cancer.

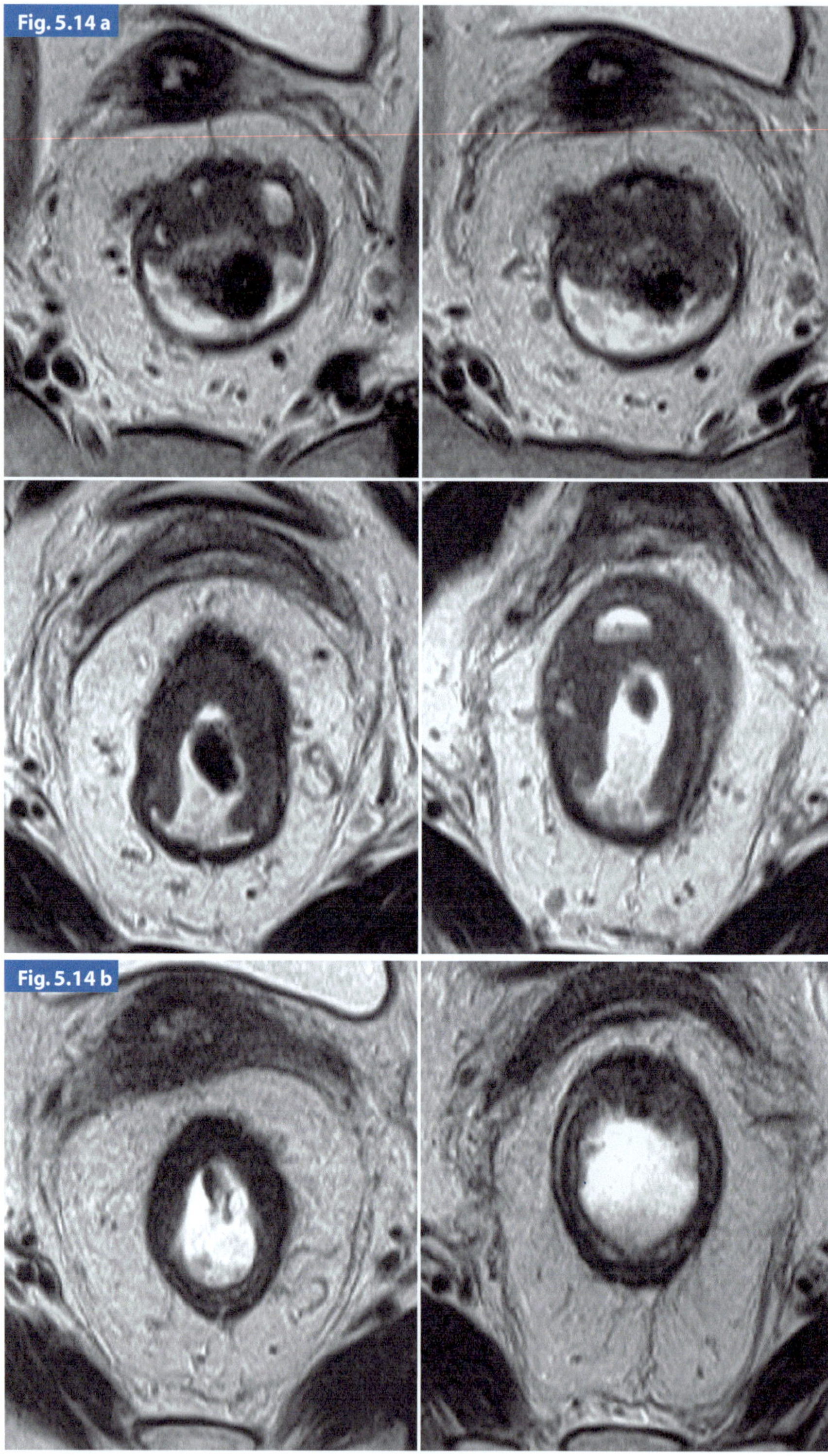

Fig. 5.14 (**a**) Pretreatment MRI. On the axial T2-TSE images, wall exceeding carcinoma of the midrectum is seen with foci of high-signal intensity corresponding to mucus lakes. (**b**) Post-neoadjuvant therapy MRI. Following chemoradiation, the tumor size decreased. Tumor fibrosis is also visible. The histopathologic stage was ypT2N0L0V0Pn0 G2.

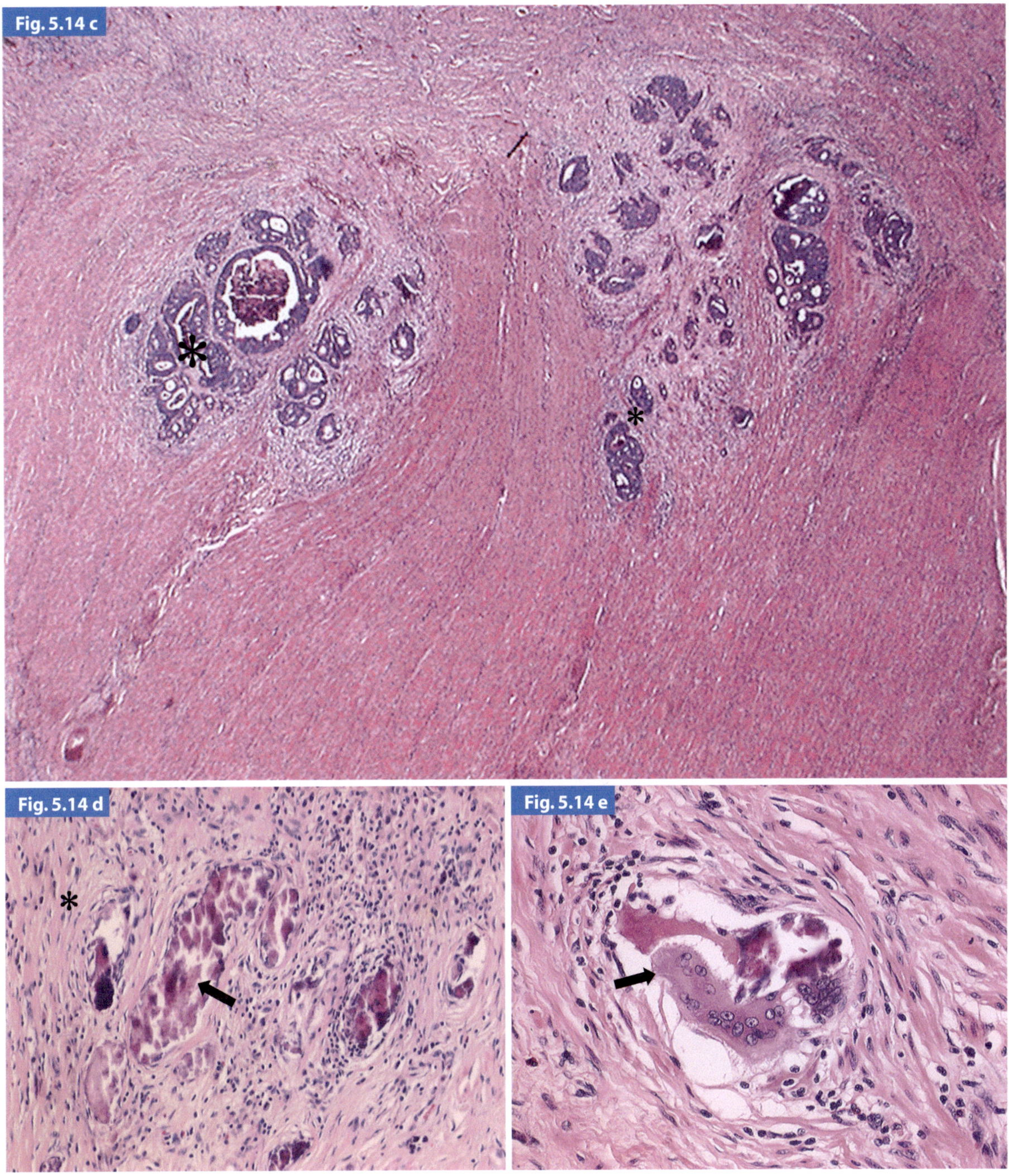

Fig. 5.14 (**c**–**e**) Coexistence of vital tumor and regressive changes following radiochemotherapy. (**c**) Foci of viable tumor within the muscularis propria (*asterisks*, H&E, ×1). (**d**) Tumor fibrosis and calcifications (*asterisk* and *arrow*, H&E, ×10). (**e**) Tumor calcification and polynucleated giant cell (*arrow*, H&E, ×20).

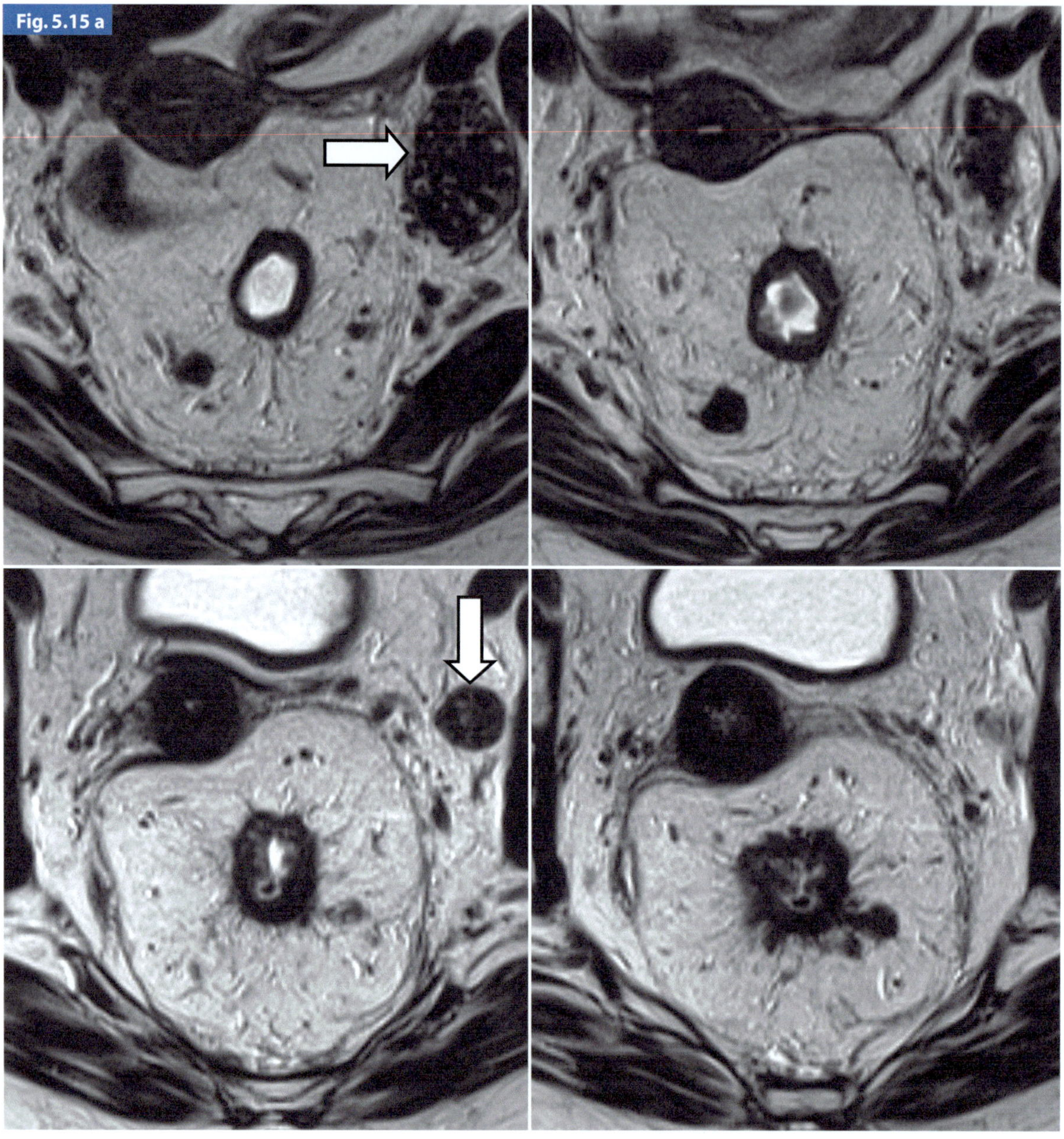

Fig. 5.15 (**a**) On the para-axial T2-TSE post-neoadjuvant chemoradiation images, a mixed signal intensity of the primary tumor can be identified, indicating tumor necrosis and fibrosis following therapy. A prediction of the degree of tumor regression is impossible. The tumor appears to directly invade the mesorectal fat. Several dark nodes are located around the tumor area. Suspicious nodes are demonstrated beyond the mesorectal fascia at the left pelvic sidewall (*arrows*). Clinically, the rectal cancer was classified as stage ycT3N2M1. The final histopathologic stage was ypT2N0L0V0R0. Surprisingly, no metastatic disease was detected in sampled left iliac nodes.

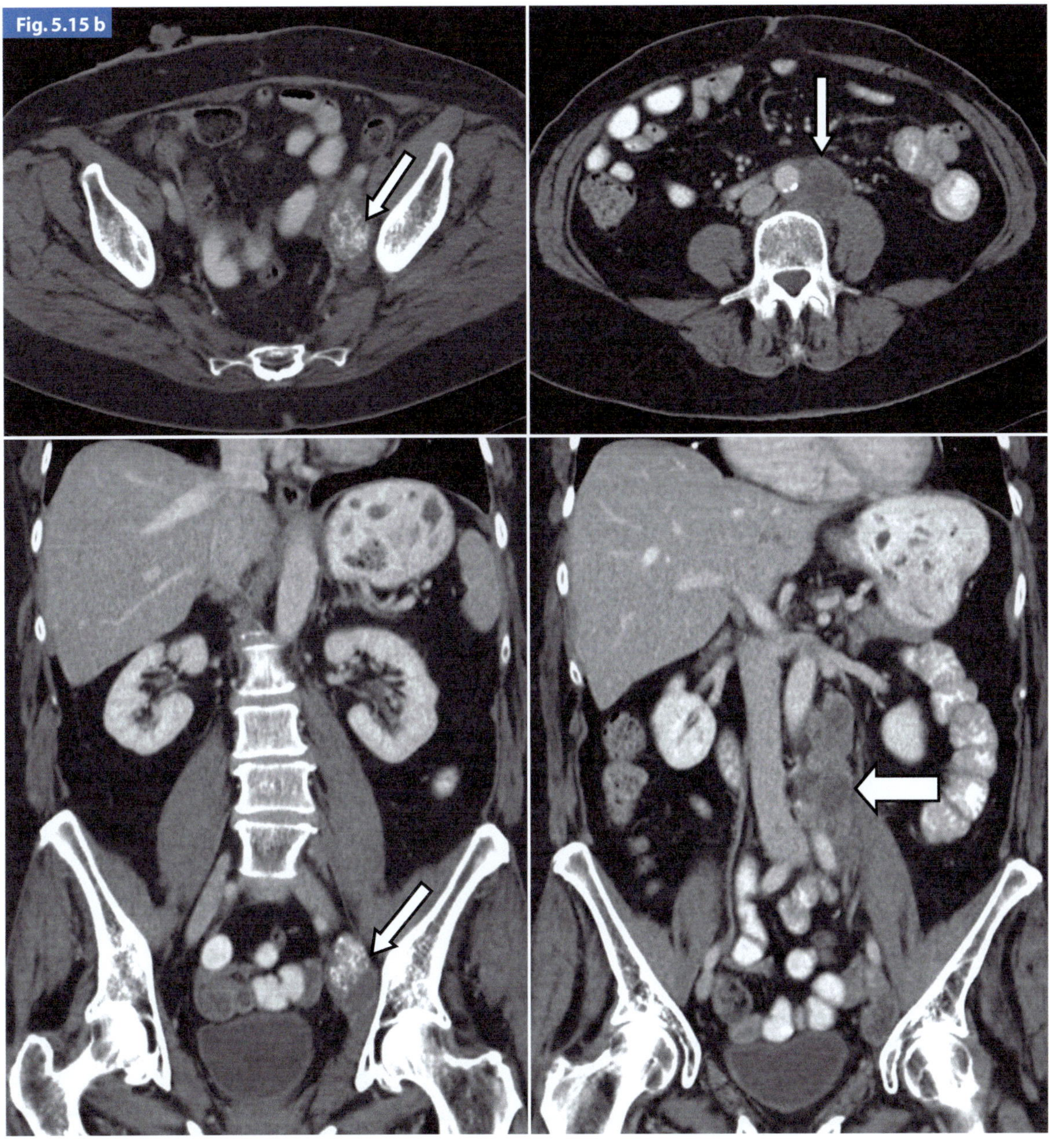

Fig. 5.15 (**b**) Follow-up abdominopelvic MSCT at 1 year after rectal cancer surgery documents progressive disease with retroperitoneal nodal spread and persistant left iliac lymph node metastasis (*arrows*).

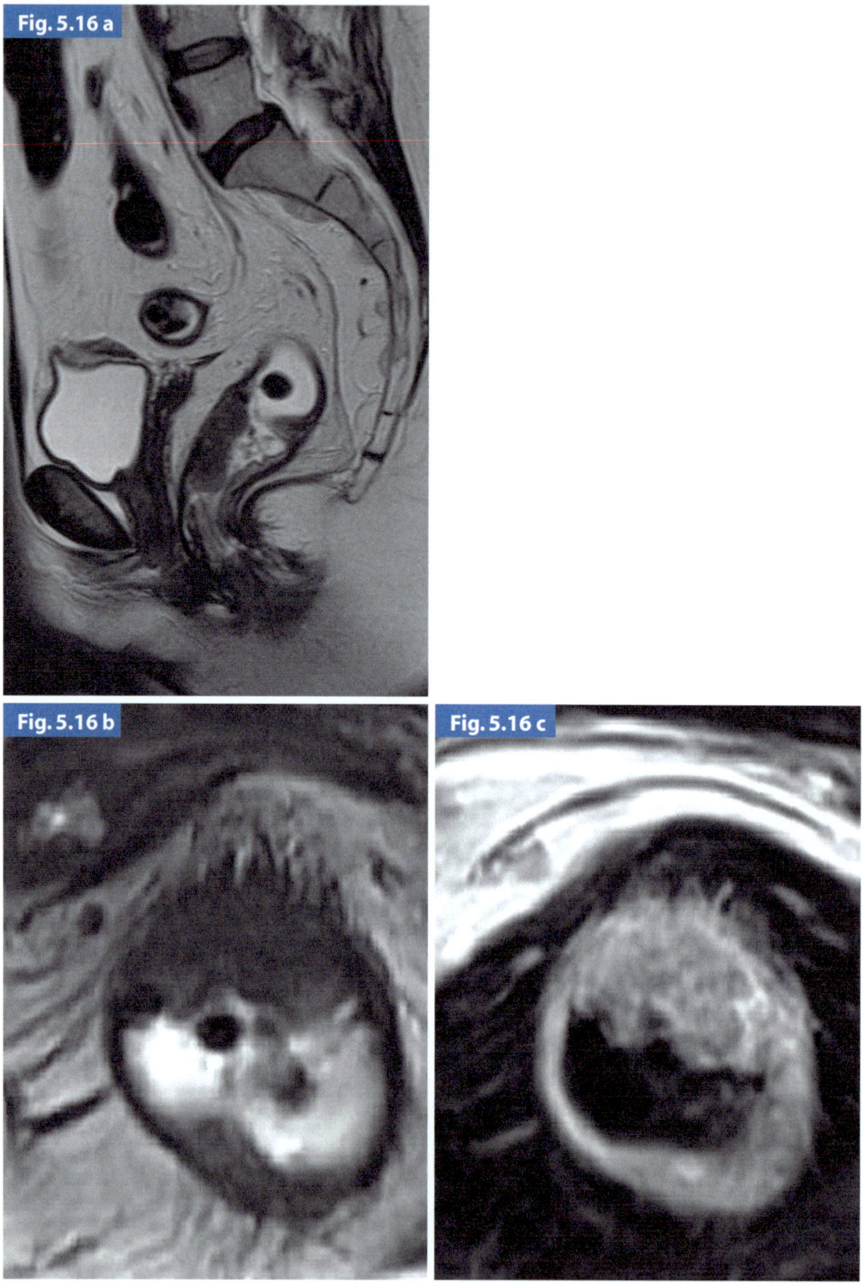

Fig. 5.16 (**a**–**c**) Pretreatment MRI. The sagittal T2-TSE image (**a**) detected an exophytic tumor of the lower and midrectum, which seems to extensively penetrate the muscle layer into the anterior aspects of the mesorectal fat depicted on the axial CISS-3D (**b**) and corresponding CE-VIBE 3D (**c**) image.

Fig. 5.16 (**d–f**) Post-neoadjuvant therapy MRI. (**d**) The sagittal T2-TSE image reveals tumor shrinkage and fibrosis identifiable as signal decrease. (**e**, **f**) The digitate mesorectal tumor extensions regressed and there is pronounced contrast-agent uptake in the treated tumor bed. Problem: Diagnosing the degree of tumor regression. The final histopathologic diagnosis was stage T2N0L0V0Pn0. Fibrosis and peritumorous inflammation were observed. (**g**) Ink drawing: Desmoplastic reaction.

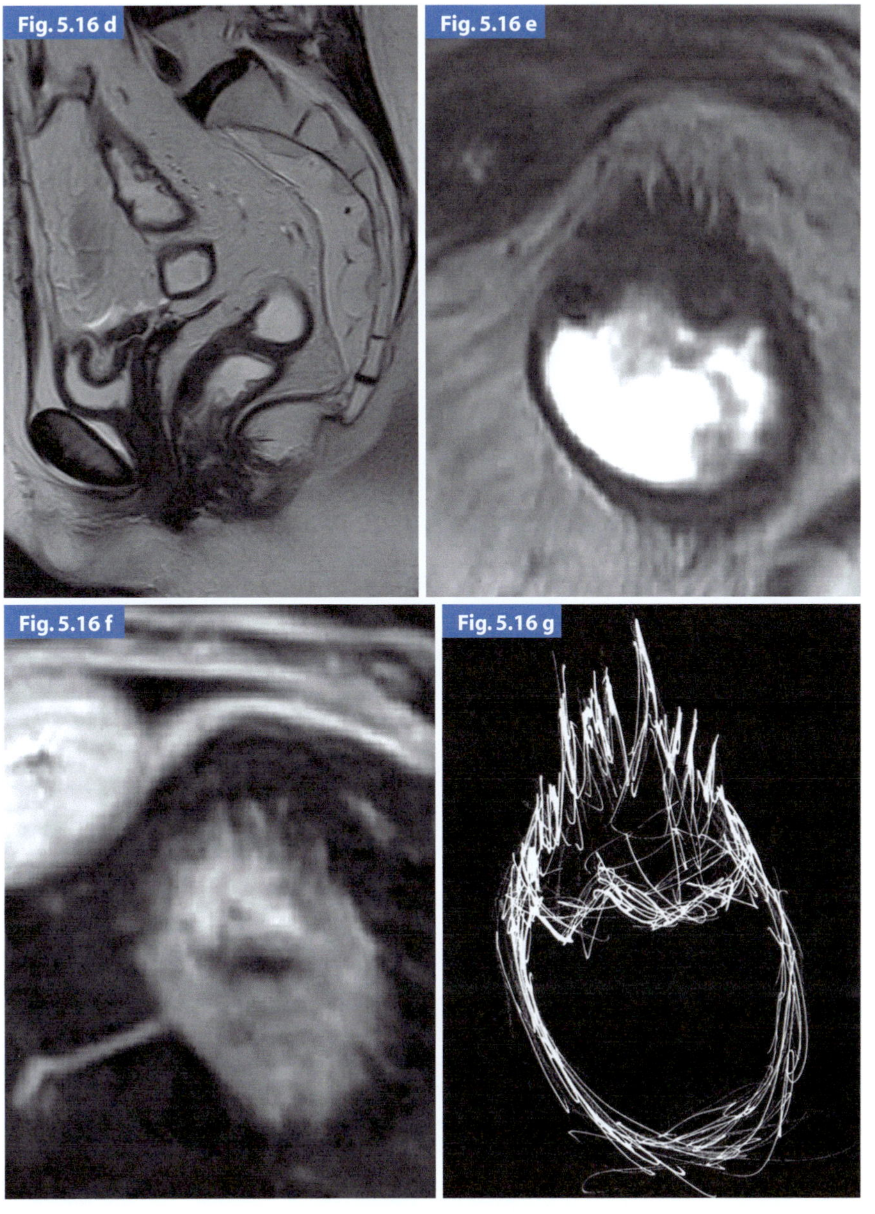

5.4 Stage T3 Rectal Cancer

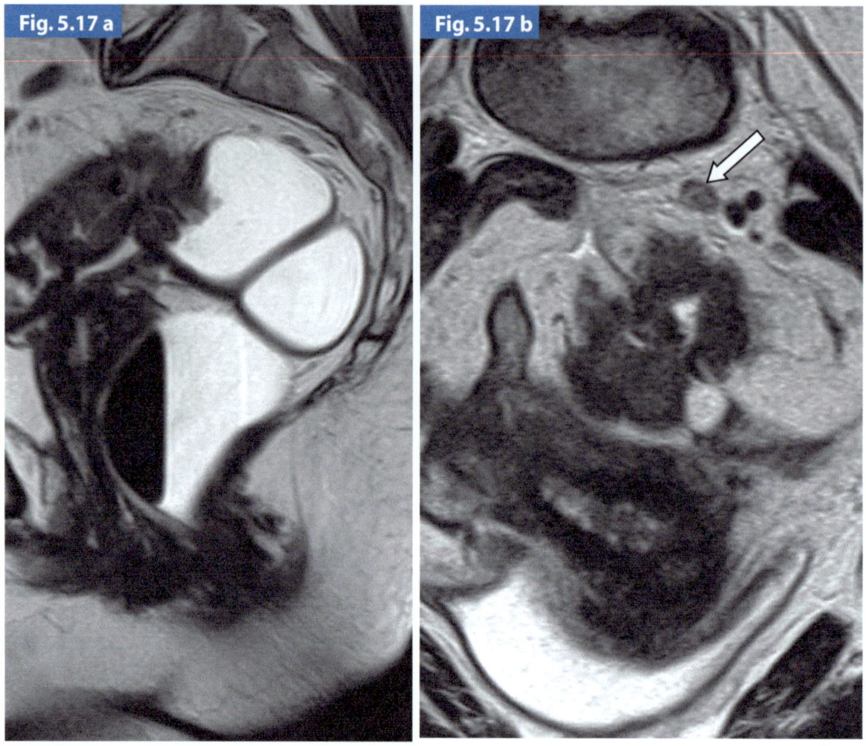

Fig. 5.17 Sagittal (**a**) and para-coronal (**b**) images reveal a wall-exceeding tumor of the upper rectum with a solitary adjacent mesorectal lymph node metastasis (*arrow*). Patient history: Diagnosis of synchronous double cancer consisting of left inflammatory breast carcinoma and hepatic metastasized moderately differentiated tubular rectal carcinoma. Deep anterior resection of the rectum and J-pouch anastomosis were performed. The histopathologic stage was pT3N1 (1/17) M1 (liver) L1V0 G2.

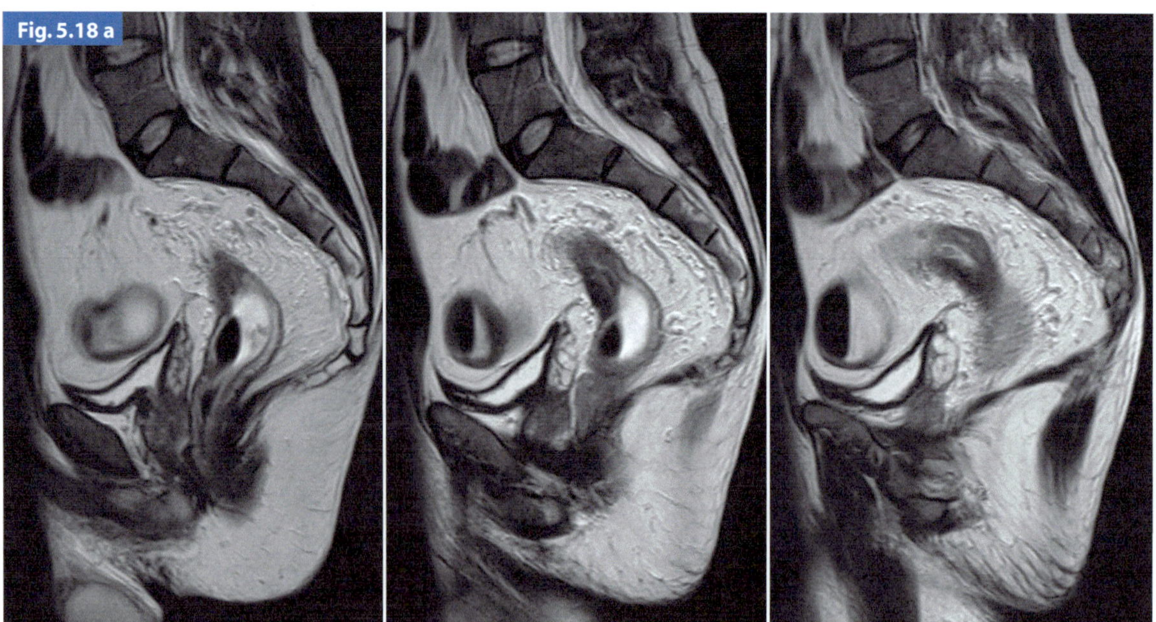

Fig. 5.18 Patient history: Longstanding ulcerative colitis. (**a**) Sagittal T2-TSE images reveal submucosal edema of the lower and midrectum due to ulcerative colitis. Additionally, fibrofatty proliferation of the mesorectum is distinguishable. Stenosis of the upper rectum is caused by a low-signal tumor.

Fig. 5.18 (**b**) Axial T2-TSE images perpendicular to the tumor axis delimit intermediate signal circular carcinoma with invasion of all rectal wall layers. At the 8-o'clock lithotomy position, the lowsignal of the muscularis propria has vanished, indicating the possibility of minimal mesorectal infiltration (*arrow*). Adjacent to the mesorectal fascia a cluster of small lymph nodes is visible. (**c**) Axial CE-VIBE 3D images demonstrate increased vessel density of the tumor area and blurred tumor margins. Proctocolectomy was performed and a stage pT3N1 rectal cancer was diagnosed.

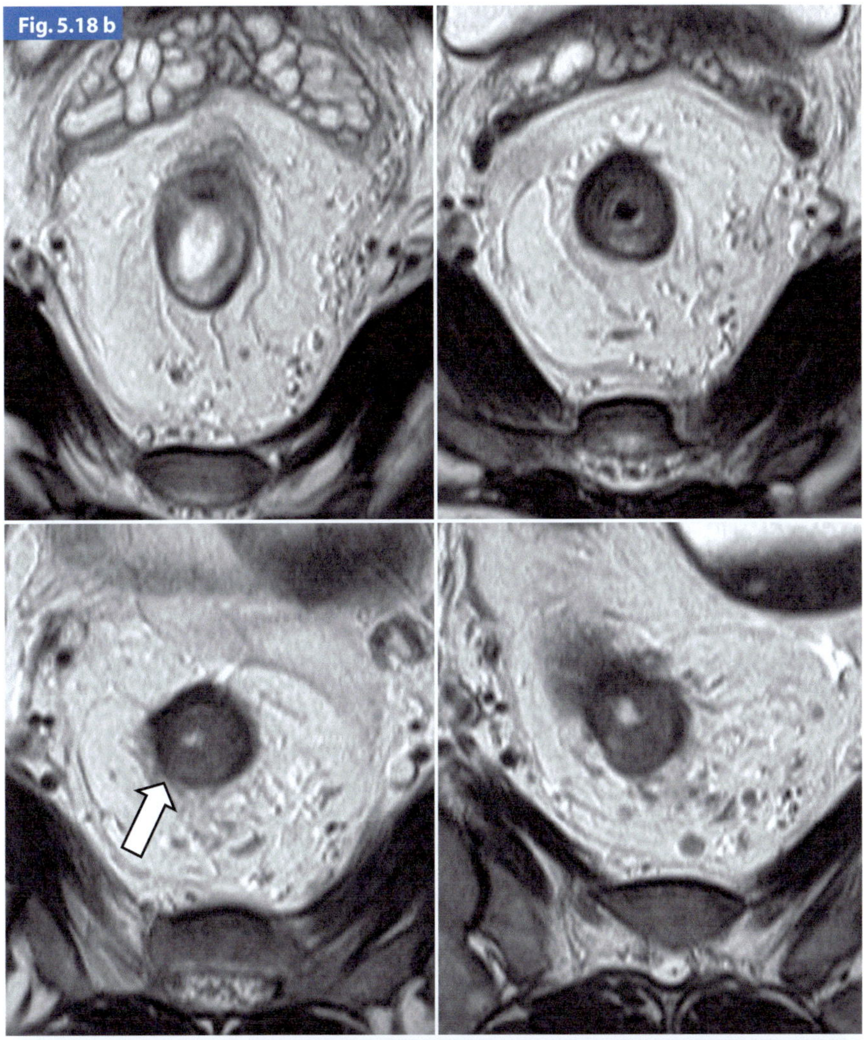

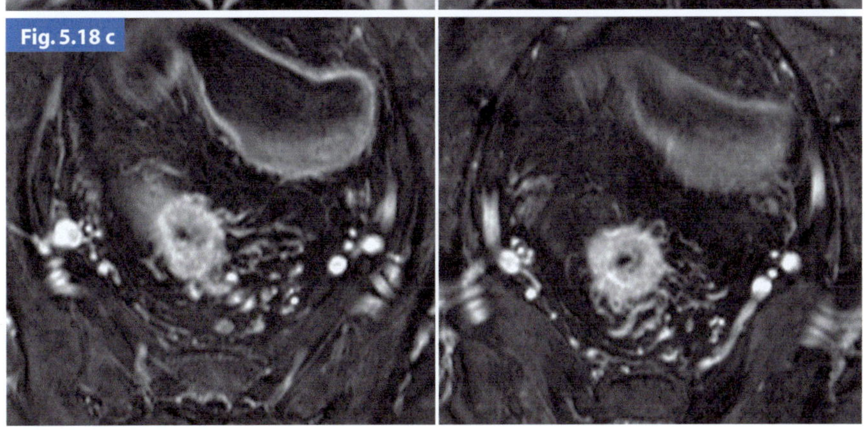

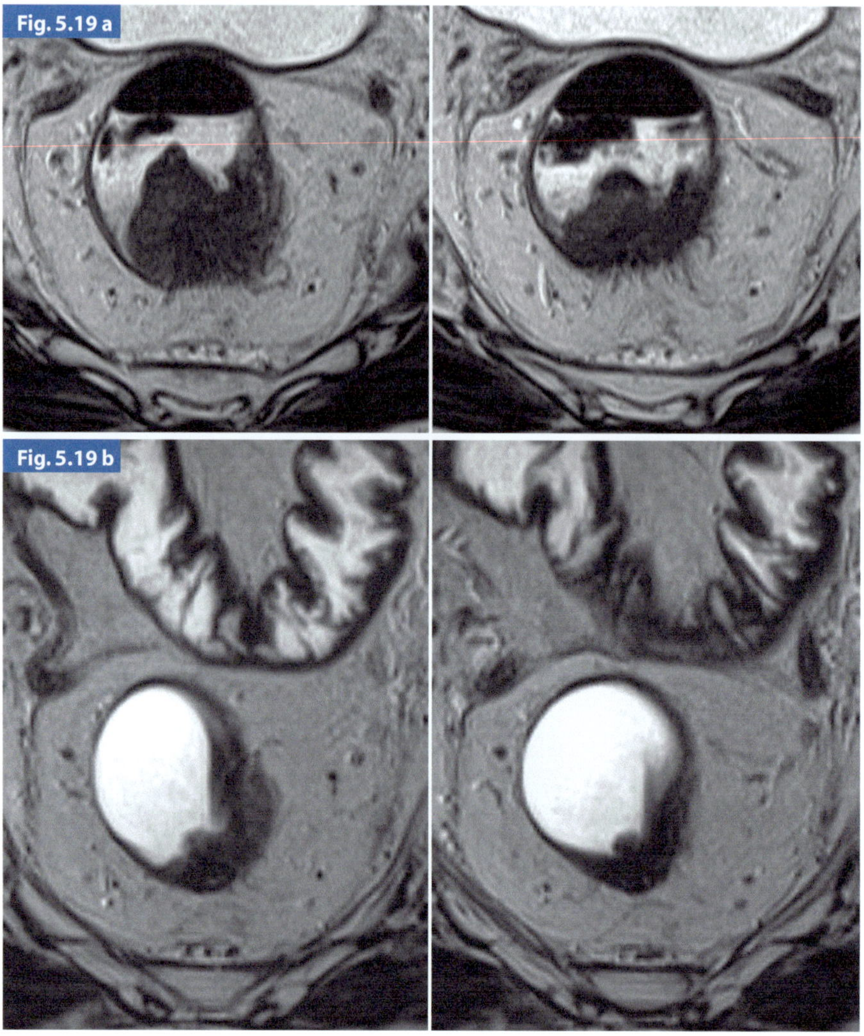

Fig. 5.19 Stage ypT0 rectal cancer. (**a**) Pretreatment MRI. Para-axial T2-TSE images from the midrectum revealing wall-exceeding carcinoma with a central ulcer. (**b**) Post-neoadjuvant therapy MRI. Para-axial T2-TSE images confirm tumor downsizing and incomplete tumor fibrosis. Surprisingly, histopathologic diagnosis indicated stage ypT0N0 rectal cancer.

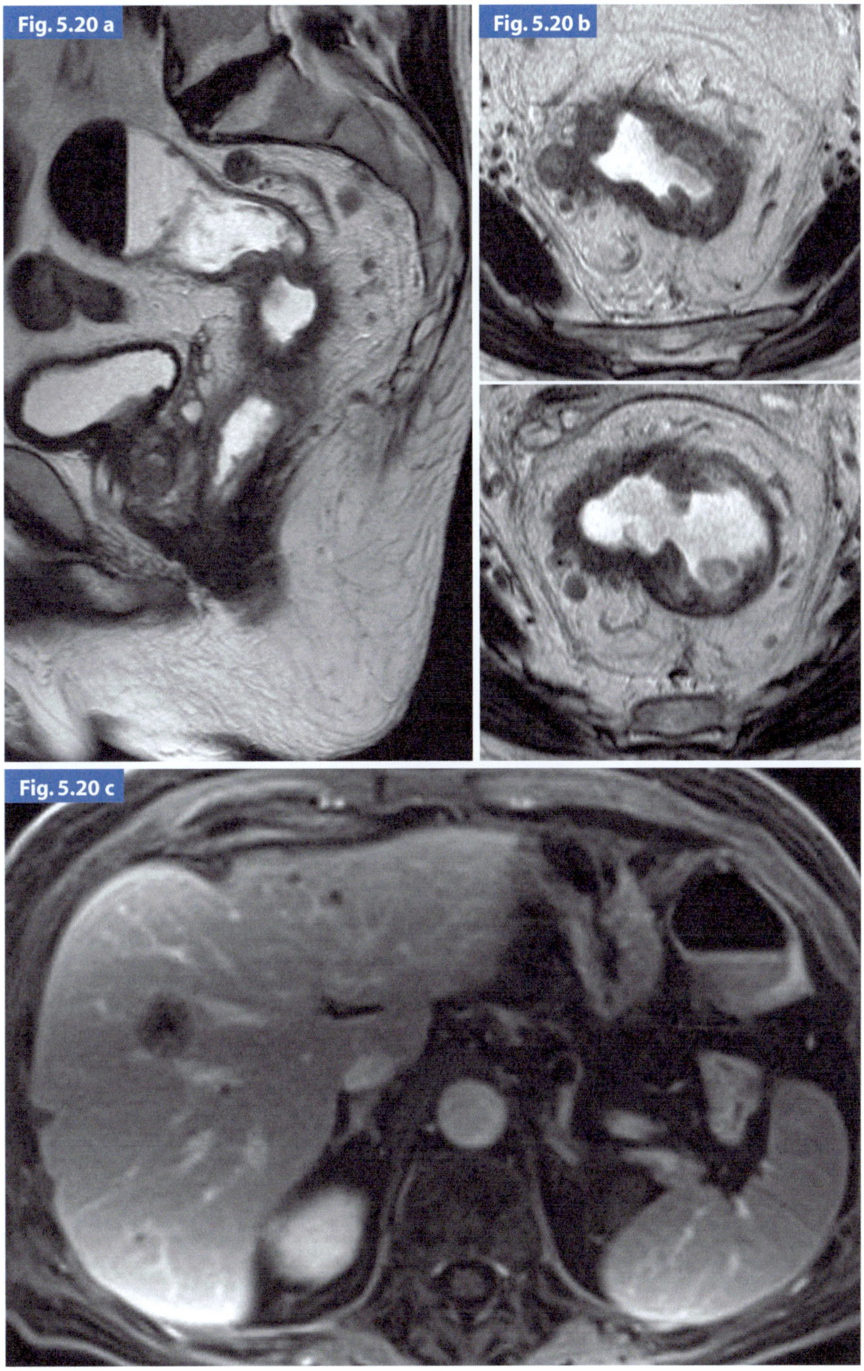

Fig. 5.20 (**a–f**) Cancer in a rectal stump after left hemicolectomy and synchronous liver metastases. (**a–c**) Pretreatment MRI. On the sagittal (**a**) and corresponding axial (**b**) T2-TSE images, rectal cancer exceeding the wall is detectable along with a central ulcer. Metastatic nodes can be seen directly adjacent to the mesorectal fascia. (**c**) During moving-table MRI, synchronous liver metastases can be observed on the axial CE-FLASH 2D image.

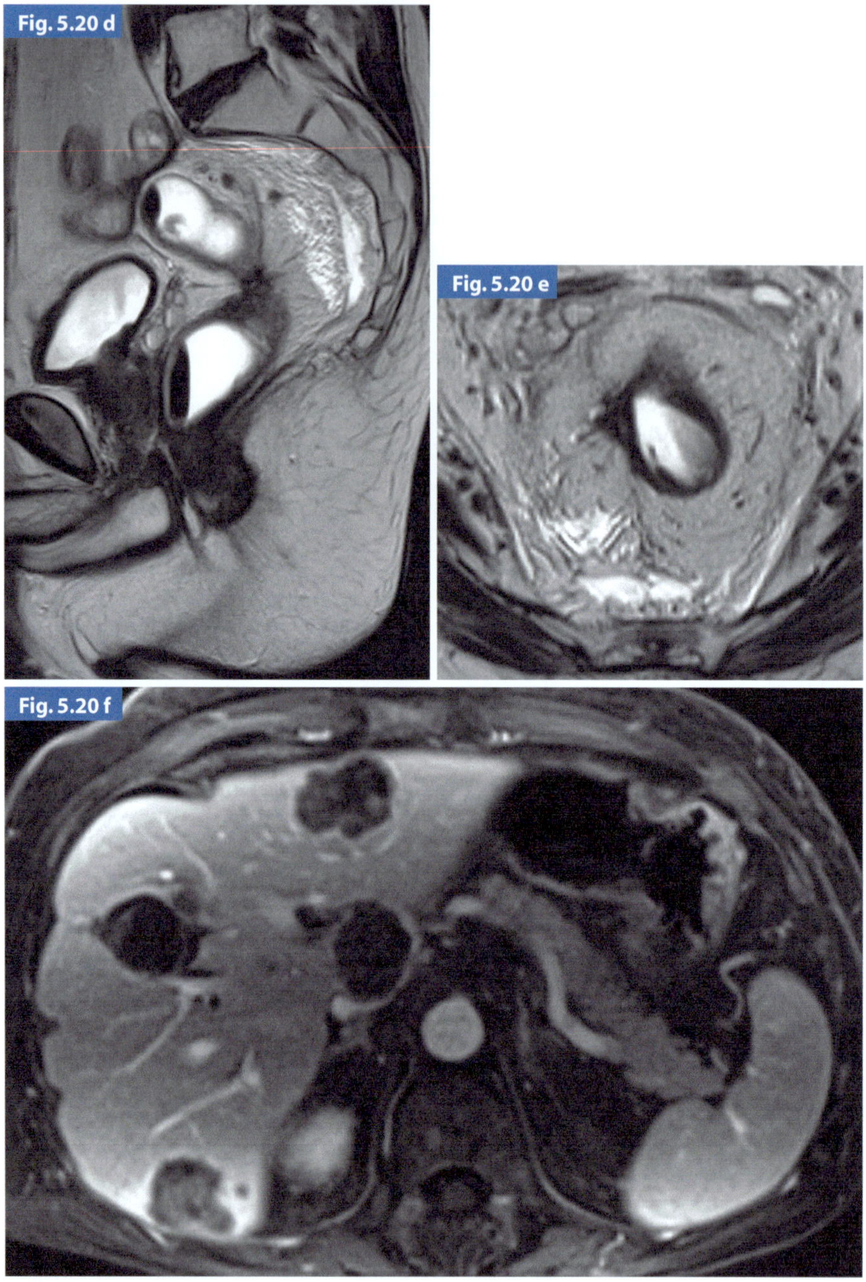

Fig. 5.20 (**d**–**f**) Post-neoadjuvant therapy MRI. Radiochemotherapy resulted in tumor shrinkage and fibrosis—the metastatic nodes almost completely disappeared and a reactive edema within the mesorectum is present (**d**, **e**). Unfortunately, progression of the liver metastases occurred, as was documented by moving-table MRI (**f**).

Fig. 5.21 a

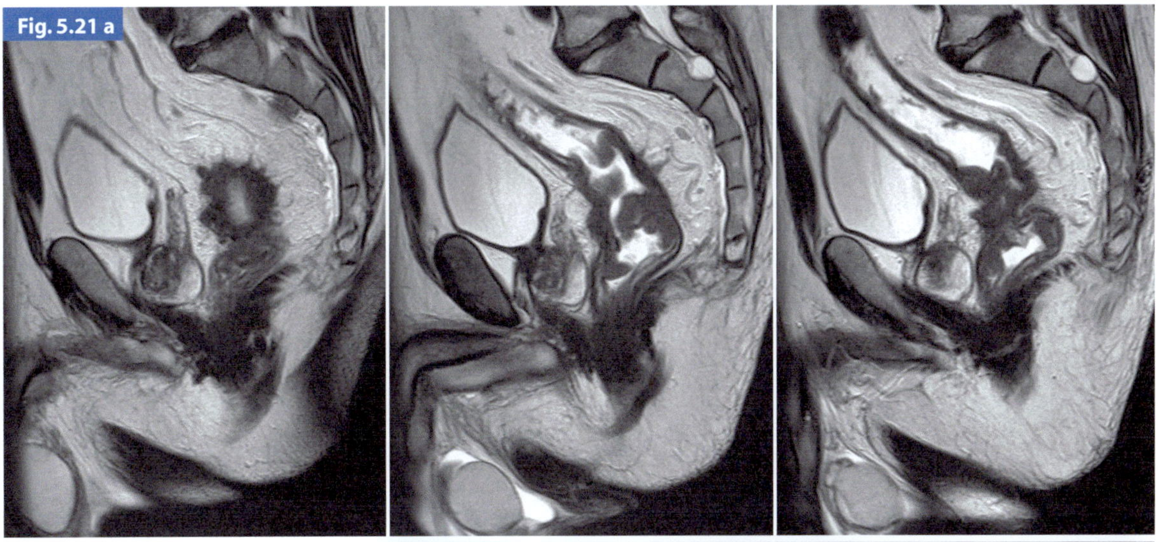

Fig. 5.21 b

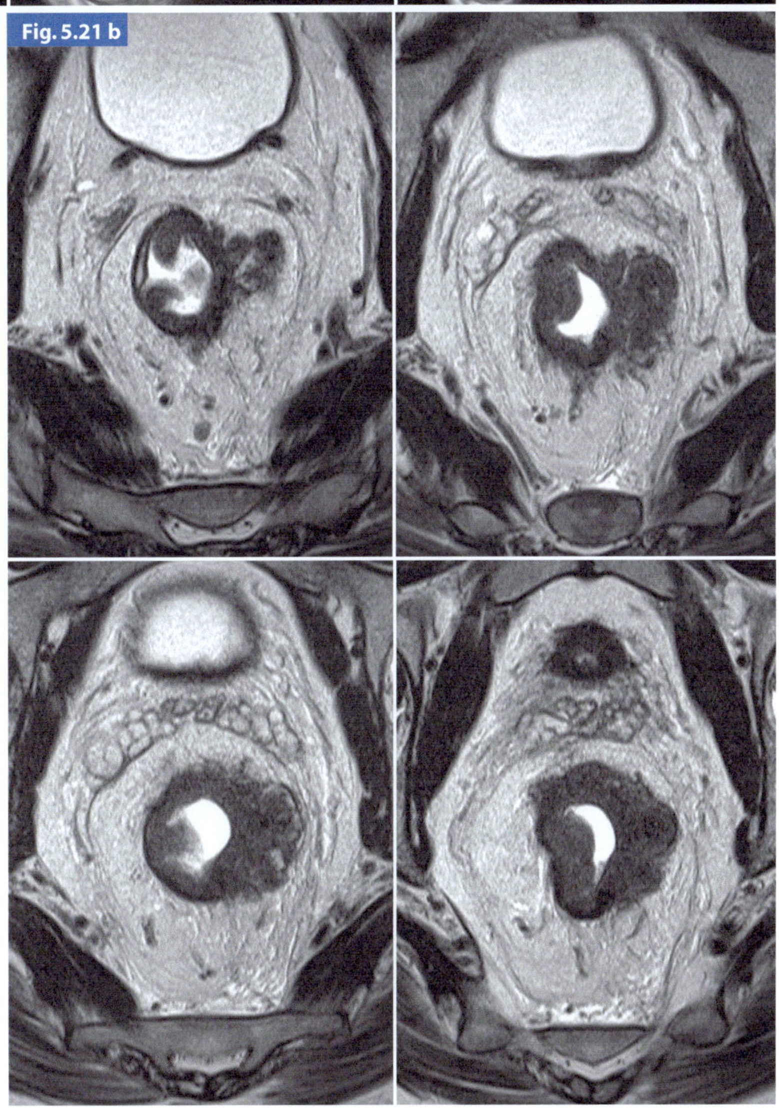

Fig. 5.21 (**a**, **b**) Pretreatment MRI. On the sagittal (**a**) and para-axial (**b**) T2-TSE images, a low-signal intensity tumor extends from the lower rectum to the midrectum. The Wide parts of the carcinoma involve all components of the rectal wall. Additionally, the tumor invades the perimuscular fat and reaches the mesorectal fascia. Neoadjuvant therapy was therefore indicated.

Fig. 5.21 (**c**–**d**) MRI following neoadjuvant therapy. Sagittal (**c**) and para-axial (**d**) T2-TSE images indicate tumor shrinkage, tumor necrosis, and fibrosis as well as thickening of the mesorectal fascia. The pathologic stage was ypT3N0V0L0Pn0 G2. (**e**) Ink drawing: Tumor necrosis.

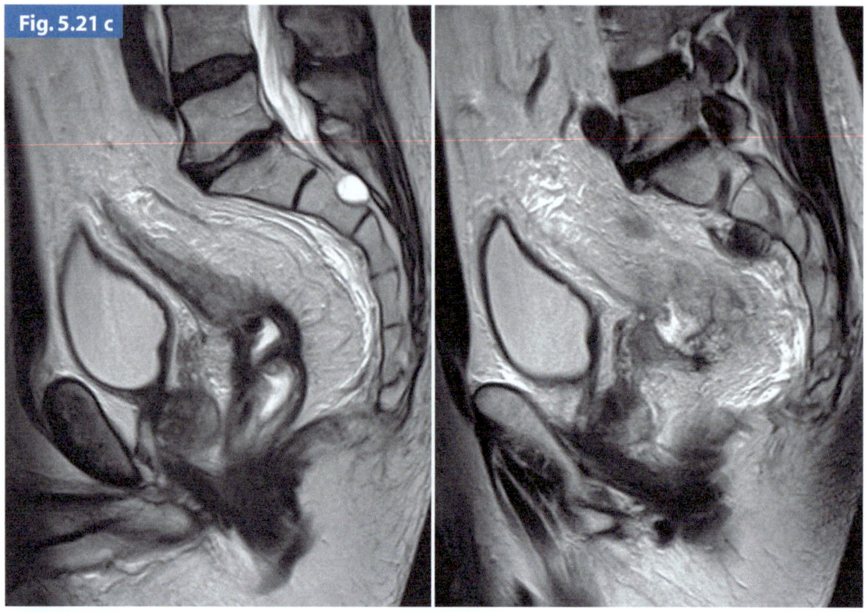

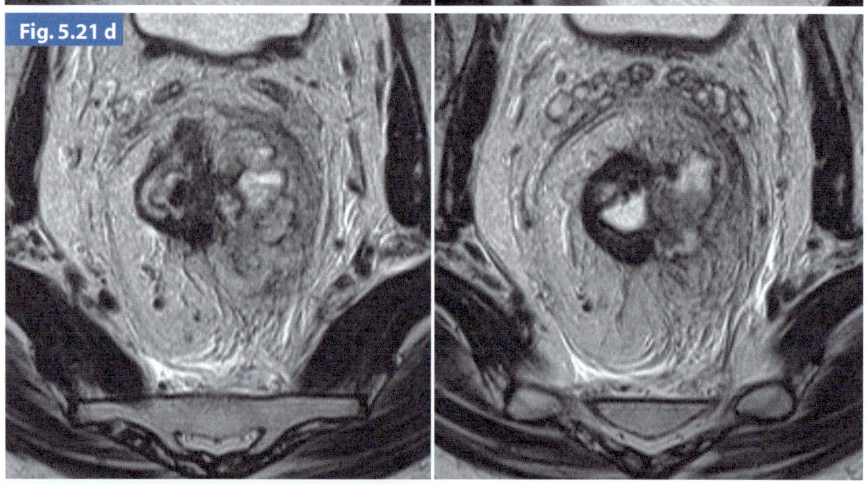

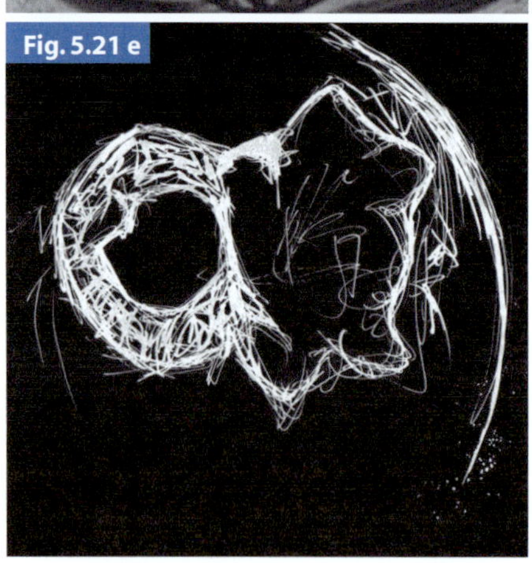

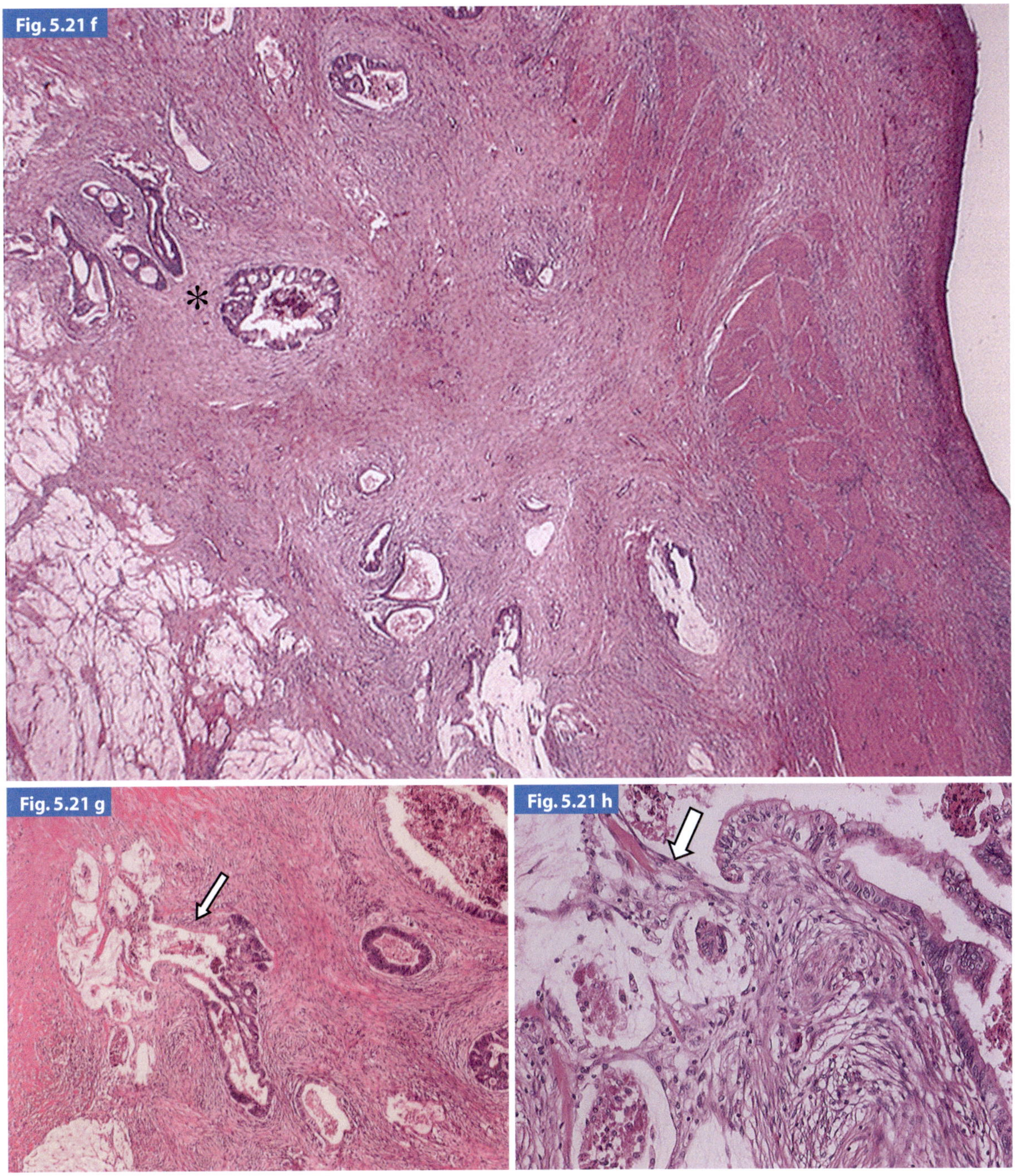

Fig. 5.21 (**f–h**) Histopathologic specimens: Partial response. (**f**) Foci of viable tumor in the perimuscular fat besides areas of tumor regression (*asterisk*, H&E, ×1). (**g**, **h**) The same specimen demonstrating partial tumor necrosis (*arrows*, H&E, ×2.5 and ×10).

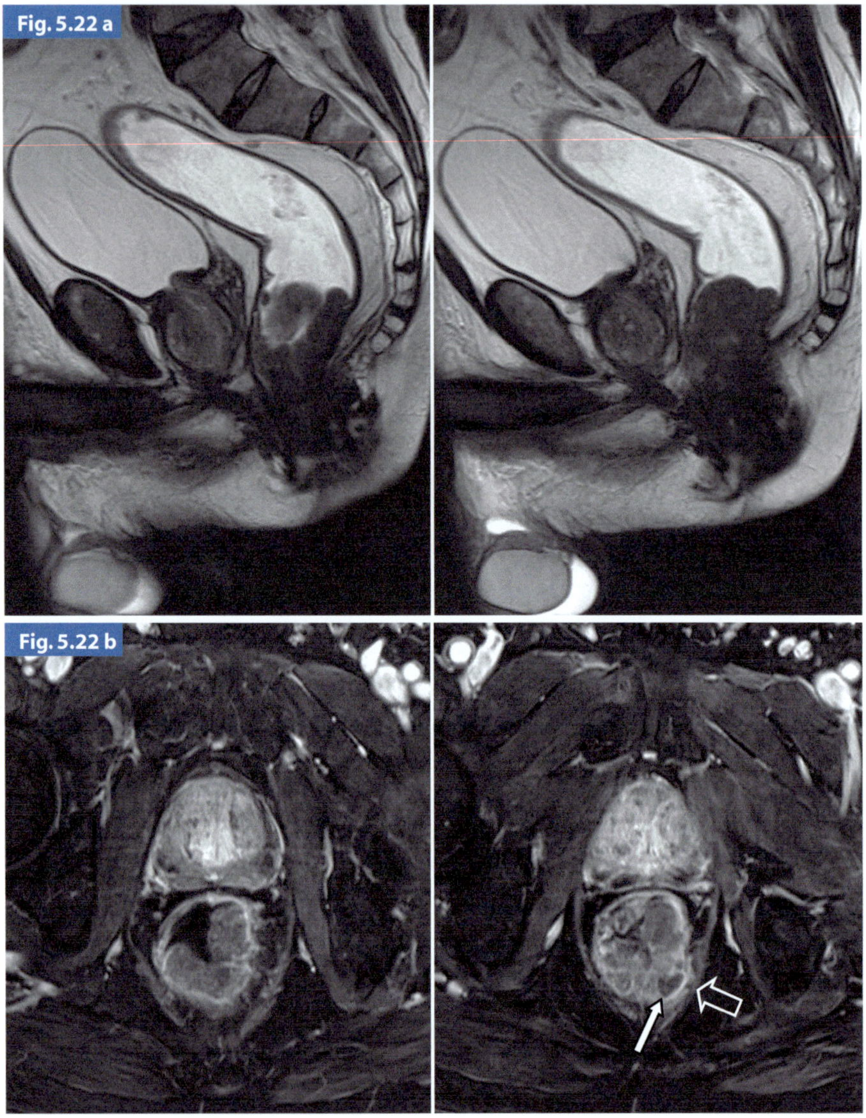

Fig. 5.22 (**a**) Sagittal T2-TSE images reveal an immediately supraanal polypoid tumor causing stenosis. (**b**) On the corresponding CE-VIBE 3D images, the circular growing tumor is penetrating the muscle layer at 5-o'clock lithotomy position and involves the lower posterior aspects of the mesorectum (*white arrow*). No signs of infiltration of the left levator ani muscle (*open arrow*). The tumor was judged as cT3N0 rectal cancer and neoadjuvant therapy was performed. Histopathology diagnosed stage ypT3N0 rectal cancer.

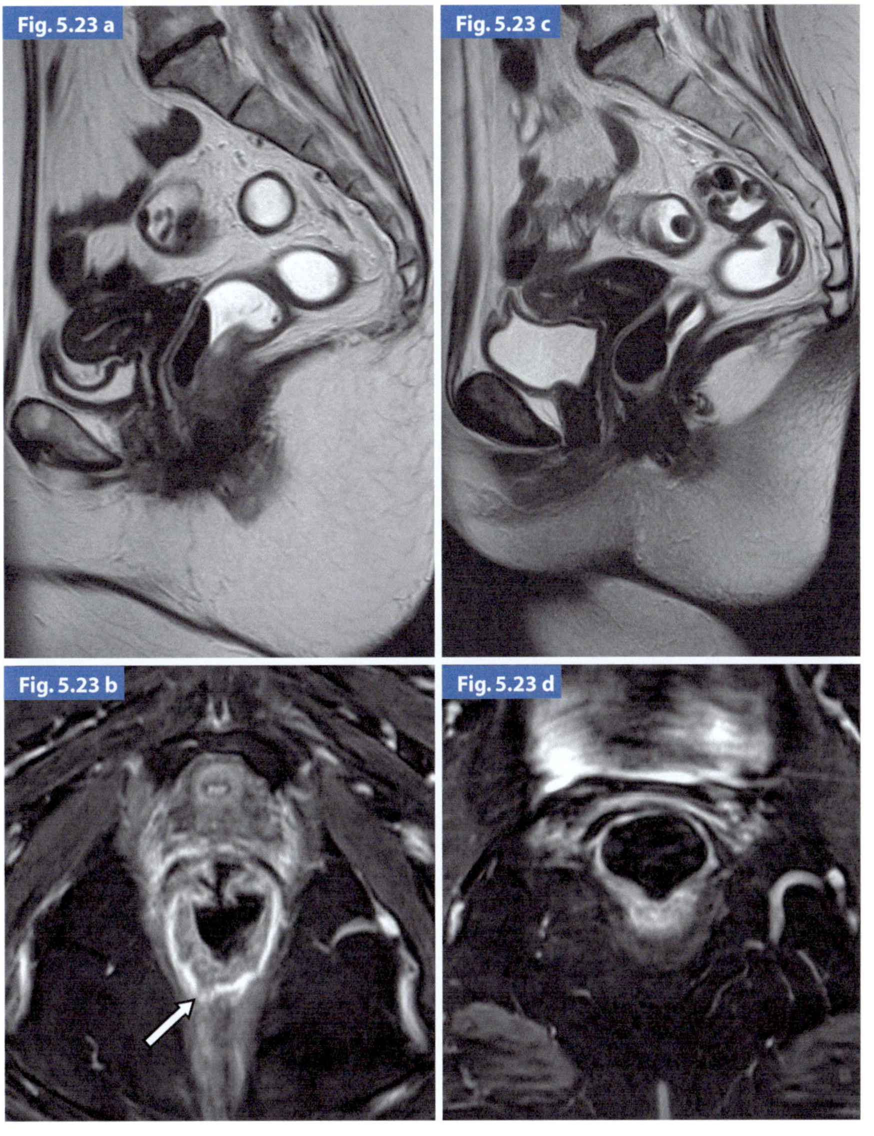

Fig. 5.23 (**a**, **b**) Pretreatment MRI. (**a**) On the sagittal T2-TSE image, a tumor is seen arising from the lower rectum. (**b**) The para-axial CE-VIBE 3D image detects wall-excision at 7-o'clock lithotomy position (*arrow*). (**c**, **d**) Post-neoadjuvant therapy MRI. (**c**) The sagittal T2-TSE image reflects tumor downsizing. (**d**) On the para-axial CE-VIBE 3D image, the residual tumor is indistinguishable from radiation-induced peritumorous inflammation. The histopathologic diagnosis was stage ypT3N0.

Fig. 5.24 a

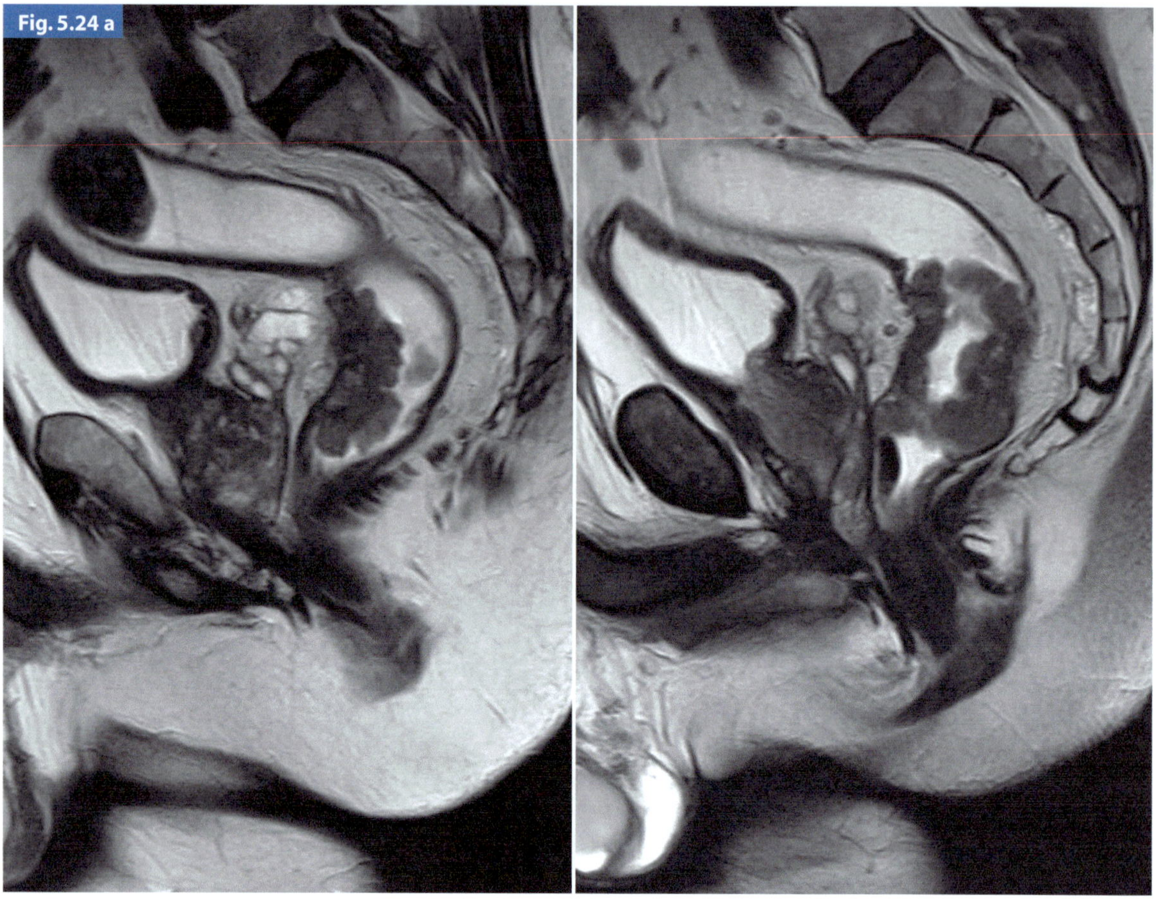

Fig. 5.24 (**a–c**) Pretreatment MRI. Representative sagittal views (**a**) of a T2-TSE sequence. An exophytic mass within the midrectum is seen causing tumor stenosis. The tumor signal is brighter than that of the surrounding normal rectal wall. CISS three-dimensional (3D) images were derived from a plane perpendicular to the tumor axis (**b**) and correspond with contrast-enhanced VIBE 3D images (**c**) The tumor invaded all layers of the rectal wall, as well as the mesorectal fat. The muscle layer of the rectal wall has a lower signal compared with the carcinoma, whereas the wall components normally show intensive contrast-enhancement and are therefore clearly distinguishable from adenocarcinoma. The streak-like tissue changes adjacent to the tumor margins are indicative of lymphangiitis but cannot be differentiated from desmoplastic reaction. At the 12-o'clock lithotomy position (magnifications, *arrows*), detection of a vessel with high-signal intensity in the T2-weighted sequence and a corresponding low-signal intensity on the CE-VIBE images is present. The signal abnormalities are caused by tumor thrombosis, which is known to be of negative prognostic value. Aside from the rectal cancer, two suspect lymph nodes can be observed within 2 mm of the mesorectal fascia (*arrow*), which is known to meet criteria for circumferential resection margin involvement. The larger node shows identical contrast-media uptake behavior as compared with the primary tumor. The clinical stage was determined to be cT3N1V2L1CRM+.

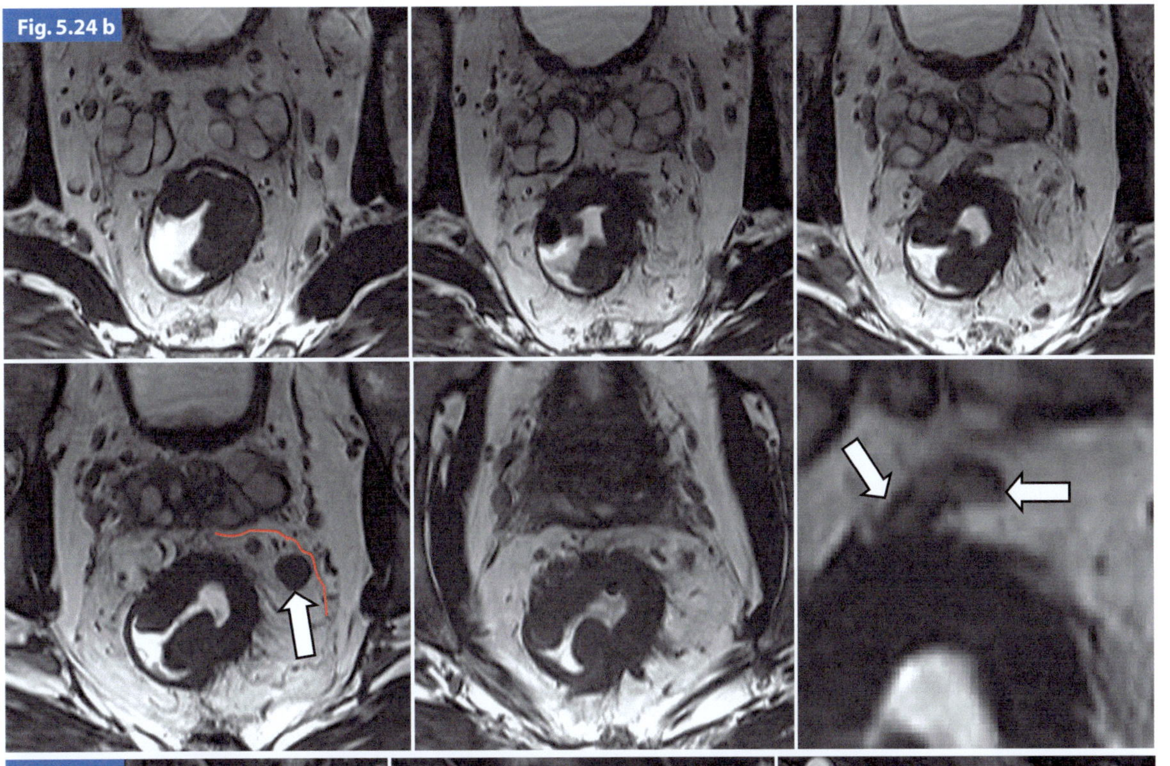
Fig. 5.24 b

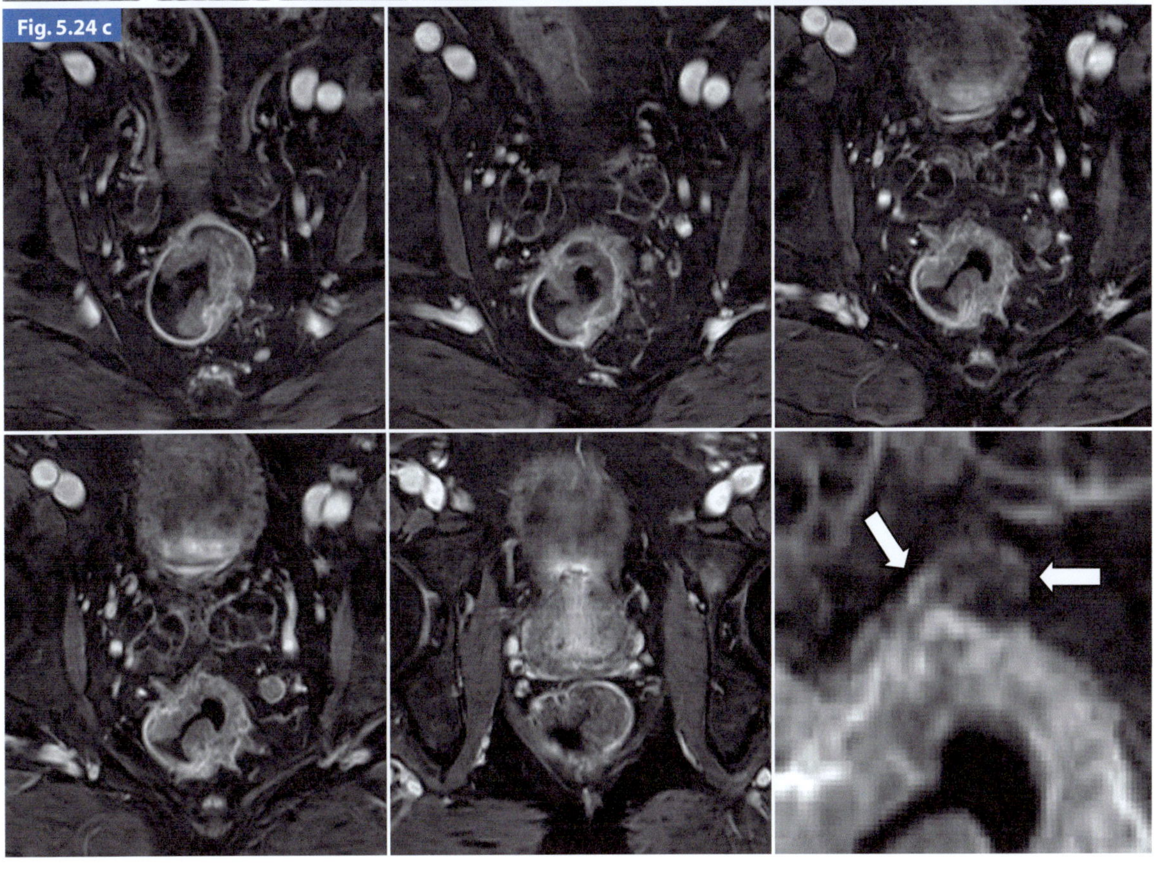
Fig. 5.24 c

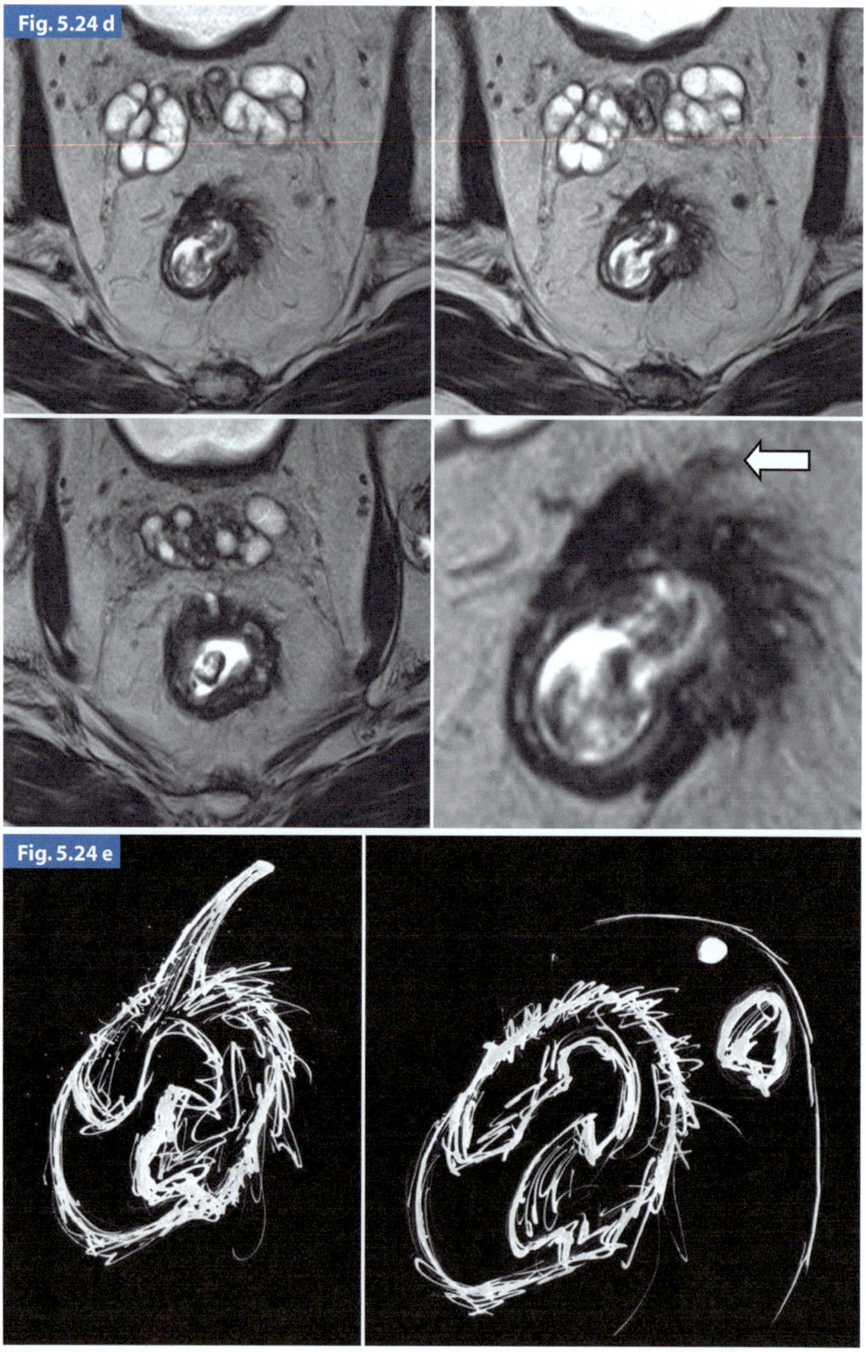

Fig. 5.24 (**d**) Post-radiochemotherapy MRI prior to surgery. Representative axial T2-SPACE images. When compared with the pretreatment MRI, tumor downsizing is evident. Problem: Is downsizing coupled with downstaging? Parts of the carcinoma show signal decrease (a sign of therapy-associated fibrosis), whereas other parts of the tumor display a high signal resulting from necrosis. However, other parts of the carcinoma have not changed intensity, indicative of residual viable tumor. The surrounding streaky changes of the mesorectal fat are of unclear relevance, but strongly suspicious of lymphangiitis. Of the former two nodes, one remains and has decreased in size and signal. The infiltrated vein at 12-o'clock persisted through therapy (*arrow*). The pathologic stage was determined as ypT3-N0V1L1R0 G2 moderately differentiated rectal cancer. Interestingly, 2 out of 12 sampled lymph nodes showed fibrosis. (**e**) Ink drawing: Extramural venous invasion, threatening of the circumferential resection margin by nodal metastases.

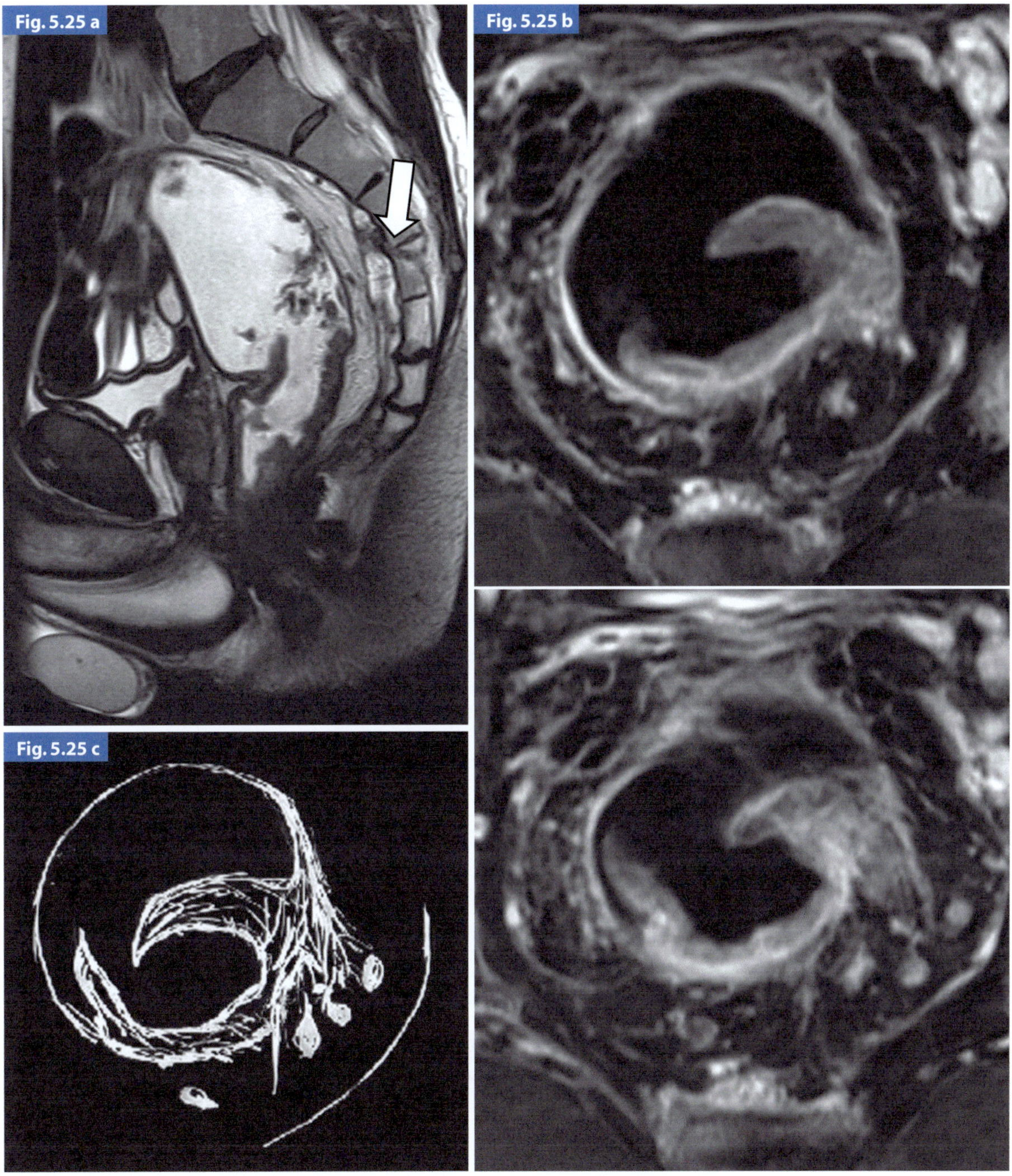

Fig. 5.25 Patient history: Incidental finding of a rectal carcinoma during diagnostic work-up of polytrauma, among others sacral fracture involving the S4 segment. (**a**) Sagittal T2-TSE image of the pretreatment MRI demonstrates the S4 fracture with presacral hematoma and a supraanal rectal tumor. (**b**) Axial CE-VIBE 3D images show wall-exceeding carcinoma with several small lymph nodes in close vicinity to the primary tumor, suspicious of nodal metastases. The definitive histopathologic staging was ypT3N2 G2. (**c**) Ink drawing: Wall-exceeding carcinoma with mesorectal nodes.

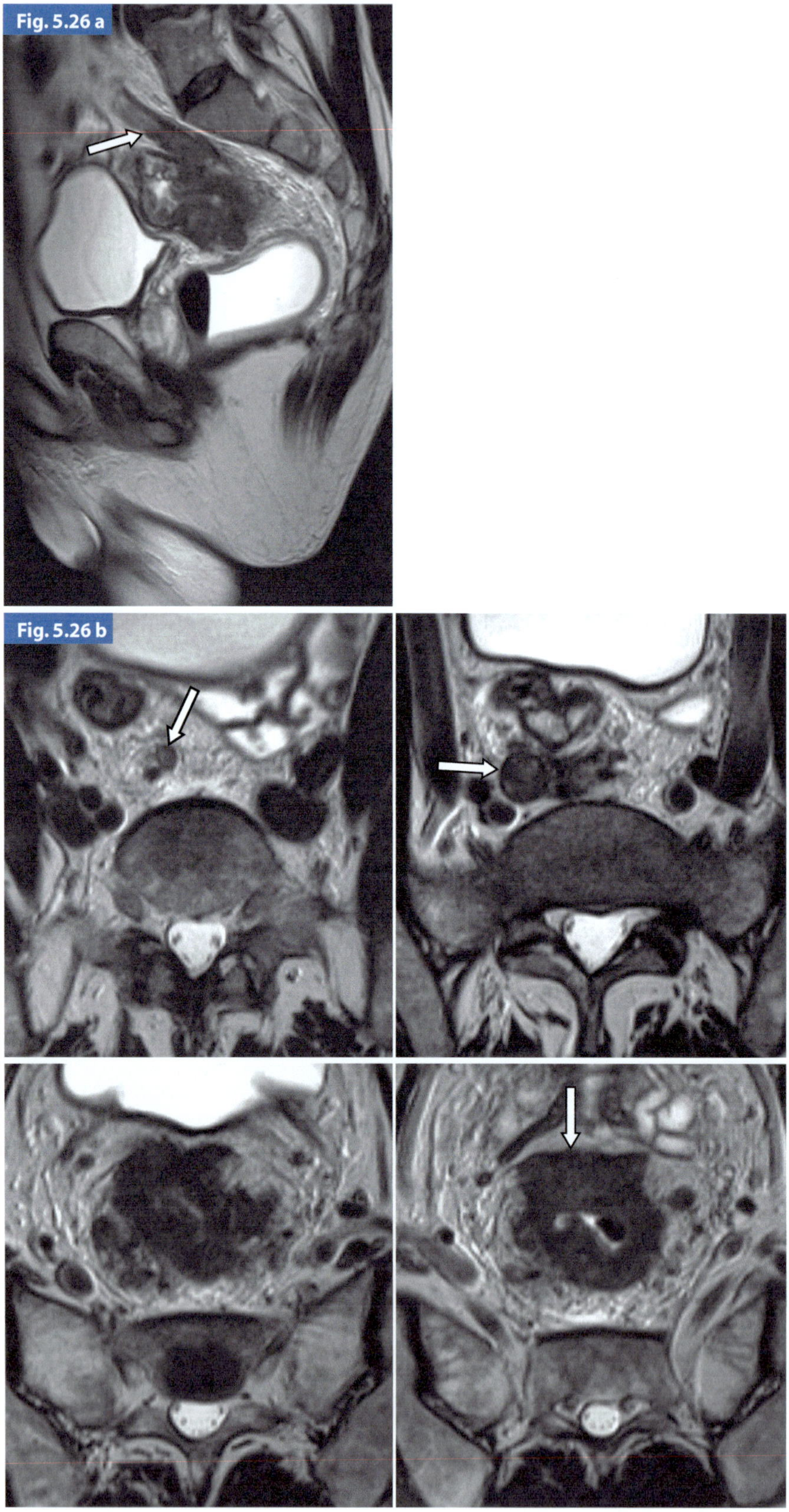

Fig. 5.26 Pretreatment MRI. (**a**) Sagittal T2-TSE image shows extensive tumor originating from the middle and upper thirds of the rectum with extramural venous invasion (*arrow*). (**b**) On the corresponding para-axial T2-TSE images, tumor thrombosis of the superior rectal vein is seen (*arrow*). Tubular tumor deposits following the superior rectal vessels are indicative of lymphangiitis and venous infiltration. Additionally, irregular-shaped tumor deposits within the mesorectum and lymph node metastasis adjacent to the mesorectal fascia are visible (*arrow*). The carcinoma involves the circumferential resection margin (*arrow*).

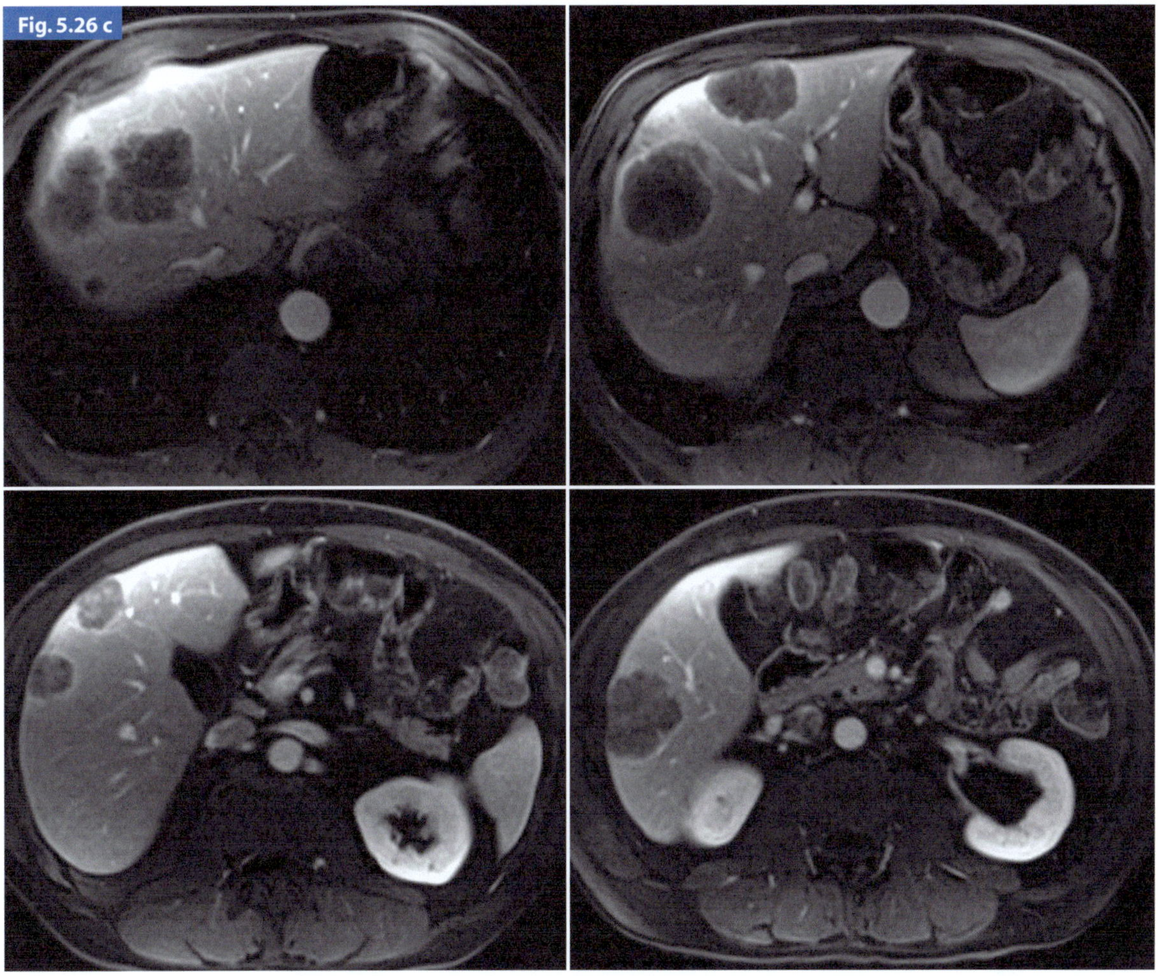

Fig. 5.26 (c) Axial CE-FLASH 2D images obtained using SMS technique revealed typical hypovascular synchronous liver metastases. The clinical stage was determined to be cT3N + L1V2CRM+.

Fig. 5.27 a

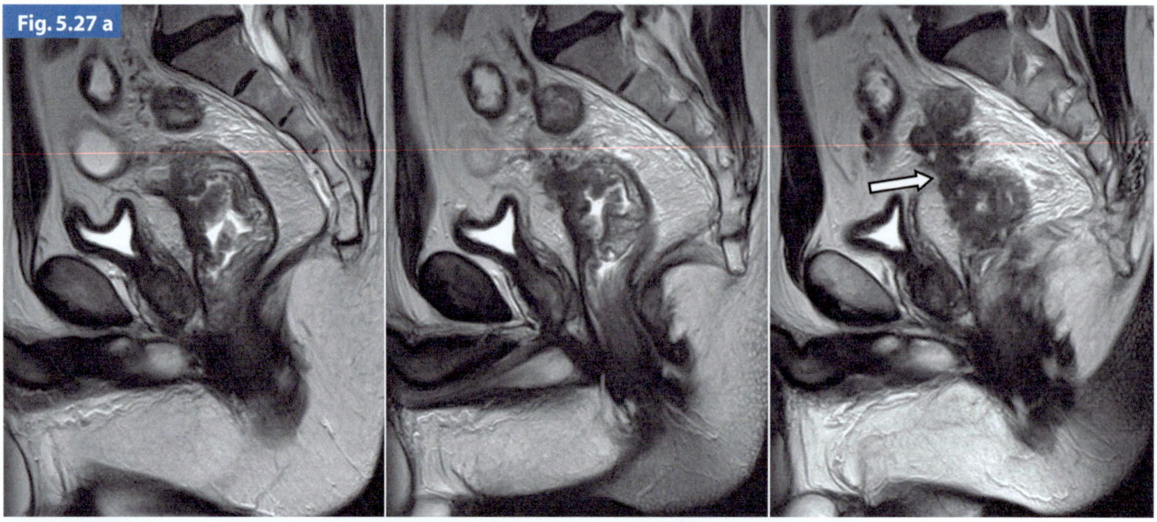

Fig. 5.27 b

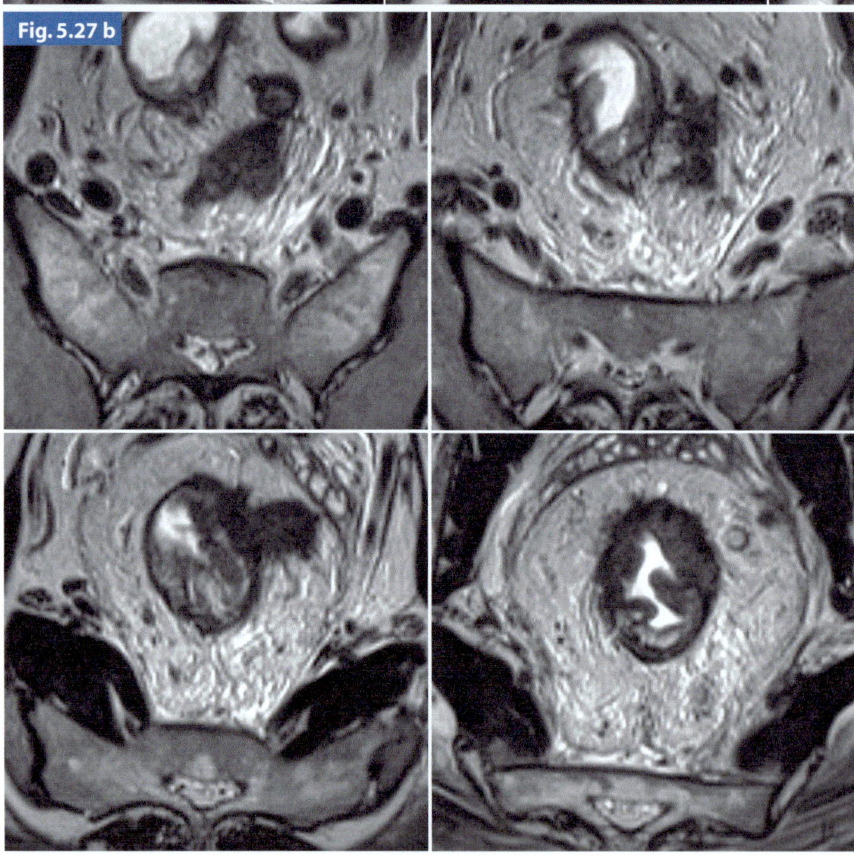

Fig. 5.27 Locally advanced rectal cancer with diffuse hepatic spread. (**a**) Sagittal T2-TSE images show a large tumor extending from the lower third into the middle third of the rectum and cord-like infiltration of the mesorectum involving the superior rectal vessels and the lymphatics (*arrow*). (**b**) Axial T2-TSE images confirmed wide infiltration of the perirectal fat as well as extensive venous involvement with multiple metastatic nodes and a mesorectal edema. Clinically, the rectal cancer was staged as cT3N2M1V2L1CRM+.

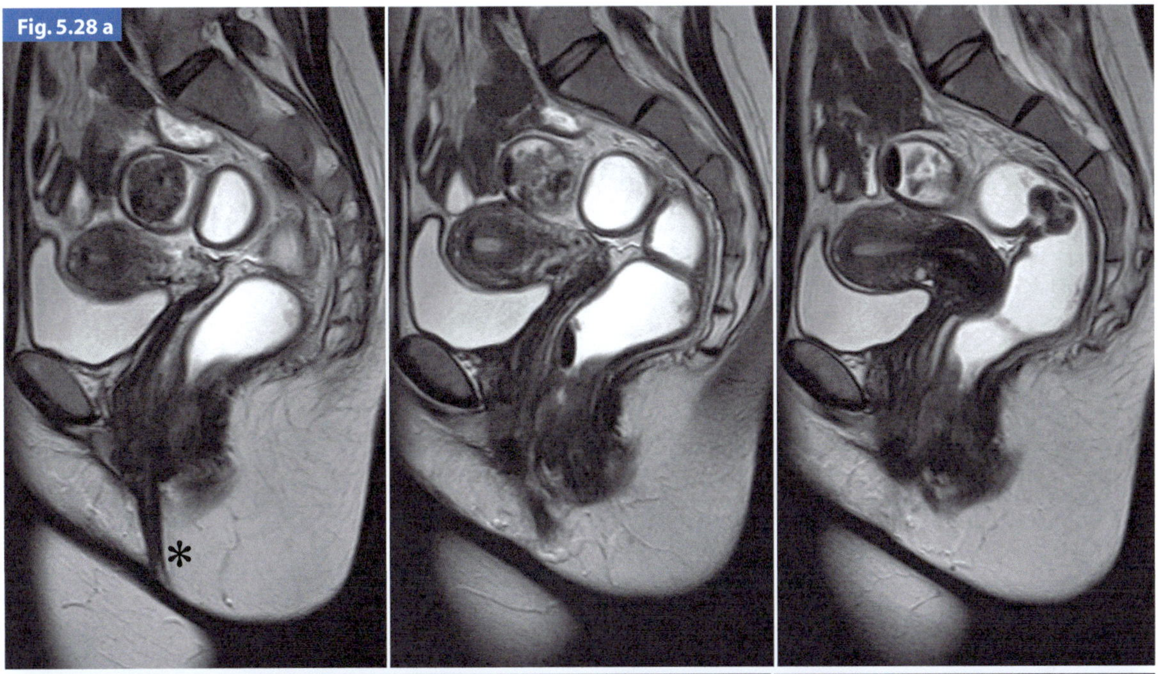

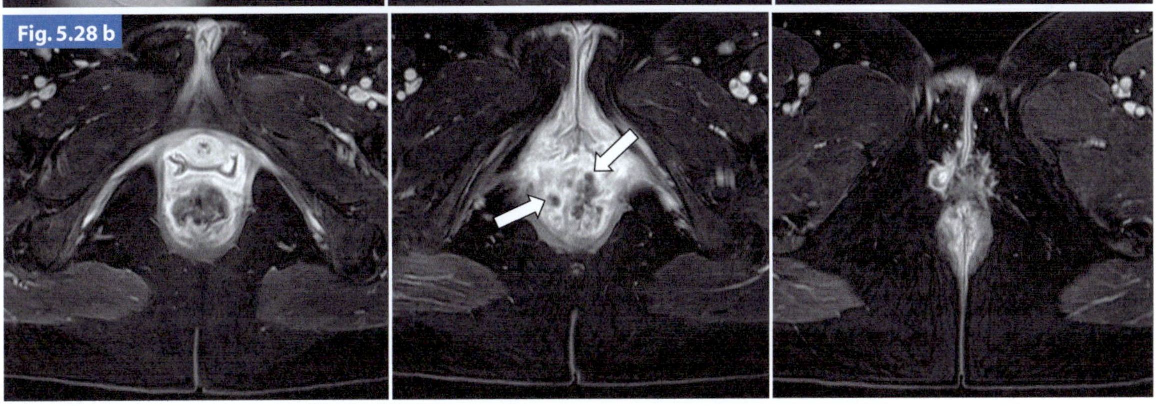

Fig. 5.28 Patient history: Pre-existing Crohn's disease with rectovaginal and rectovulval fistulas. (**a**) Sagittal T2-TSE images reveal a fistula channel to the right-sided vulva (*asterisk*) and tumor formation within the anal channel and lower rectum. (**b**) Axial CE-VIBE 3D images reveal a hypovascular anorectal tumor between 9- and 3-o'clock lithotomy positions involving the internal openings of the rectovaginal and rectovulval fistulas (*arrows*). Problem: Origin and infiltration depth of the carcinoma. According to the image criteria, a differentiation between anal and rectal cancer is impossible. A discrimination of tumor infiltration via the pre-existing fistulas from active inflammation is also inconceivable. Abdominoperineal resection, including the posterior wall of the vagina, was carried out and histopathology reveal stage pT3N0 rectal cancer. Additionally, suppurative inflammation was diagnosed.

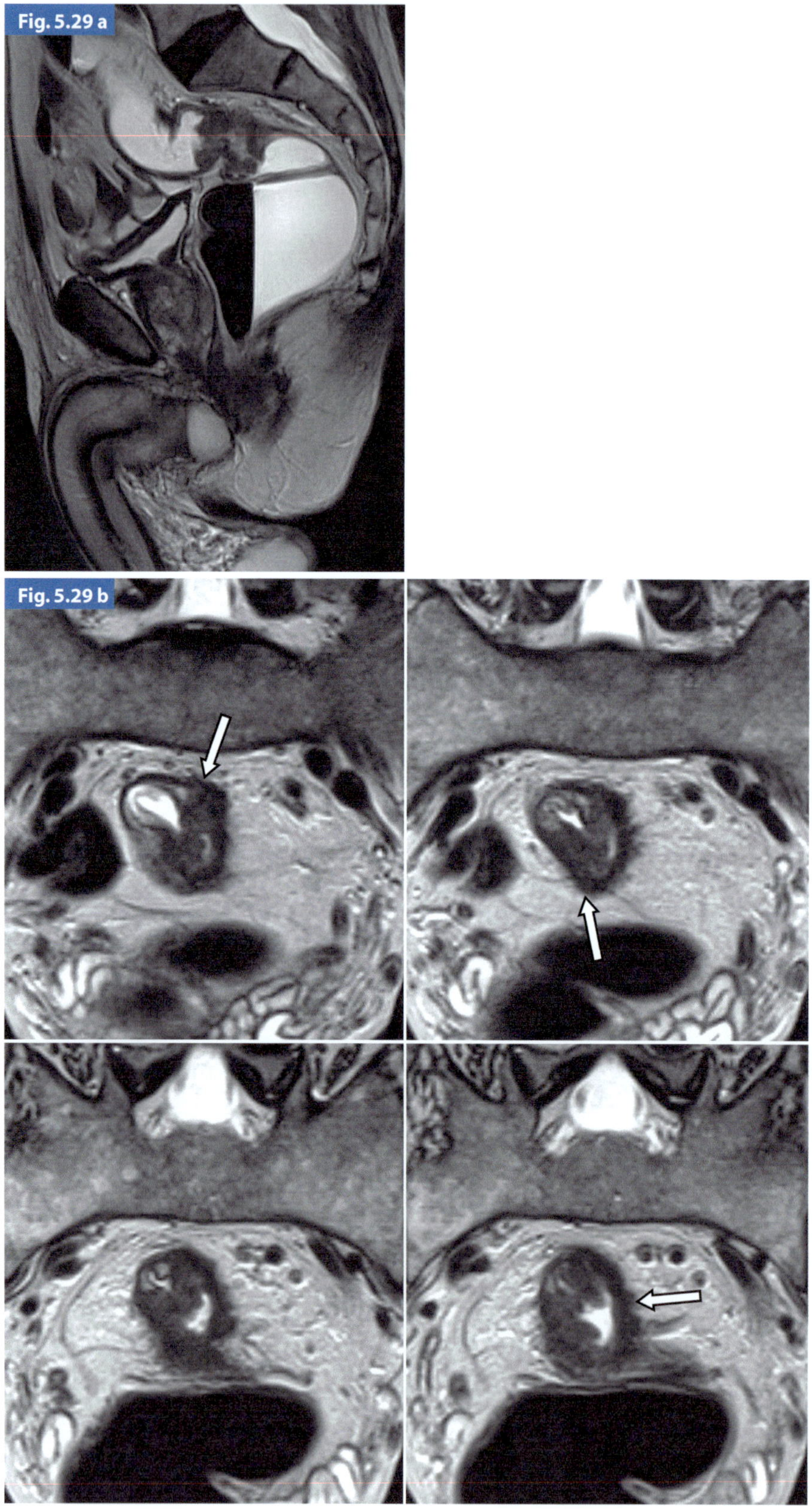

Fig. 5.29 Stage T3 rectal cancer with pulmonary metastasis. (**a**) Sagittal T2-BLADE imaging reveals a tumor that exceeds the wall of the rectosigmoid. (**b**) On the para-coronal T2-TSE images, the tumor signal extends to the surrounding mesorectal fat (*arrows*). No signs of nodal spread are indicated.

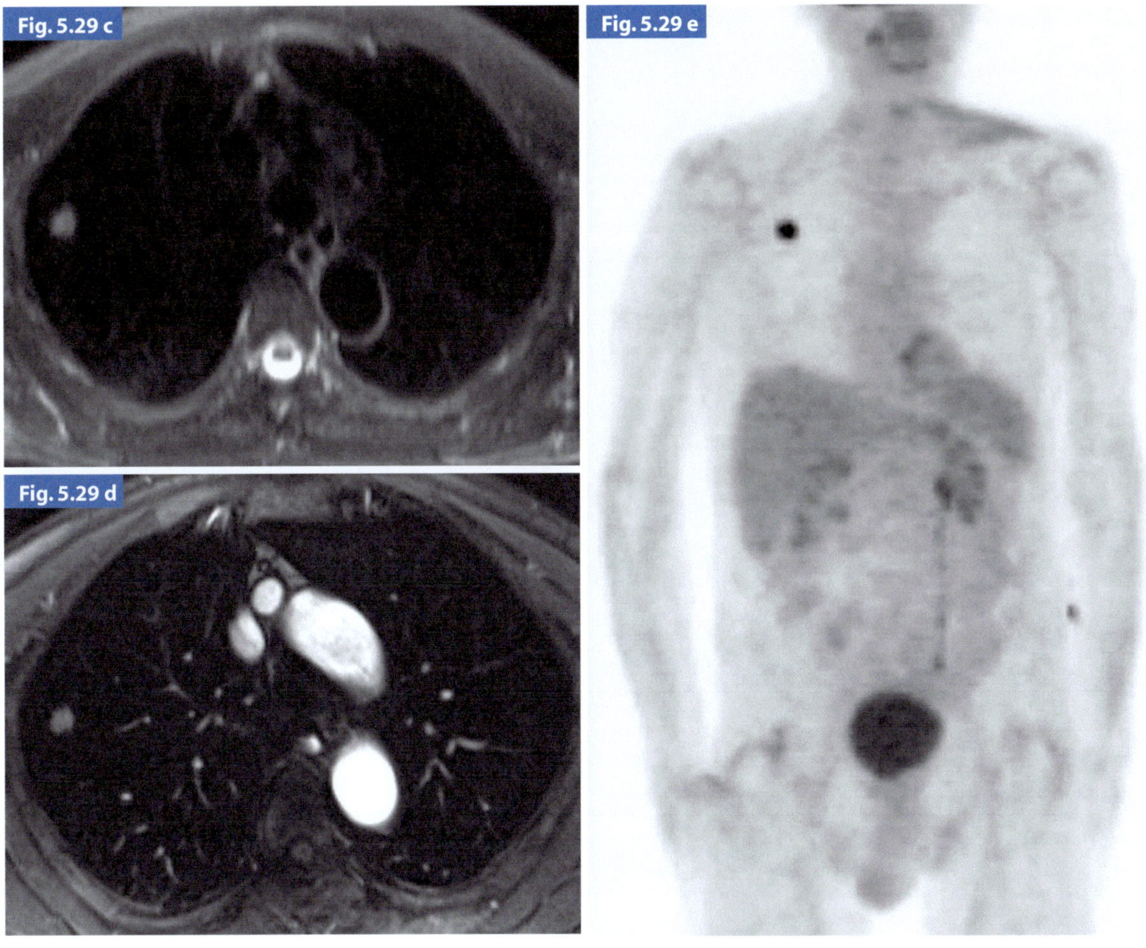

Fig. 5.29 (**c**, **d**) Axial free-breathing TIRM image (**c**) and the corresponding breath-hold CE-FLASH 2D image (**d**) derived from SMS moving-table M-staging show a solitary lung metastasis in the right upper lobe. (**e**) Corresponding FDG-PET examination confirmed the solitary lung metastasis. Deep anterior rectum resection was carried out and the final histopathologic diagnosis was stage pT3N0 rectal cancer.

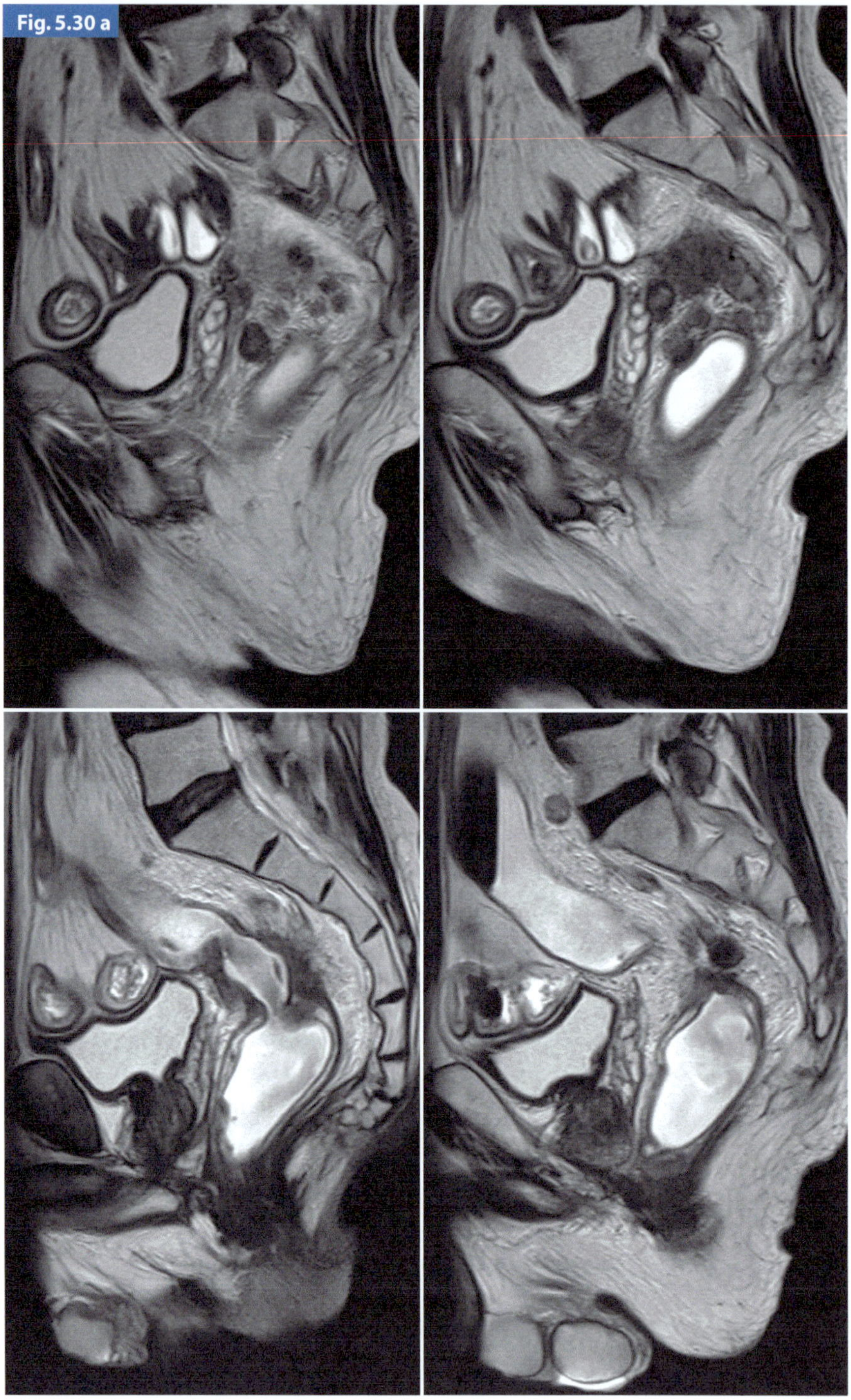

Fig. 5.30 (**a**) Sagittal T2-TSE images illustrate advanced carcinoma of the midrectum with mesorectal lymph node metastases. Metastatic nodes can be seen along the superior rectal vessels.

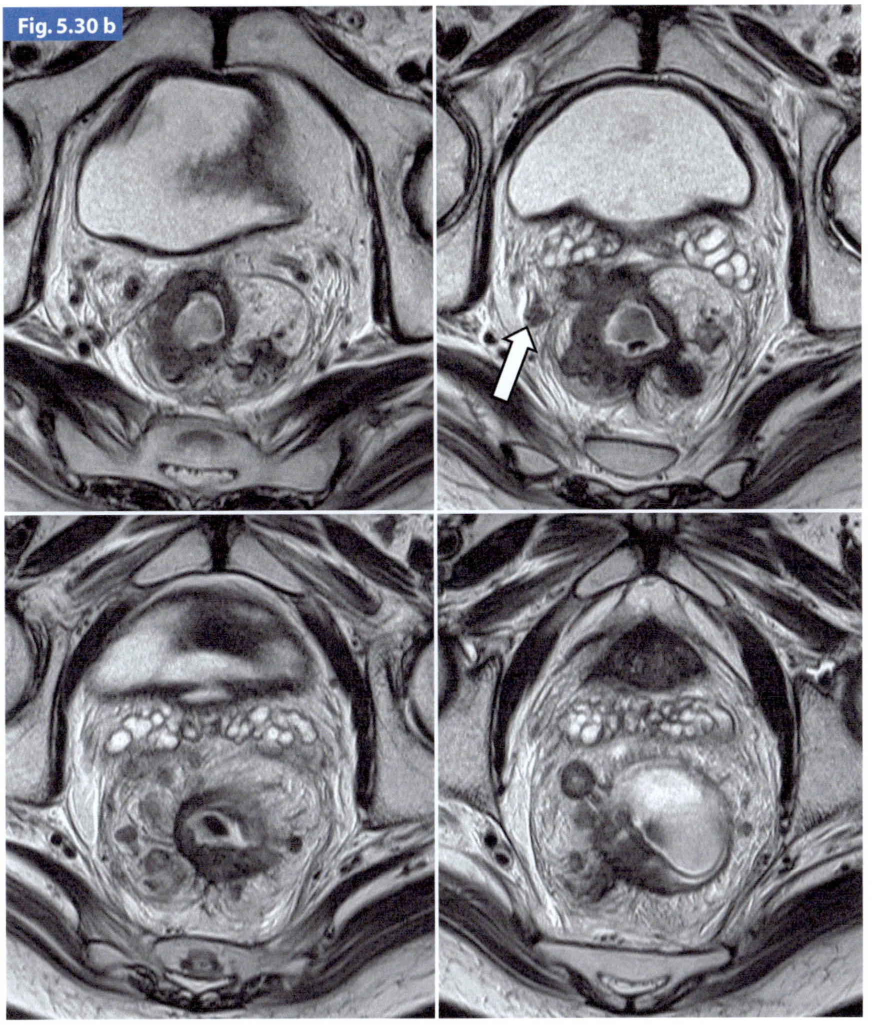

Fig. 5.30 (**b**) Axial T2-TSE images demonstrate circumferential resection margin involvement by both direct infiltration of the carcinoma and lymph node metastases. The right seminal vesicles show normal signal but there is tumor spread along the right internal iliac vessels (*arrow*).

Fig. 5.31 a

Fig. 5.31 b

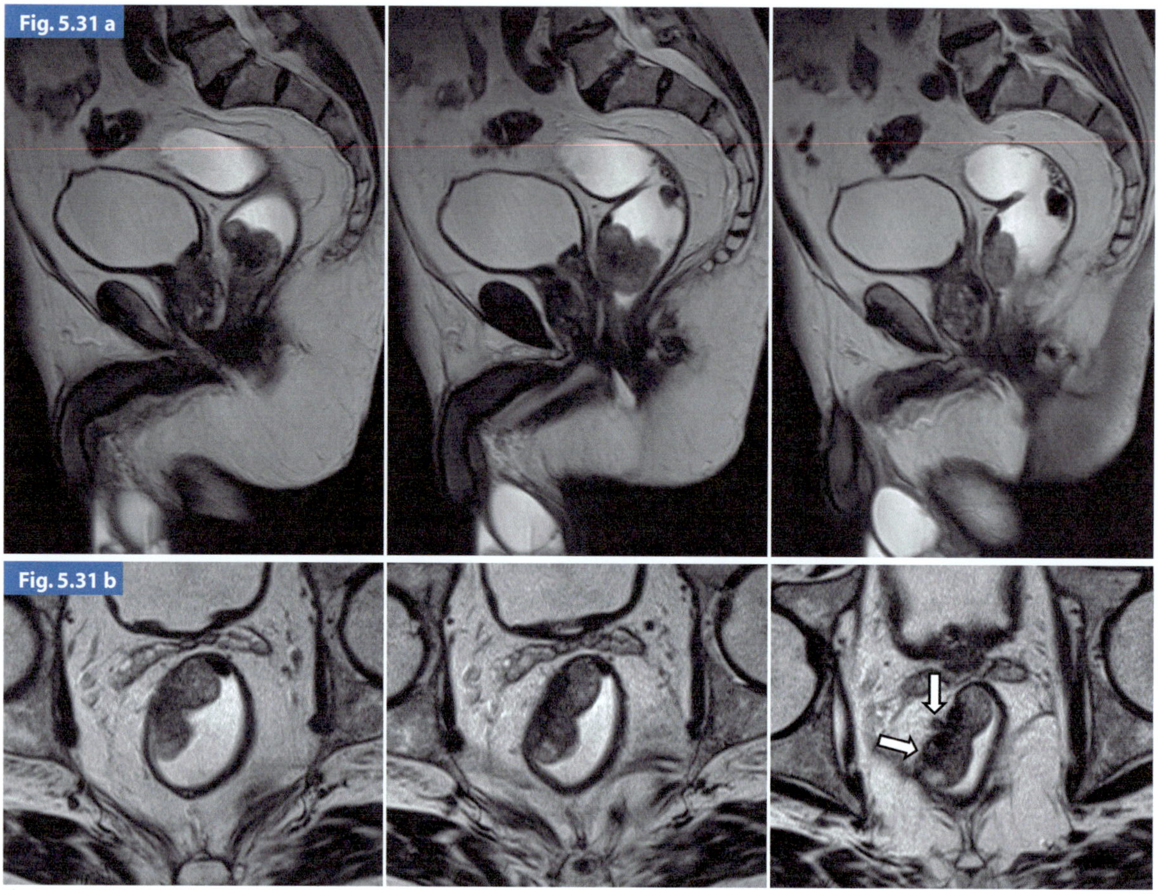

Fig. 5.31 (**a**) Sagittal T2-TSE images reveal a polypoid tumor at the junction of lower and midrectum. (**b**) Axial T2-TSE images show a hyperintense foci within the underlying low-signal muscle layer and a tumor deposit beyond the muscularis propria (*arrows*) characteristic of stage T3 rectal cancer. Histopathologic diagnosis was stage pT3N0L0V0Pn0 G2 rectal carcinoma.

Fig. 5.32 Stage ypT0 rectal cancer. (**a**) Sagittal T2-TSE images show an exophytic tumor of the lower third of the rectum. (**b**) On the corresponding para-axial T2-TSE images, the tumor signal is replacing the normal low-signal intensity of the muscle layer. Moreover, the outlines of muscularis propria in the region of the tumor appear irregular and characteristic of minor perimuscular fat infiltration. A single mesorectal node is present in close proximity to the tumor. In the light of these findings, cT3N1 rectal cancer was diagnosed and neoadjuvant chemoradiation was performed. The histopathologic examination of the specimen resulted in stage ypT0N0L0V0Pn0 rectal cancer.

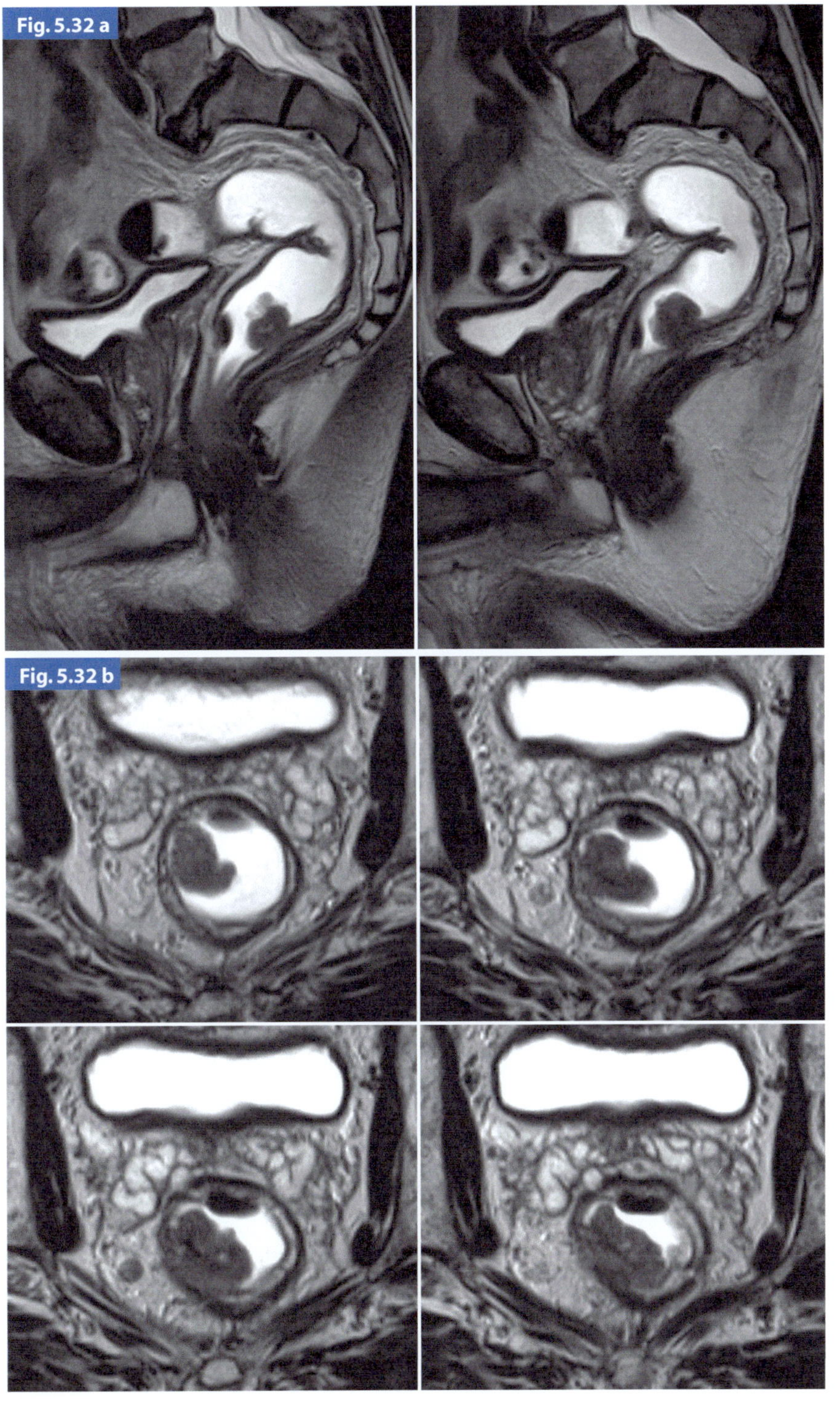

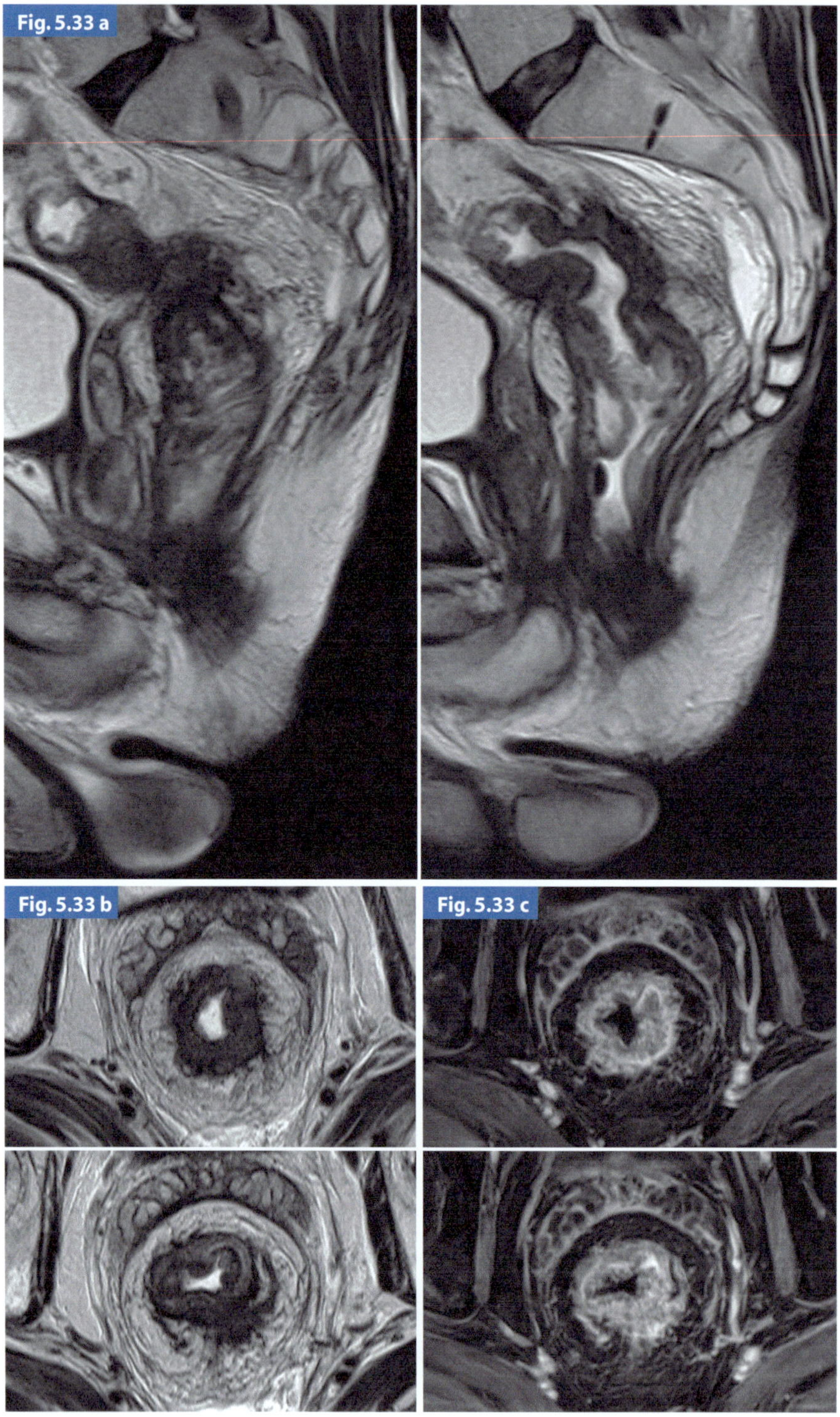

Fig. 5.33 Post-neoadjuvant radiochemotherapy MRI. Sagittal (**a**) and para-axial (**b**) T2-TSE images and corresponding para-axial (**c**) CE-VIBE 3D images reveal advanced carcinoma of the mid and upper rectum involving the mesorectal fat as well as extramural venous invasion. The tumor was clinically staged as ycT3N0V2M1. Patient history: Extensive rectal cancer with hepatic spread. The patient suffered from tumor cachexia, chronic obstructive pulmonary disease, and pulmonary hypertension. Surgery was rejected because of these comorbid conditions.

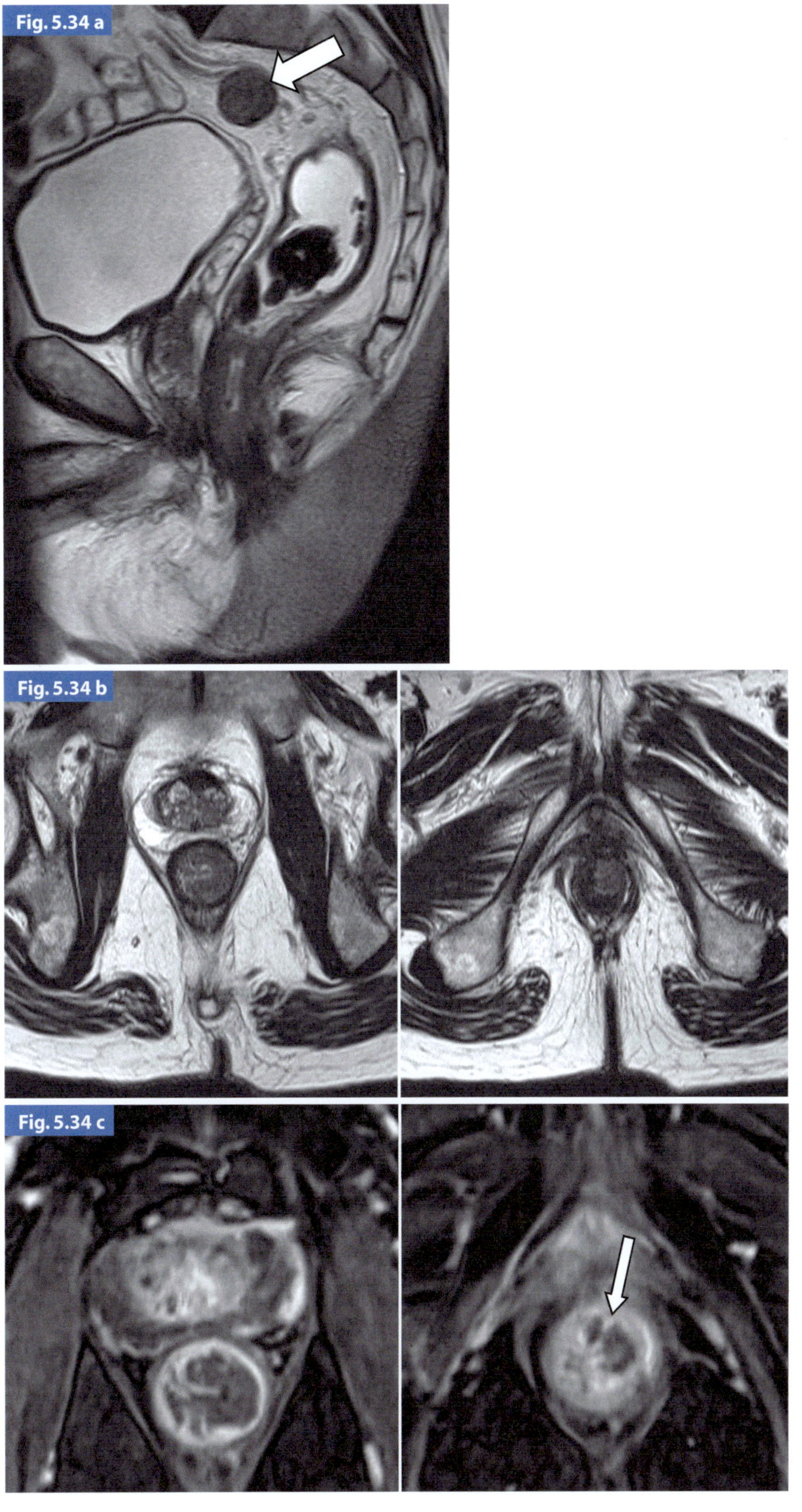

Fig. 5.34 Stage ypT0 rectal cancer. (**a**–**c**) Pretreatment MRI. Sagittal (**a**) and corresponding axial (**b**) T2-TSE images exhibit an intermediate signal tumor of the lower rectum between the 11- and 7-o'clock lithotomy positions. There are no signs of infiltration of the levator muscle and puborectalis sling. Lymph node metastasis within the upper mesorectum is present (*arrow*). (**c**) The axial CE-VIBE 3D images reveal invasion of the anorectal junction and the upper internal anal sphincter muscle (*arrow*). On contrast-enhanced imaging studies, the internal anal sphincter muscle (which is composed of smooth muscle fibers) has a significantly higher signal than the levator, puborectalis, and external anal sphincter muscles (which are composed of striated muscle fibers). The clinical stage was determined to be cT3N1.

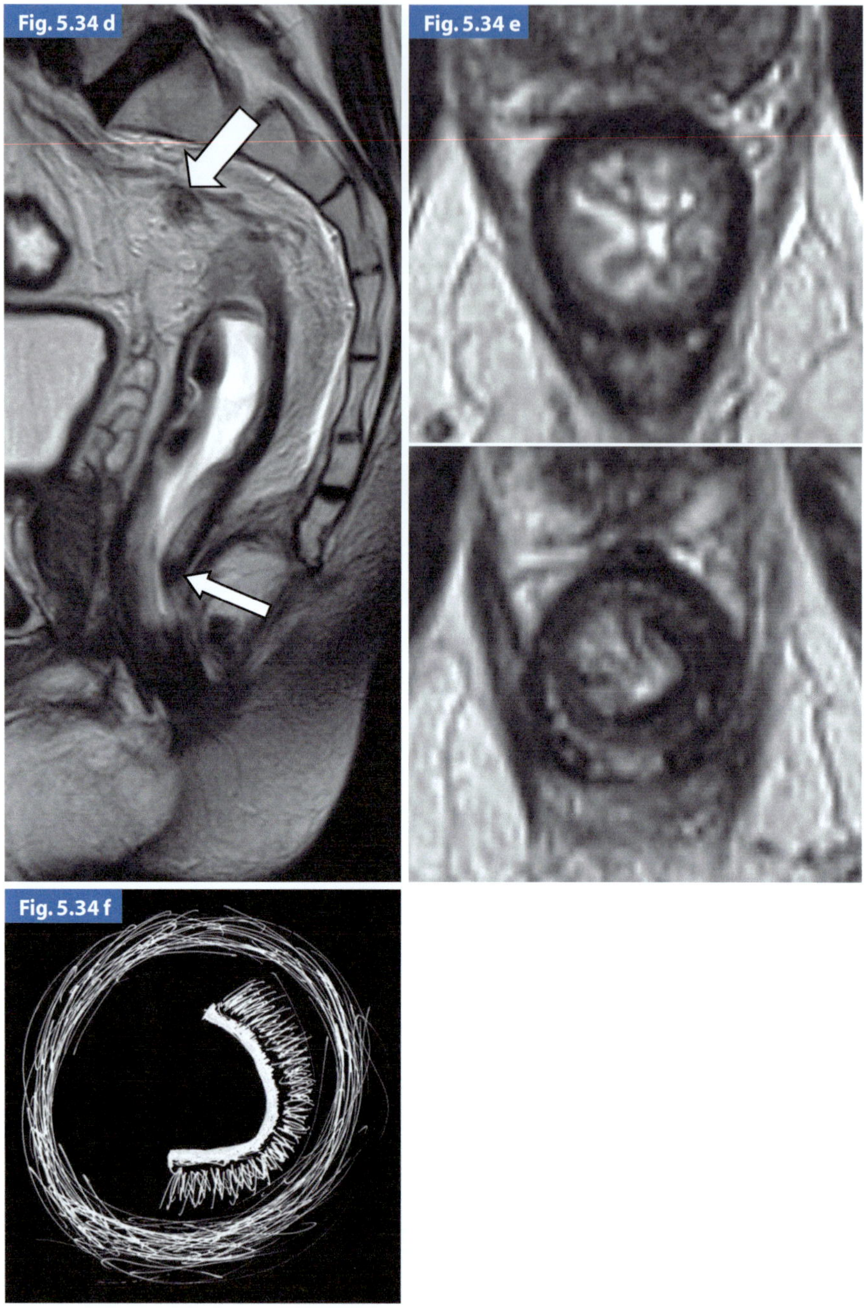

Fig. 5.34 (**d**, **e**) Post-neoadjuvant therapy MRI. Sagittal (**d**) and para-axial (**e**) T2-TSE images clearly demonstrate tumor shrinkage and regression of the solitary nodal metastasis with fibrosis (*arrows*). Immediately above the tumor bed, normal anatomy of the rectal wall can be seen: the mucosal layer represents a thin hypointense line, the submucosal layer comprises intermediate- to high-signal intensity, and the muscle layer shows low-signal intensity. In the area of the treated tumor, scar formation is detectable as a low-signal band with thickening of the mucosa. Rectoscopy confirmed the imaging findings of a circumscribed scar with no signs of residual tumor. Clinically, the tumor was staged as ycT0N0. Deep anterior resection with J-pouch anastomosis was performed. Histopathology diagnosed a stage ypT0N0L0V0 rectal carcinoma. (**f**) Ink drawing: Tumor fibrosis.

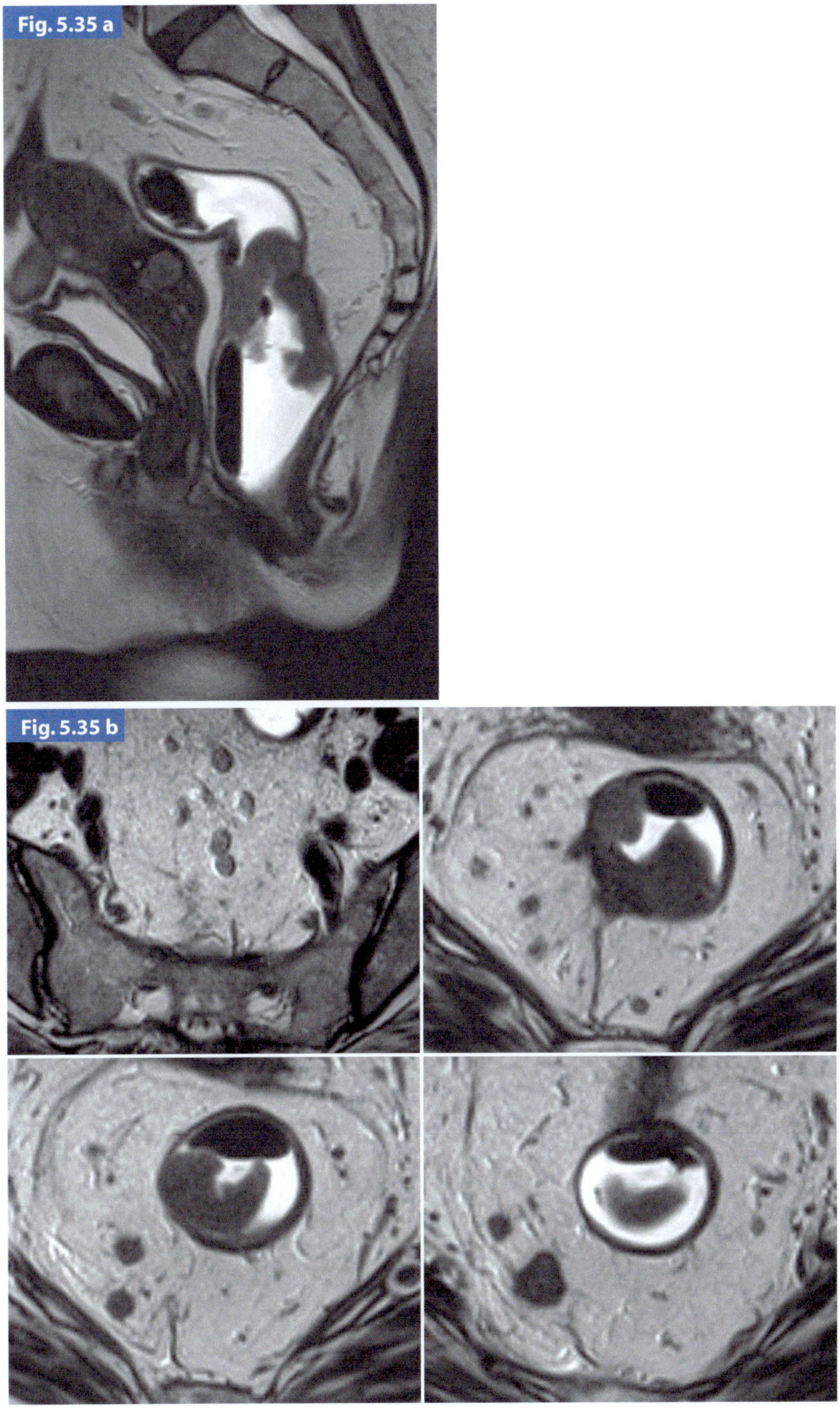

Fig. 5.35 Lymph node status. (**a**) Sagittal T2-TSE image displays stenosing carcinoma of the midrectum. (**b**) Para-axial T2-TSE images with the following findings: oval-shaped lymph nodes accompanying the superior rectal vessels; a group of small nodes with irregular borders present at the level of the wall-exceeding rectal cancer in addition to mesorectal nodes round in shape; and an enlarged node with inhomogeneous SI involving the CRM at 8 o'clock lithotomy position. The combination of enlarged or grouped mesorectal nodes, irregular contours, and signal inhomogeneities is highly indicative of nodal metastasis.

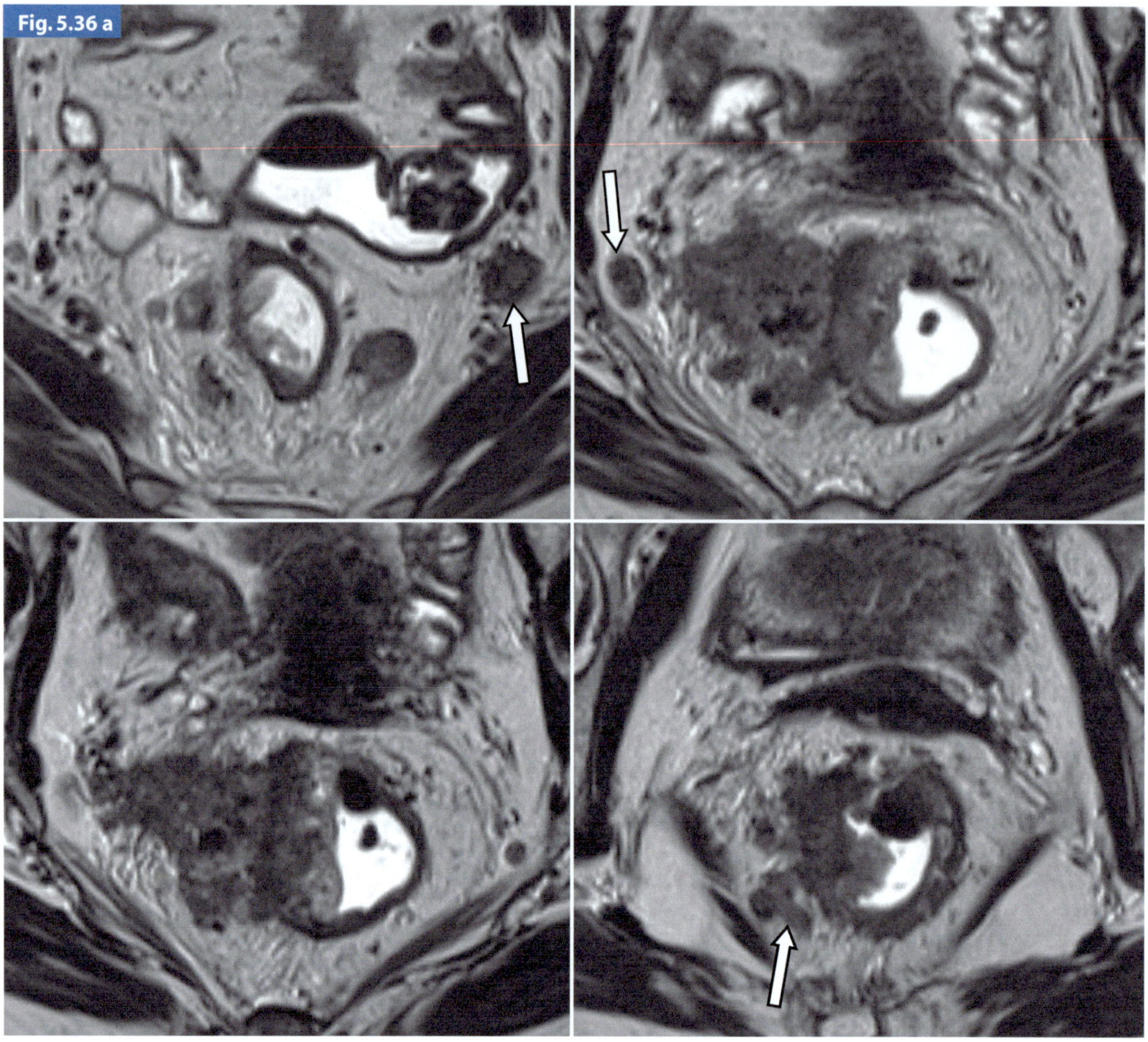

Fig. 5.36 (**a**) Para-axial T2-TSE images reflect advanced rectal tumor exceeding the right lateral aspects of the mesorectal fascia towards the iliac vessels. Multiple involved mesorectal nodes are present as well as extramural venous invasion (*arrow*) and tumor spread to iliac nodes on both sides (*arrows*). (**b**) Para-coronal T2-TSE images depict the distal parts of the mesorectal fascia (*arrow*) in close proximity to the levator ani muscle. The breaching of the mesorectal fascia is particularly well documented when this imaging plane is added. (**c**) Ink drawing: Rectal cancer crossing the mesorectal fascia.

Fig. 5.36 b

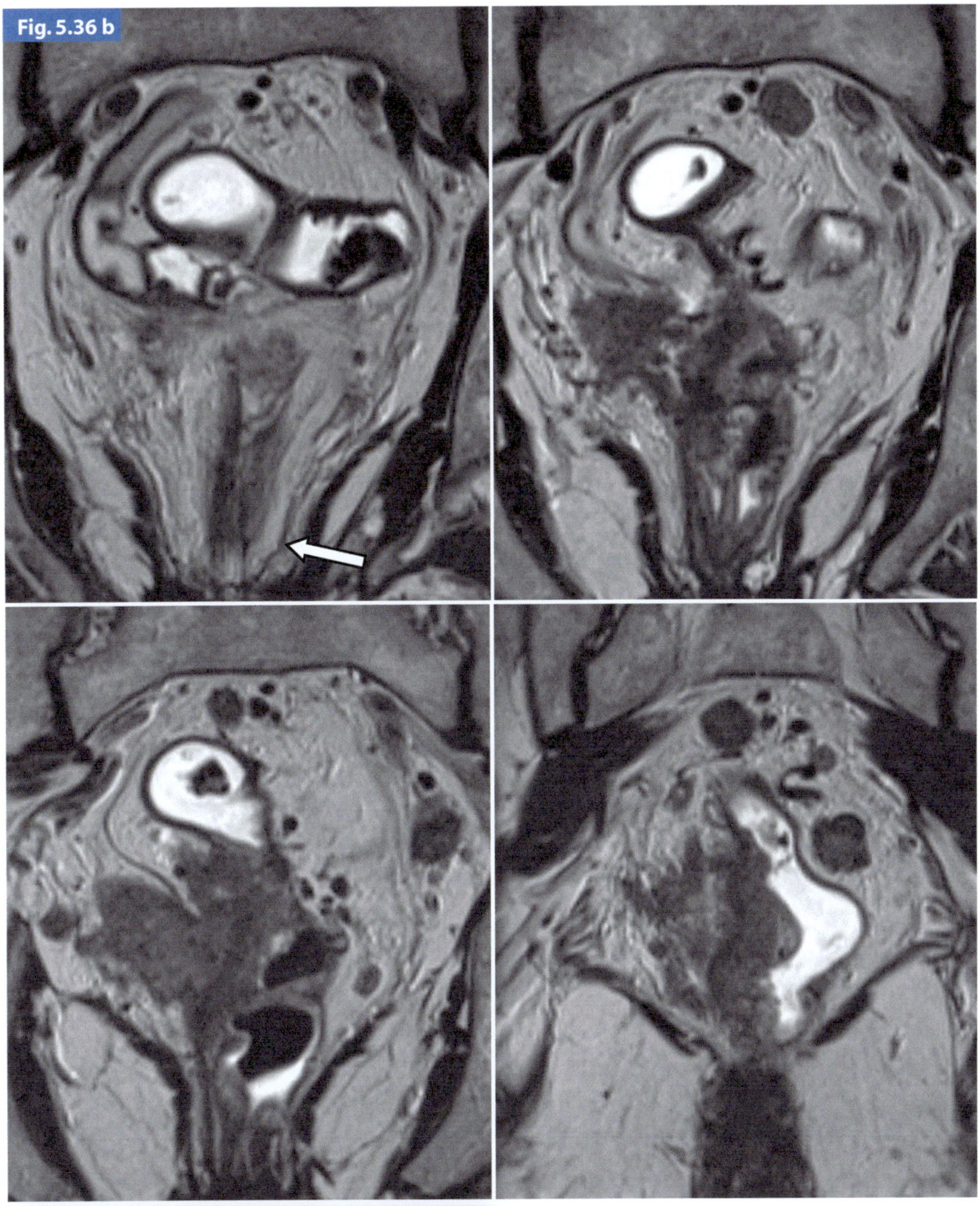

Fig. 5.36 c

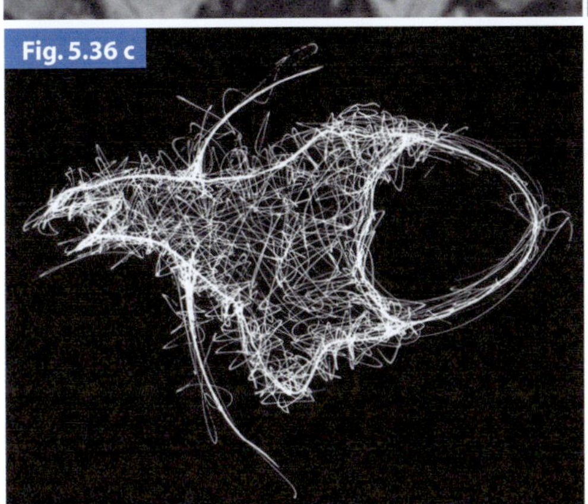

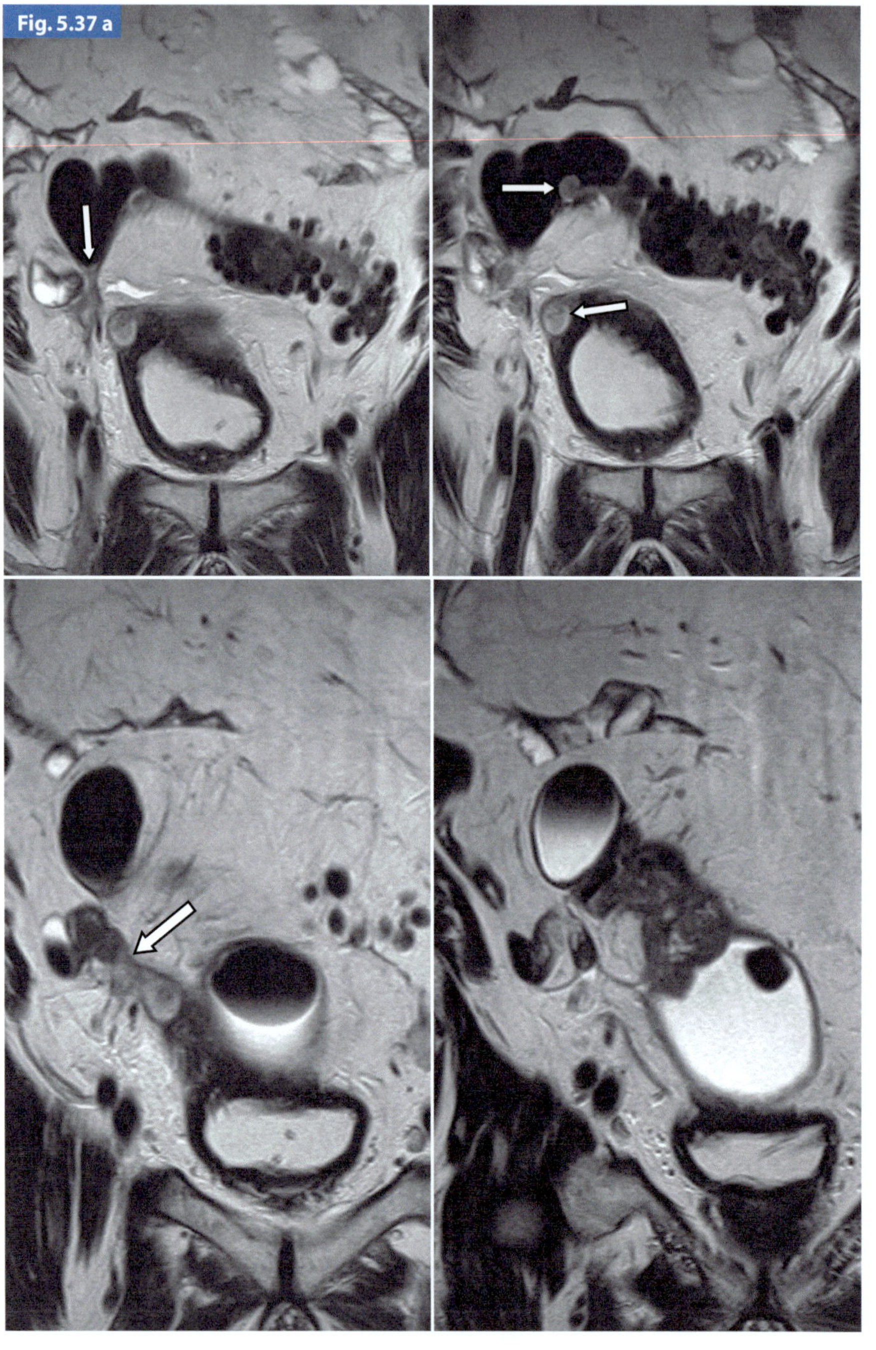

Fig. 5.37 (**a**) Stage T3 sigmoid cancer. Coronal T2-TSE images show a fistula between the roof of the bladder, the sigmoid colon, and the appendix (*arrows*). The images also reveal sigmoid cancer, a small polyp (*arrow*), and diverticulosis. Ileocecal and sigmoid resection were performed. Histopathology confirmed both a sigmoidoappendiceal and appendicovesical fistula caused by chronic appendicitis. The tumor stage was pT3N0.

5.5 Stage T4 Rectal Cancer

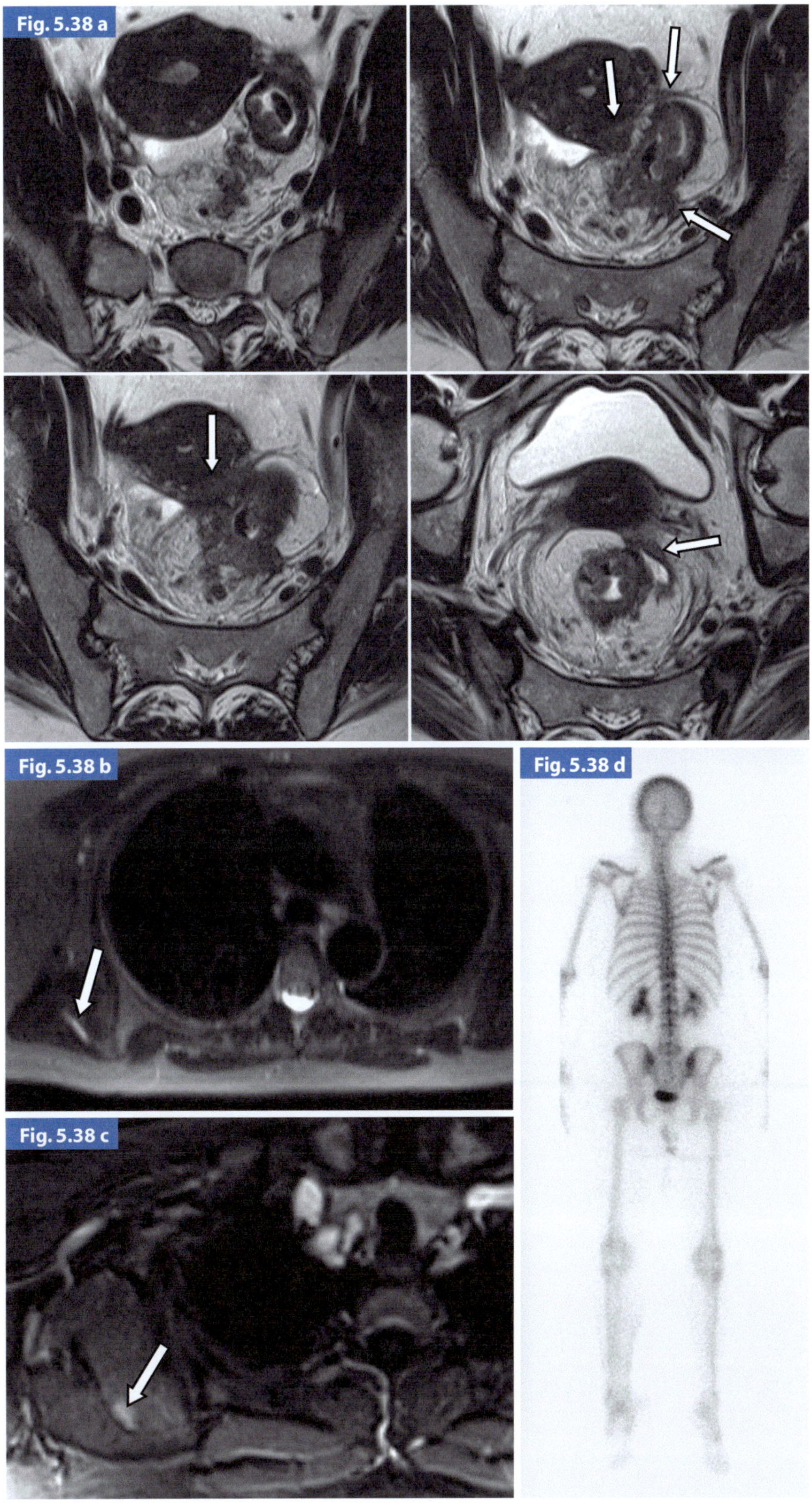

Fig. 5.38 (**a**) Para-axial T2-TSE images demonstrate advanced tumor of the upper and midrectum with involvement of the uterine neck, the peritoneal reflection, the visceral peritoneum, and the left dorsolateral circumferential resection margin (*arrows*), and ascites within the rectouterine pouch. Additionally, mesorectal tumor deposits are evident. Interestingly, both T4 criteria—organ involvement and peritoneal infiltration—are present in this case. Histopathology diagnosed stage ypT4N1 G2 rectal cancer. Axial free-breathing TIRM (**b**) and corresponding axial breath-hold CE-FLASH 2D (**c**) images derived from SMS moving-table MRI staging 6 months postsurgery show bone metastasis of the right scapula (*arrows*) as confirmed by scintigraphy (**d**).

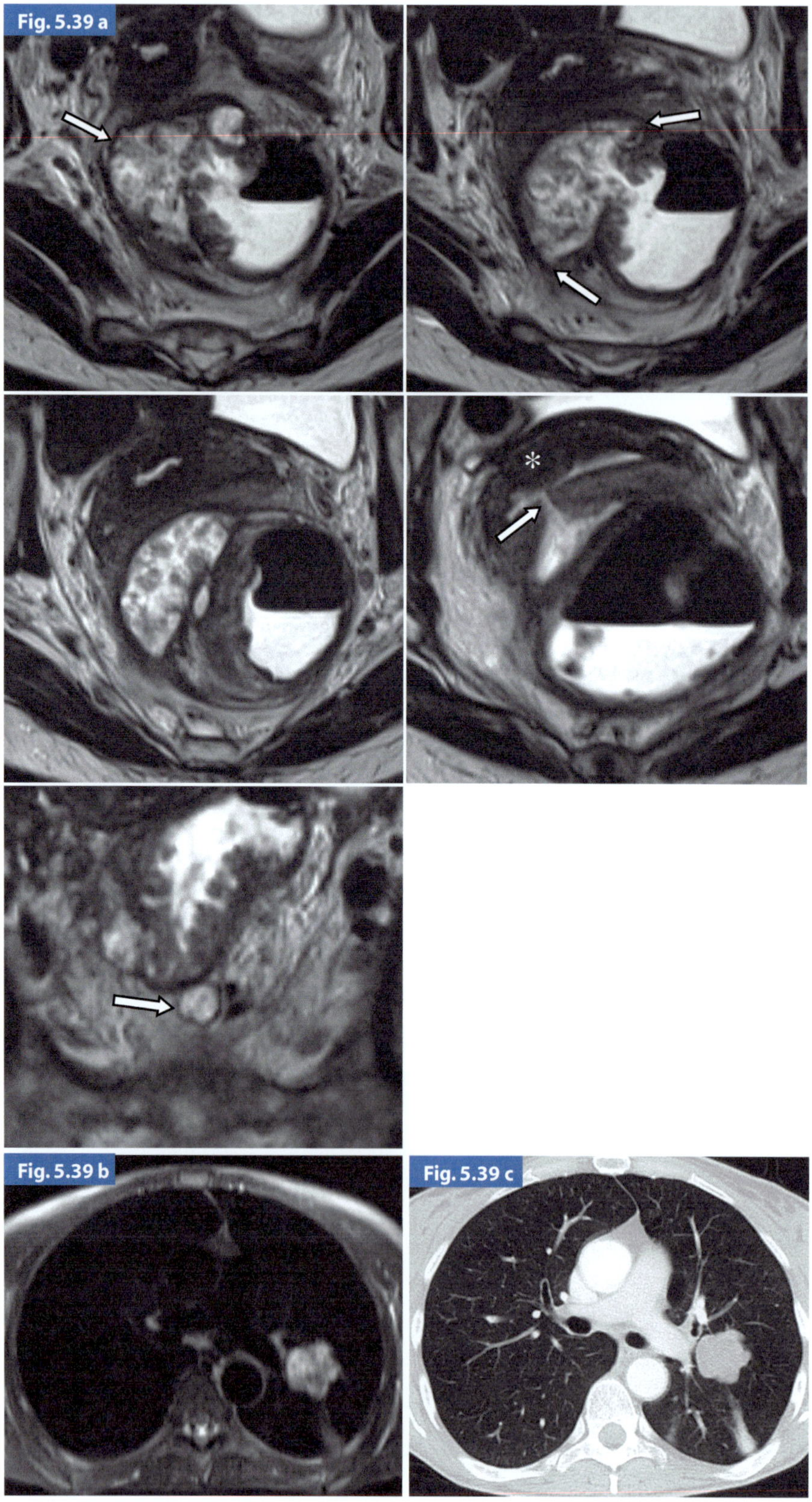

Fig. 5.39 (**a**) On the para-axial T2-TSE images, tumor perforation between 9- and 10-o'clock lithotomy position into the mesorectum is seen with abscess formation (*arrows*). The posterior vaginal wall is thickened and a tumor-vaginal fistula is present (*arrow*). Additionally, there is nodular thickening of the uterine cervix (*asterisk*). In the vicinity of the perforated tumor, bright-signal lymph node metastases are visible (*arrow*). (**b**) The free-breathing axial TIRM image of the SMS moving-table staging detected pulmonary metastasis in the left upper lobe, and was confirmed by MSCT (**c**). Emergency operation was carried out and histopathology diagnosed stage pT4N2 G3 rectal cancer with infiltration of the vagina and uterine cervix.

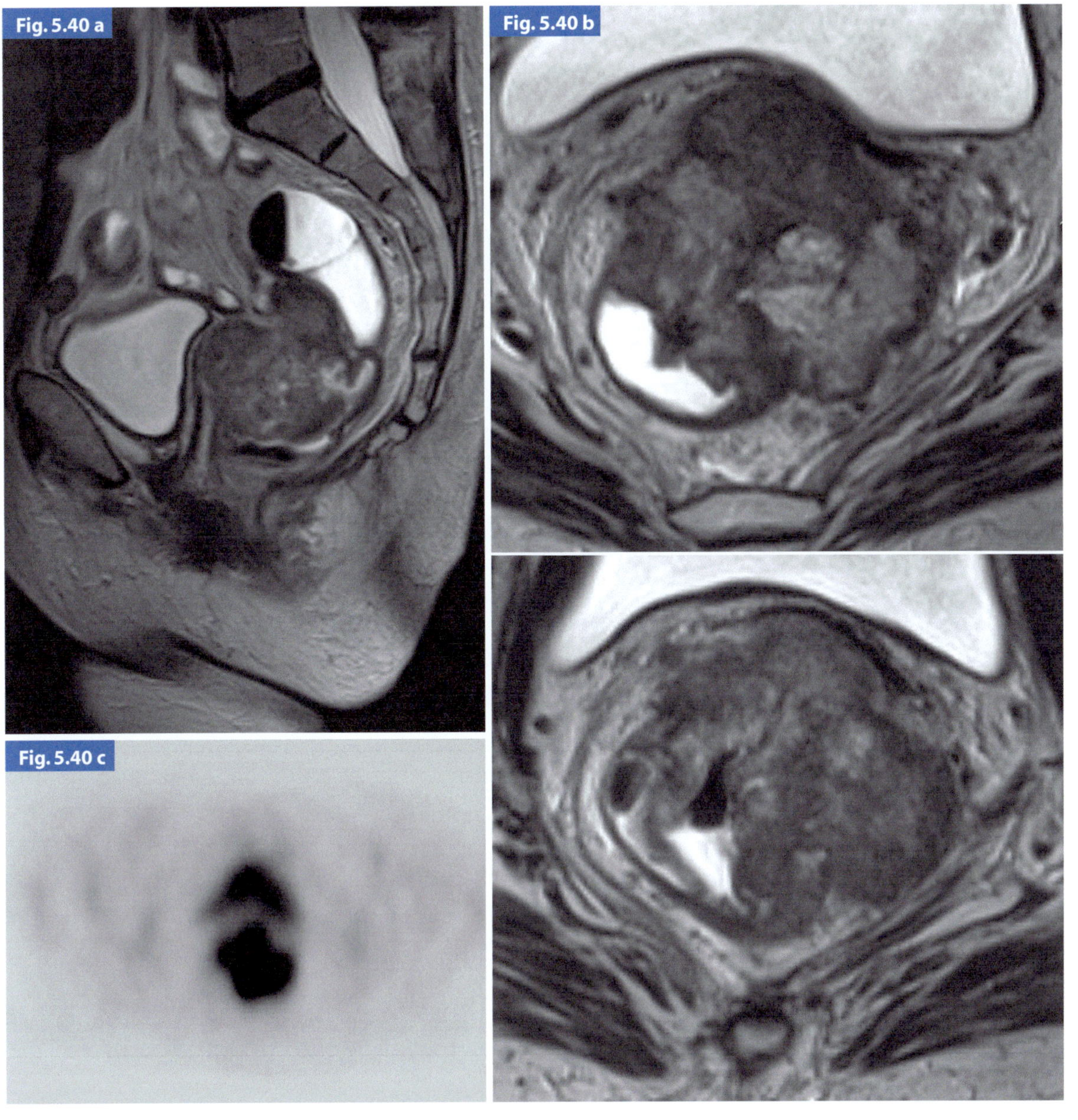

Fig. 5.40 Mucinous rectal cancer. Sagittal (**a**) and para-axial (**b**) T2-TSE images show an extensive tumor of the lower and midrectum with adherence to the vaginal stump and involvement of the mesorectal fascia. Inhomogeneous tumor signal is present with hyperintense areas suspicious of mucin lakes. (**c**) The corresponding PET image revealed high FGD-avidity of the tumor. The axial T2-TSE image (**d**) and the corresponding axial CE-FLASH 2D images (**e**) obtained during moving-table MRI depict an ileal loop with circumscribed moderate wall thickening (*arrows*) characteristic of peritoneal carcinosis. (**f**) During PET, a second FDG-avid lesion was detected adjacent to the bladder roof (*arrow*). Histopathologic examination of the biopsies verified mucinous adenocarcinoma. The tumor was classified as cT4N1M1. As a result of her poor general conditions, the patient currently receives palliative chemoradiation.

Fig. 5.40 d

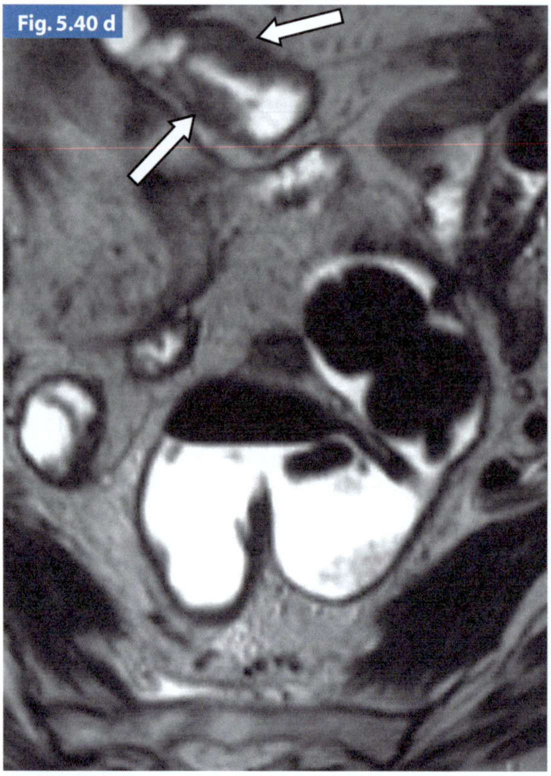

Fig. 5.40 e

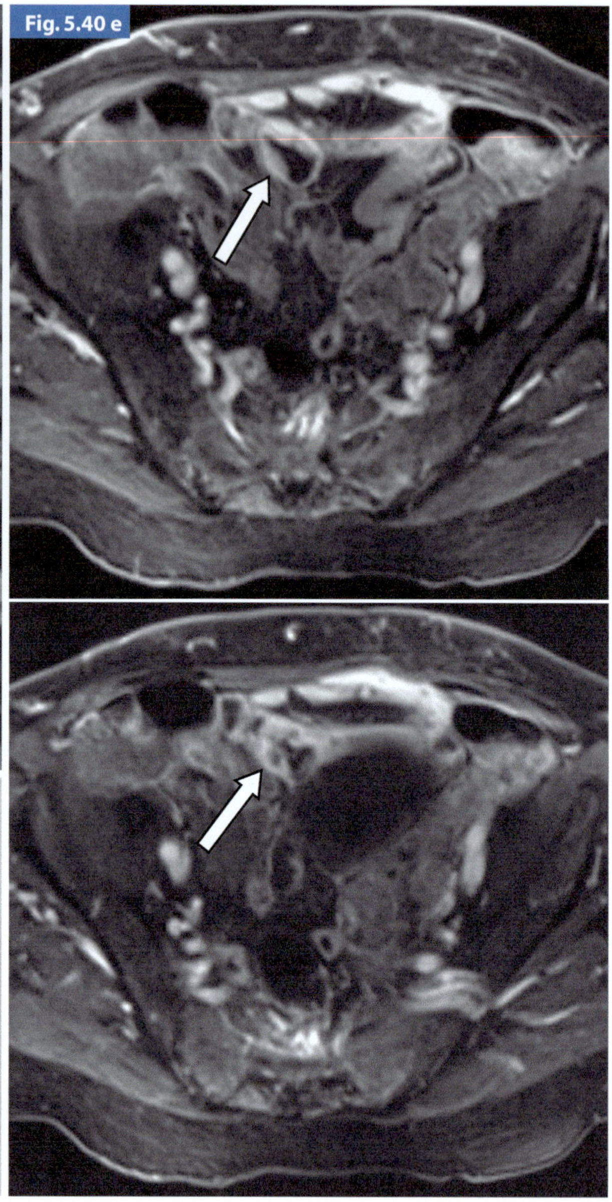

Fig. 5.40 f

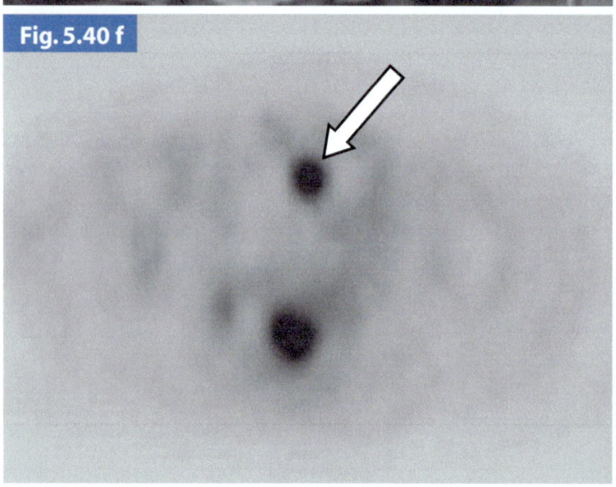

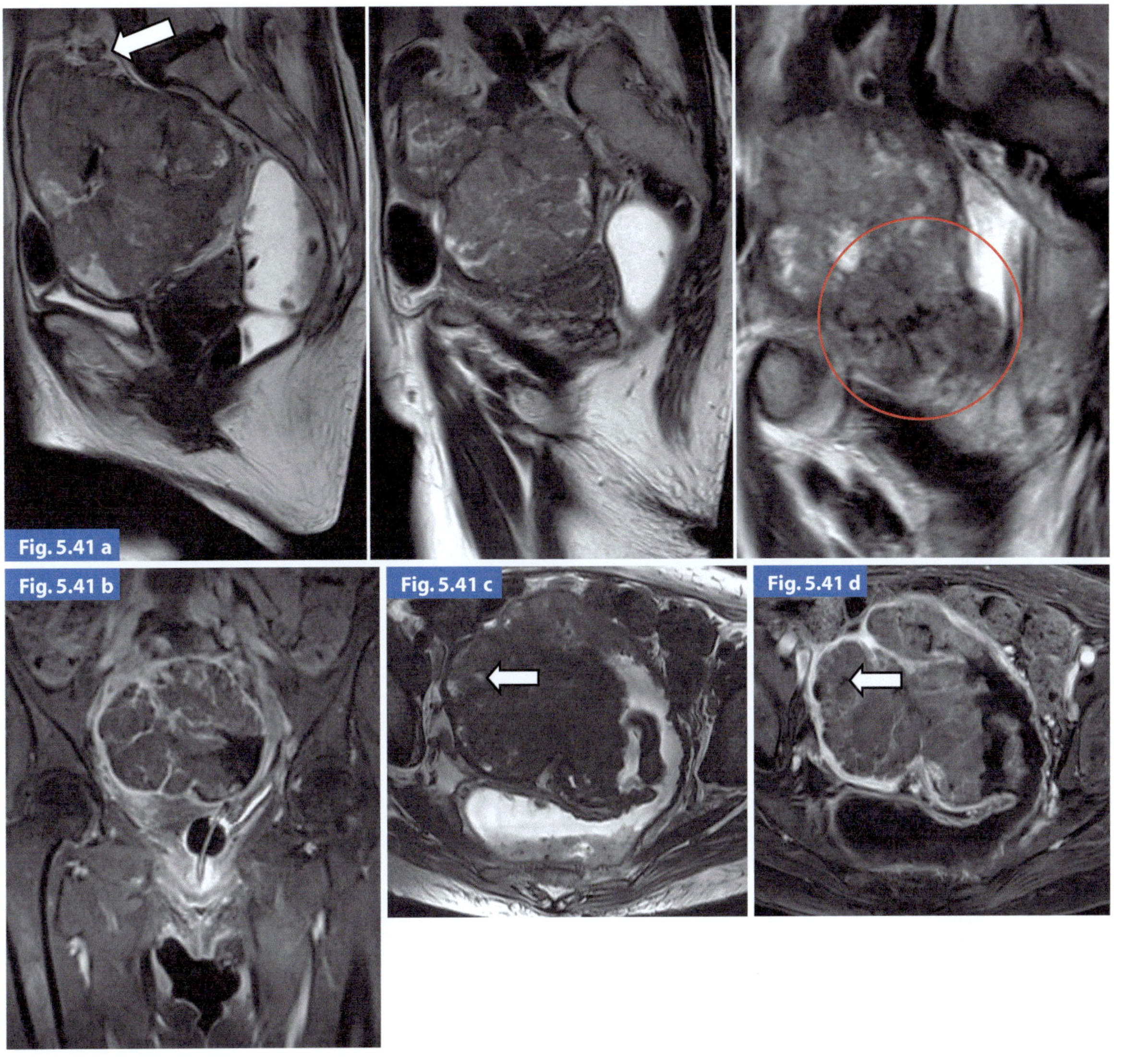

Fig. 5.41 Stage T4 sigmoid cancer. (**a**) Sagittal T2-TSE images show a large tumor mass occupying the lumen of the sigmoid colon with adjacent nodes (*arrow*). The right adnexa is involved and cannot be separated from the primary tumor (*red circle*). (**b**– **d**) Coronal CE-VIBE 3D (**b**), axial CISS-3D (**c**), and axial CE-VIBE 3D images (**d**) show that wide parts of the carcinoma are confined to the sigmoid wall. The tumor shows small necrotic foci (*arrows*). The histopathologic examination resulted in a stage T4N1M1 (adnexa) poorly differentiated sigmoid adenocarcinoma.

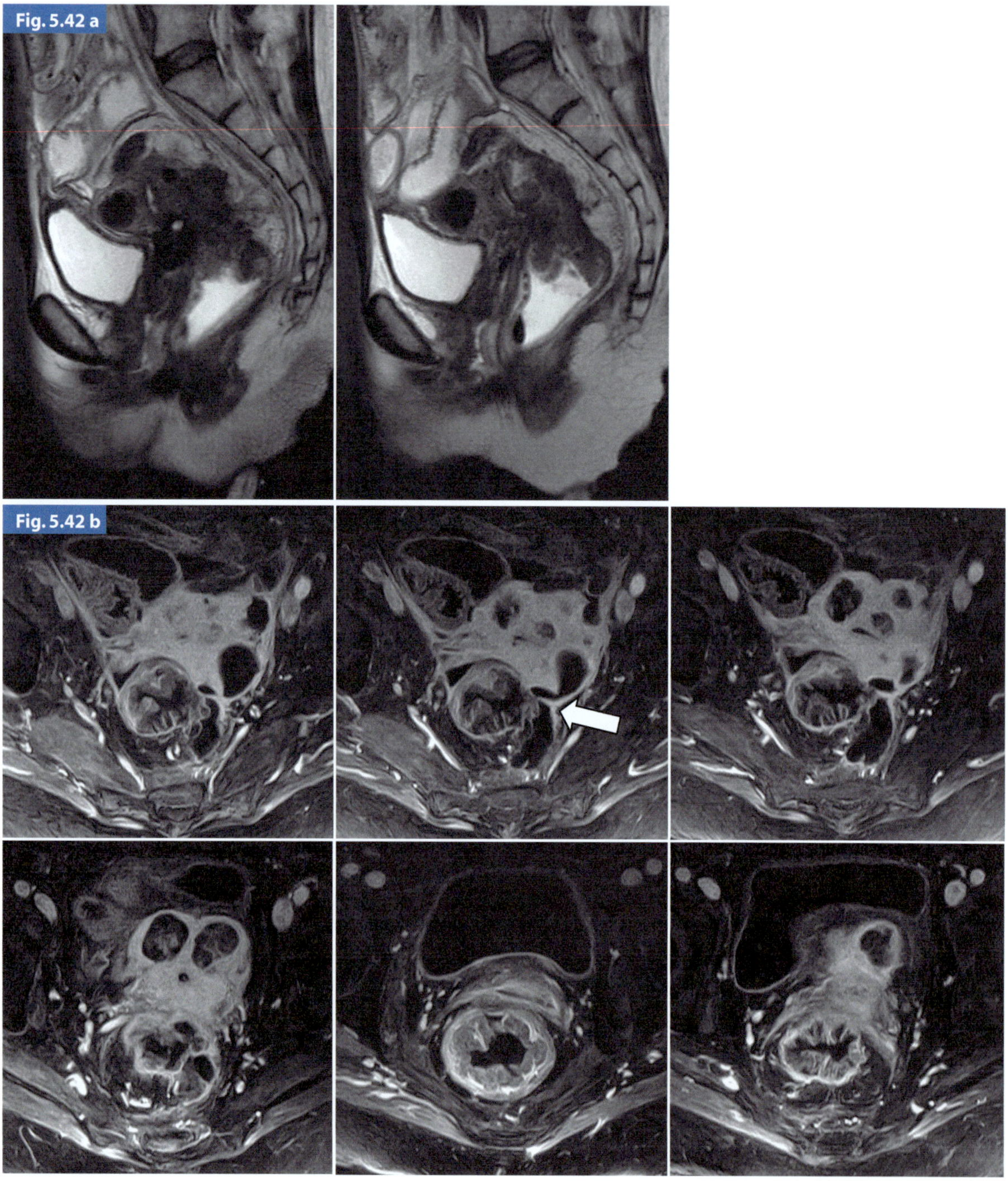

Fig. 5.42 Stage T4 rectal cancer and left-sided pyosalpinx. Patient history: Pulmonary metastatic disease from clinical stage T4 rectal cancer, acute abdomen. (**a**) On the sagittal T2-TSE images, an advanced tumor of the mid and upper rectum is visible with direct infiltration of the uterus and vagina. (**b**) Axial CE-VIBE 3D images show an ill-defined, contrast-enhancing mass with irregular borders and fluid-filled inclusions involving the left adnexa and the uterus. In addition, uterine myomas can be detected. Tumor perforation into the mesorectum is seen at 3-o'clock lithotomy position (*arrow*) with abscess formation. There is communication of the rectal cancer with the enhancing tumor-like mass. Emergency surgery was carried out and confirmed left-sided pyosalpinx and pelvic peritonitis. Therefore, ovariectomy and peritoneal lavage were performed. Additionally, the perforated rectal carcinoma that truly invaded the uterus and vagina was explored and descendostoma was created.

Fig. 5.43 a

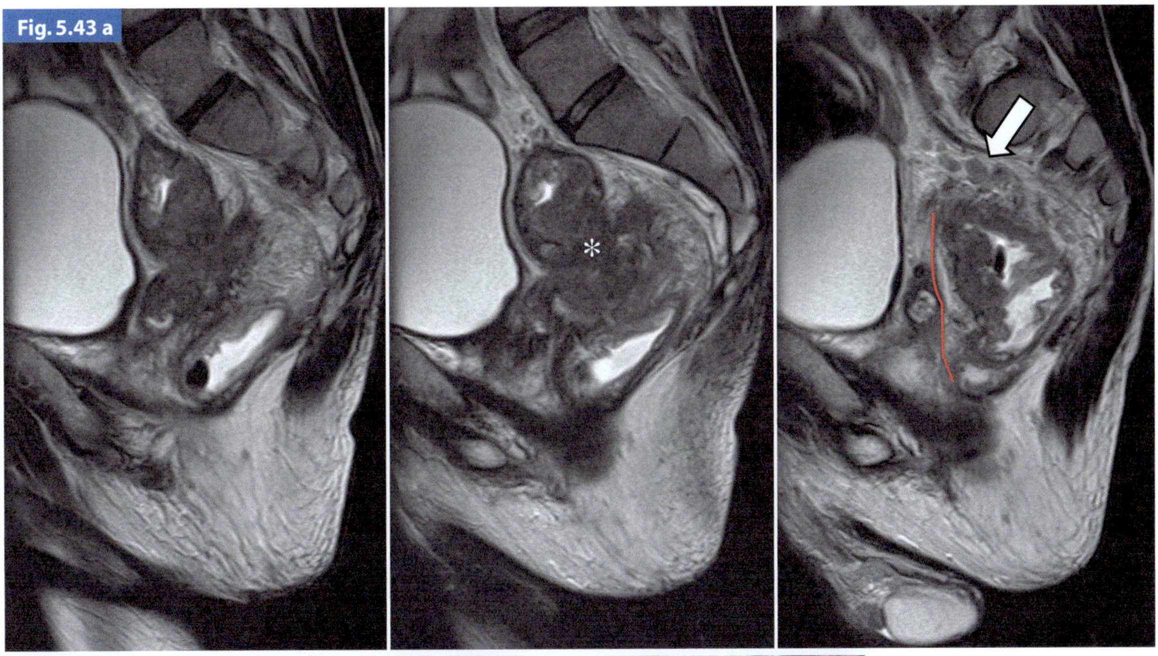

Fig. 5.43 b

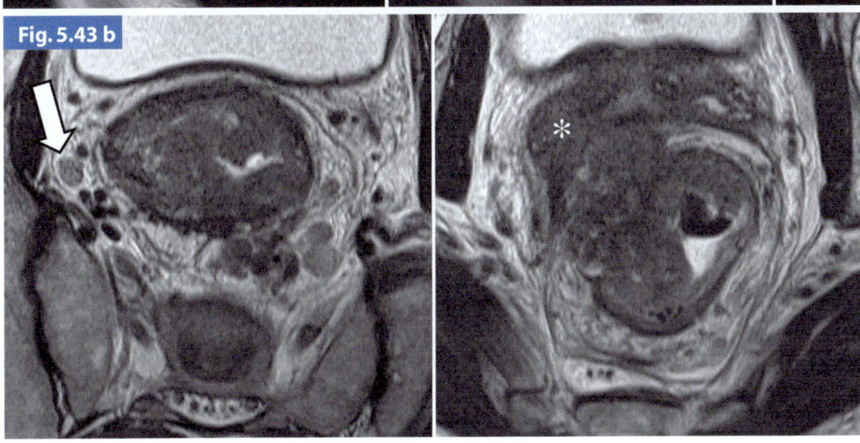

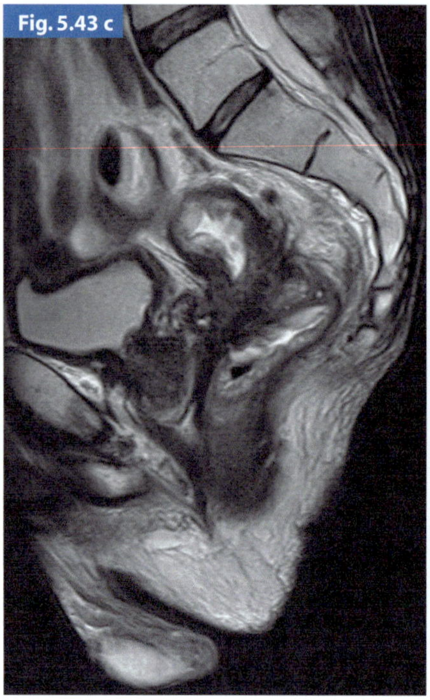

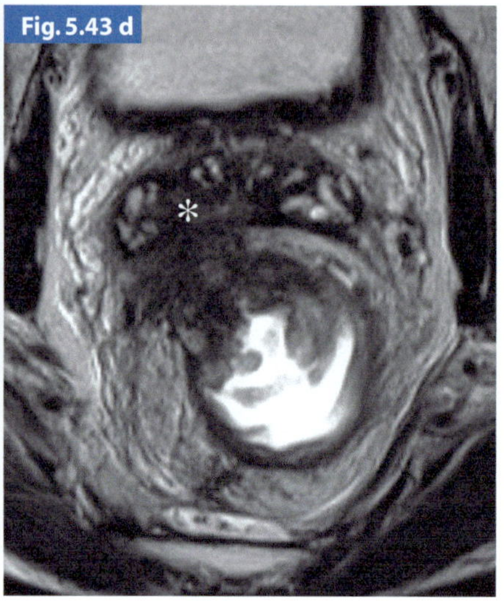

Fig. 5.43 Stage ypT3 rectal cancer. (**a**, **b**) Pretreatment MRI. On the sagittal T2-TSE images (**a**), depiction of advanced carcinoma of the midrectum (*asterisk*) exceeding Denonvilliers' fascia (*red line*) was seen. Note the cluster of lymph nodes inside the mesorectum (*arrow*). The corresponding axial T2-TSE images (**b**) show direct invasion of the right seminal vesicles (*asterisk*). In addition, a suspicious lymph node is located outside the mesorectal fascia close to the right internal iliac vessels (*arrow*). (**c**, **d**) Post-radiochemotherapy MRI. Sagittal (**c**) and axial (**d**) T2-TSE images. After neoadjuvant therapy tumor downsizing and regression of the pathologic mesorectal nodes can be noticed. The suspected iliac nodes completely disappeared. Constantly, the tumor penetrates the mesorectal fascia and stationary seems to infiltrate the seminal vesicles (*asterisk*). On the basis of the imaging findings the rectal carcinoma was clinically judged as ycT4. Surprisingly, histopathology revealed stage ypT3N1L1V0Pn0CRM + G2 rectal cancer. Interesting aspects concerning this case: Only parts of the carcinoma decreased in signal following radiochemotherapy, indicative of partial tumor fibrosis. The signal changes of the seminal vesicles were produced by marked desmoplastic reaction. The circumferential resection margin was involved.

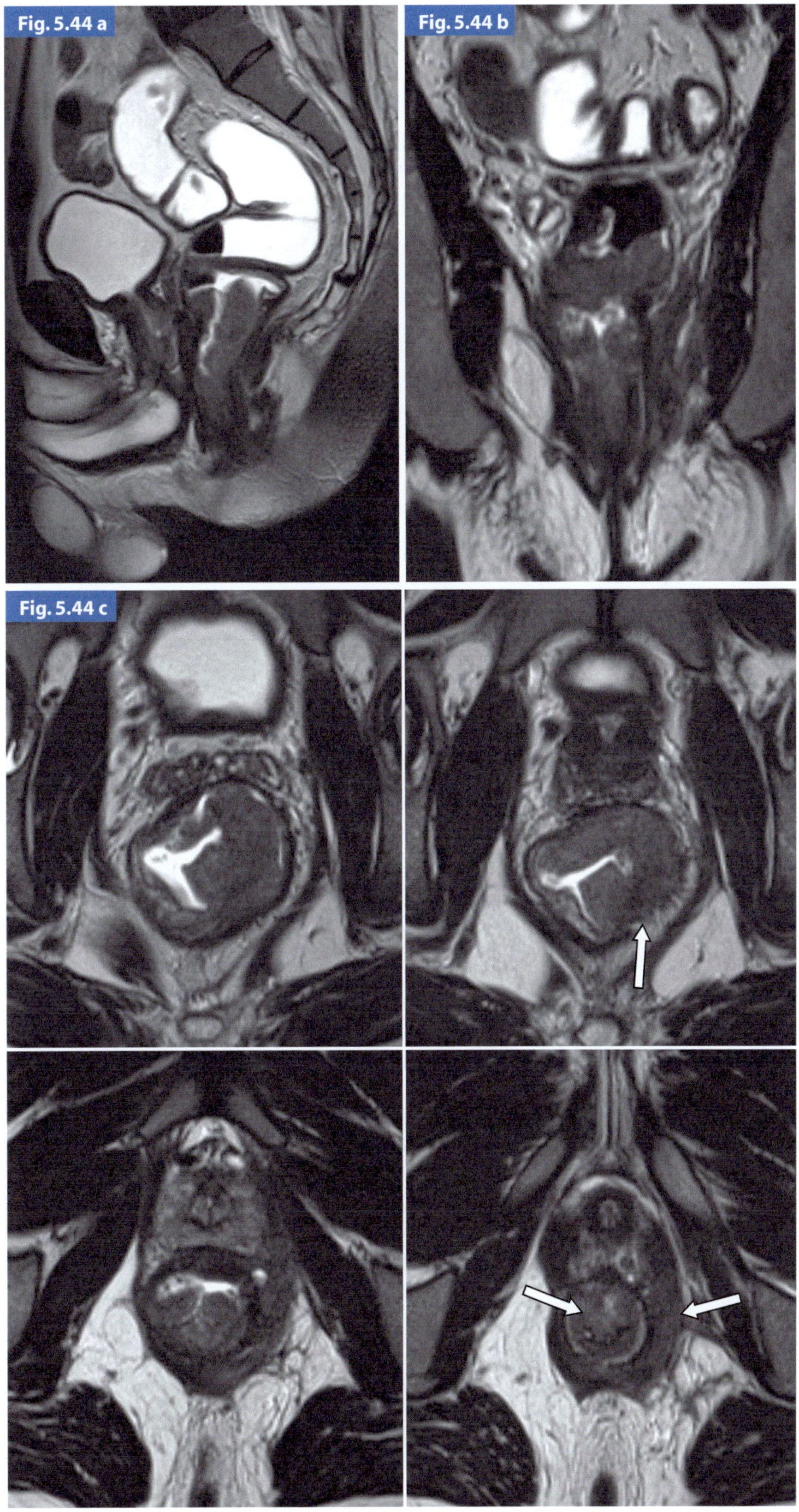

Fig. 5.44 Sagittal (**a**) and coronal (**b**) T2-TSE images show luminal tumor growth in the lower rectum and anal channel in addition to a conspicuous thickening of the left levator ani muscle. (**c**) Para-axial T2-TSE images display extension of the tumor signal into the perimuscular fat (*arrow*), the left levator ani muscle (*arrow*), and the anal channel (*arrow*). On the basis of the above mentioned findings, a low-lying stage T4 rectal cancer could be diagnosed.

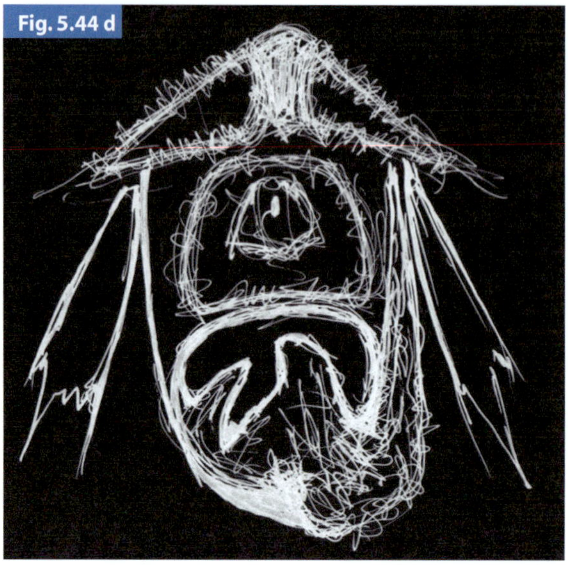

Fig. 5.44 (**d**) Ink drawing: Levator ani muscle infiltration.

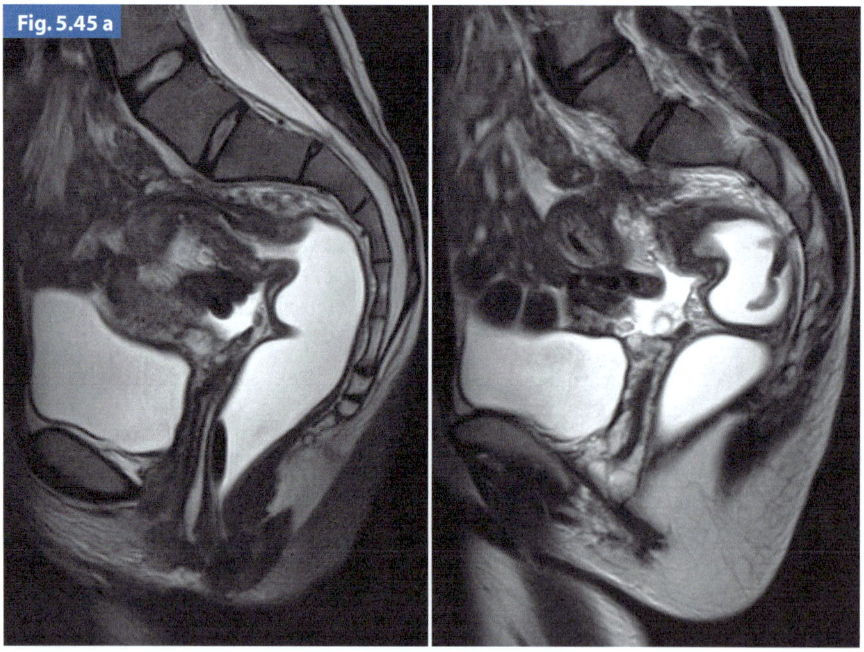

Fig. 5.45 On the sagittal (**a**) T2-TSE images advanced tumor o the upper rectum and rectosigmoid is visible.

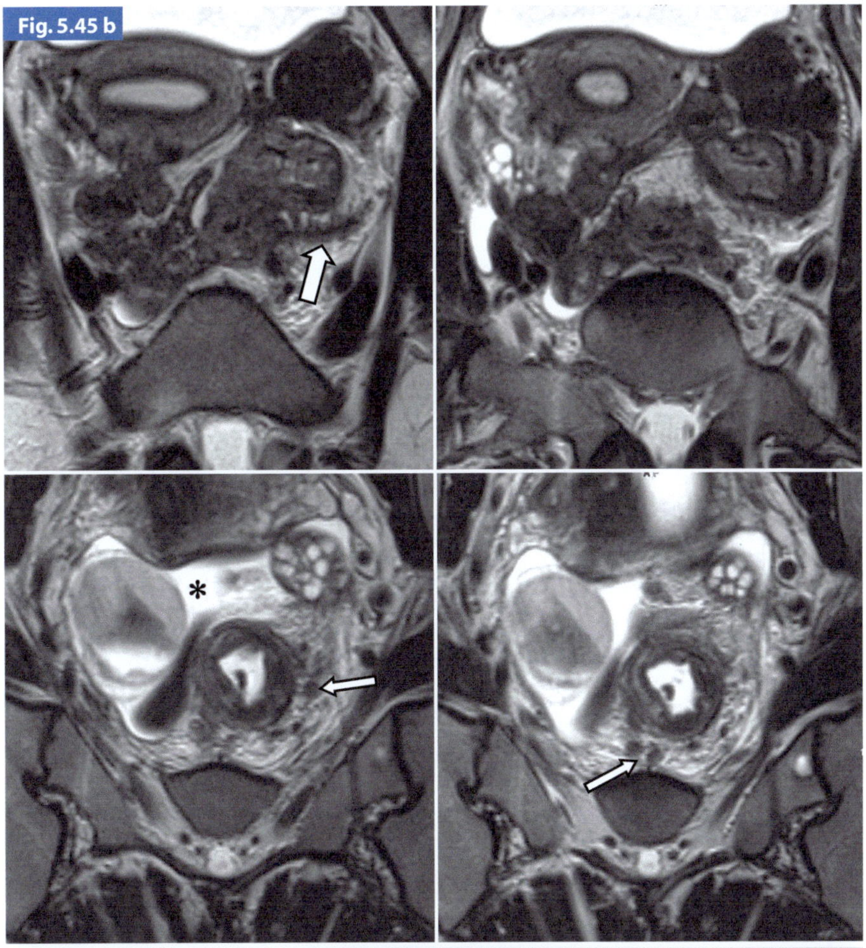

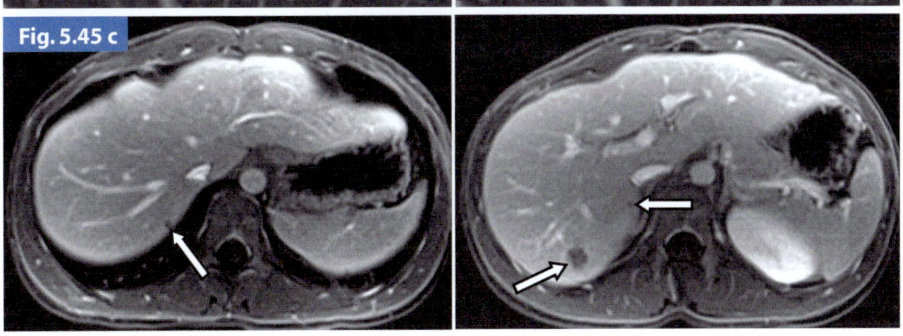

Fig. 5.45 Para-axial (**b**) T2-TSE images display direct tumor infiltration of the peritoneum (*arrow*) with ascites (*asterisk*). The wall-exceeding tumor is accompanied by several irregularly shaped mesorectal nodes indicative of metastatic spread (*thin arrows*) Additionally, a chocolate cyst of the right ovary is present.Detection of liver metastases during Sliding Multislice axial moving table M-satging using breath-hold CE-FLASH 2D (**c**, *arrows*). With respect to these findings the tumor was clinically staged as cT4N2M1 rectal cancer. Patient history: A 23-year old female with initial diagnosis of rectal cancer followed by diagnostic work-up at the beginning of August 2007. Neoadjuvant radiochemotherapy was planned and an ileostomy was created on August 15th. Peritoneal carcinosis was detected during surgery and metastatic spread to the liver was confirmed. The therapeutic strategy had to be changed based on the new findings, and a palliative deep anterior resection of the rectum, resection of cancer-afflicted jejunal and ileal segments, and lower abdominal peritonectomy were carried out on August 31. Rapid progressive disease was observed intraoperatively. Histopathology diagnosed stage pT4N2M1 (liver, peritoneum) L1V1Pn1 G3 rectal adenocarcinoma.

5.6 Negative Prognostic Factors

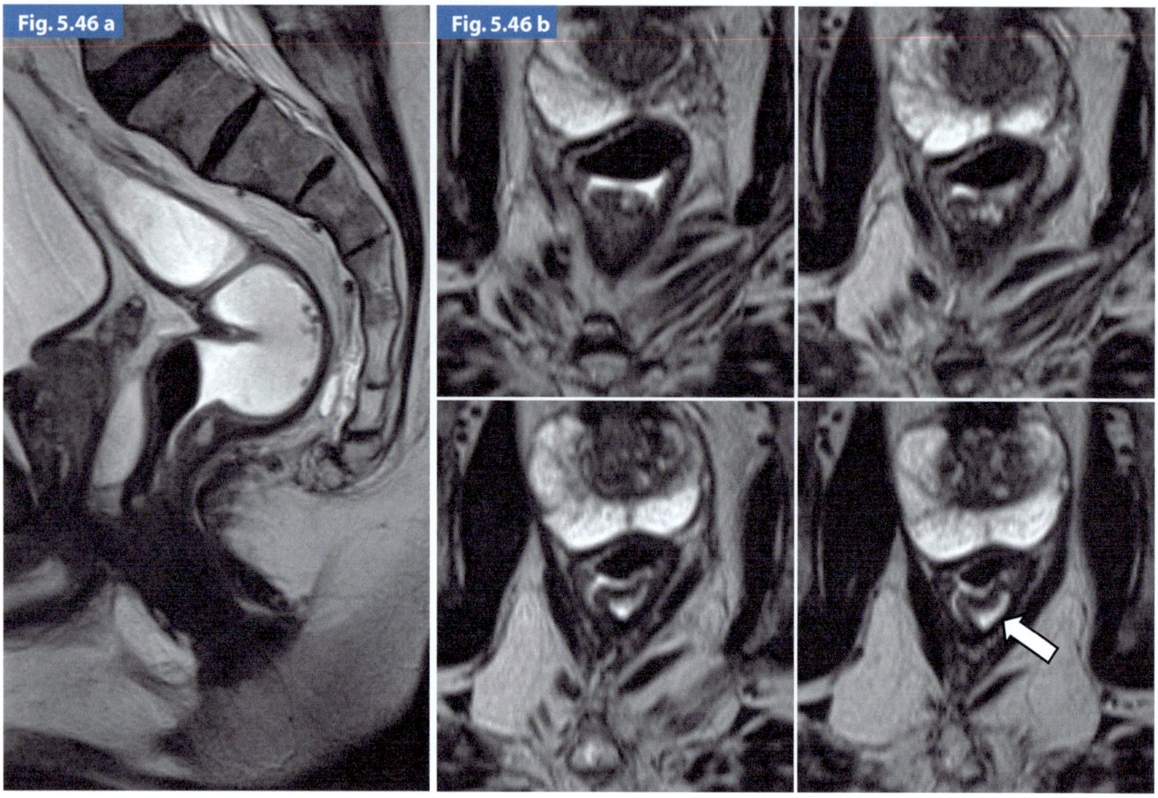

Fig. 5.46 Stage T2 rectal cancer. (**a**) Sagittal T2-TSE images reveal a tumor of the lower rectum. (**b**) Para-axial T2-TSE images show a polypoid rectal tumor reaching the muscle layer with signal-rich inclusions within the submucosa (*arrow*) indicative of mucus lakes resulting from mucinous adenocarcinoma. Histopathology staged the tumor as pT2N0L0V0 G2 mucinous adenocarcinoma.

Fig. 5.47 (**a**–**c**) Stage T2 rectal cancer. (**a**) Sagittal T2-TSE images reveal a tubulovillous adenoma of the midrectum with conspicuous cystic changes. (**b**) On the corresponding axial T2-TSE images, these high-signal components can also be observed near the polyp stalk, which is located between the 3 and 4 o'clock lithotomy positions. Fluid isointense areas within an adenoma are highly suggestive of malignant transformation. They correspond to mucus lakes resulting from mucin pooling in the tumor stroma. Histopathology diagnosed stage pT2N0L0V1Pn1 mucinous adenocarcinoma developed from a tubulovillous adenoma.

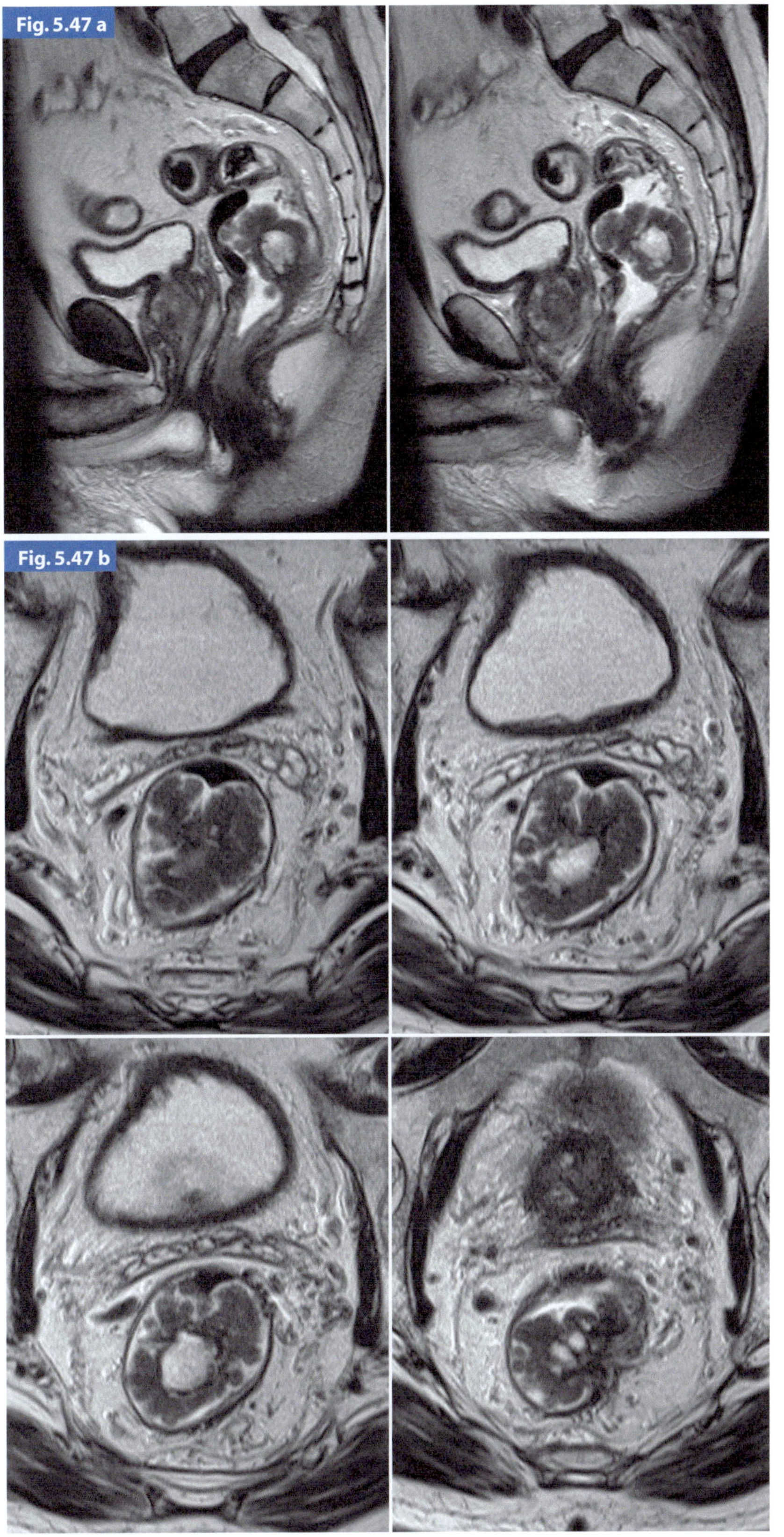

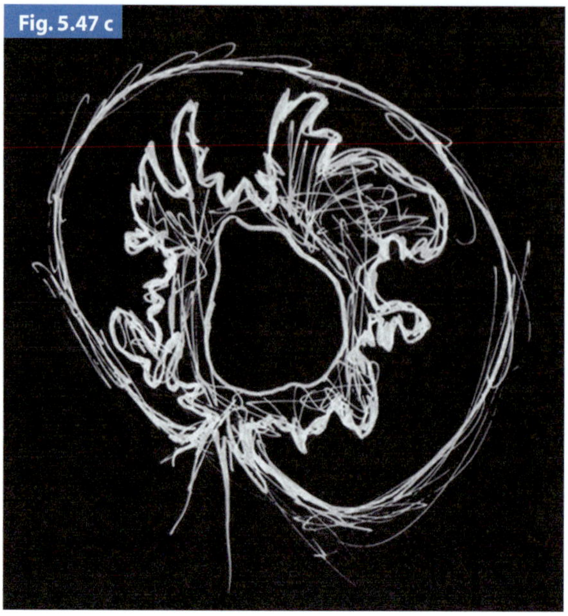

Fig. 5.47 (c) Ink drawing: Mucinous carcinoma within a tubulovillous adenoma.

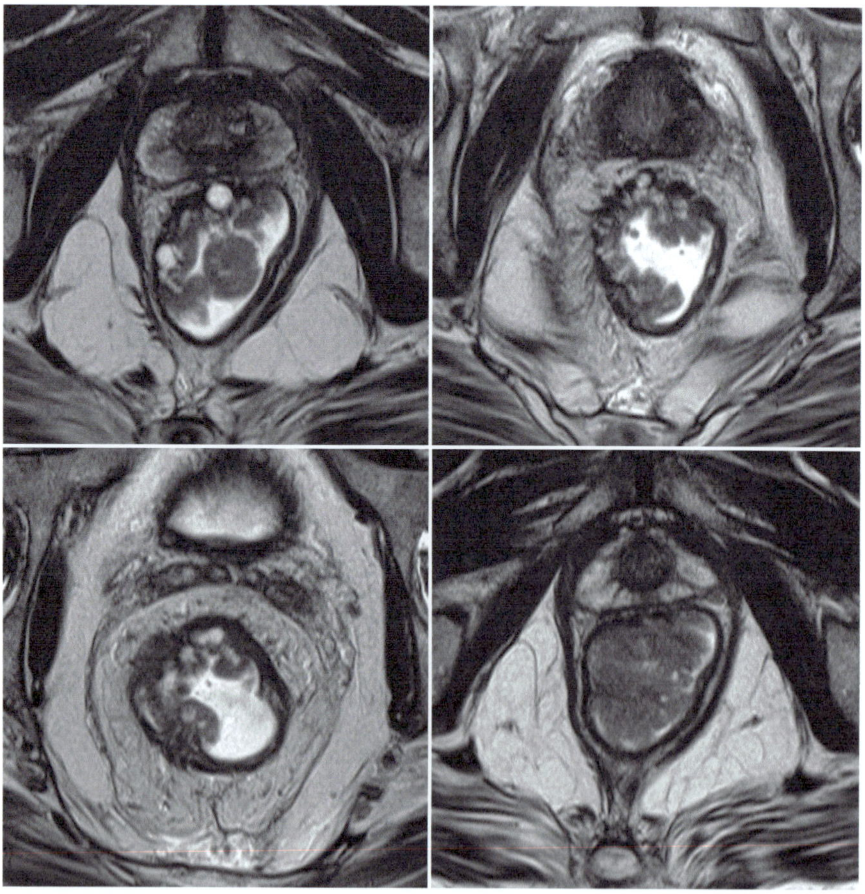

Fig. 5.48 Stage T3 rectal cancer. Axial T2-TSE images reveal signal characteristics of a mucinous adenocarcinoma of the rectum. The exophytic tumor contains foci of high-signal intensity representing mucus lakes. In addition, the carcinoma is penetrating the muscle layer into the mesorectal fat in spots. The histopathologic examination revealed stage pT3N2 moderately differentiated mucinous adenocarcinoma.

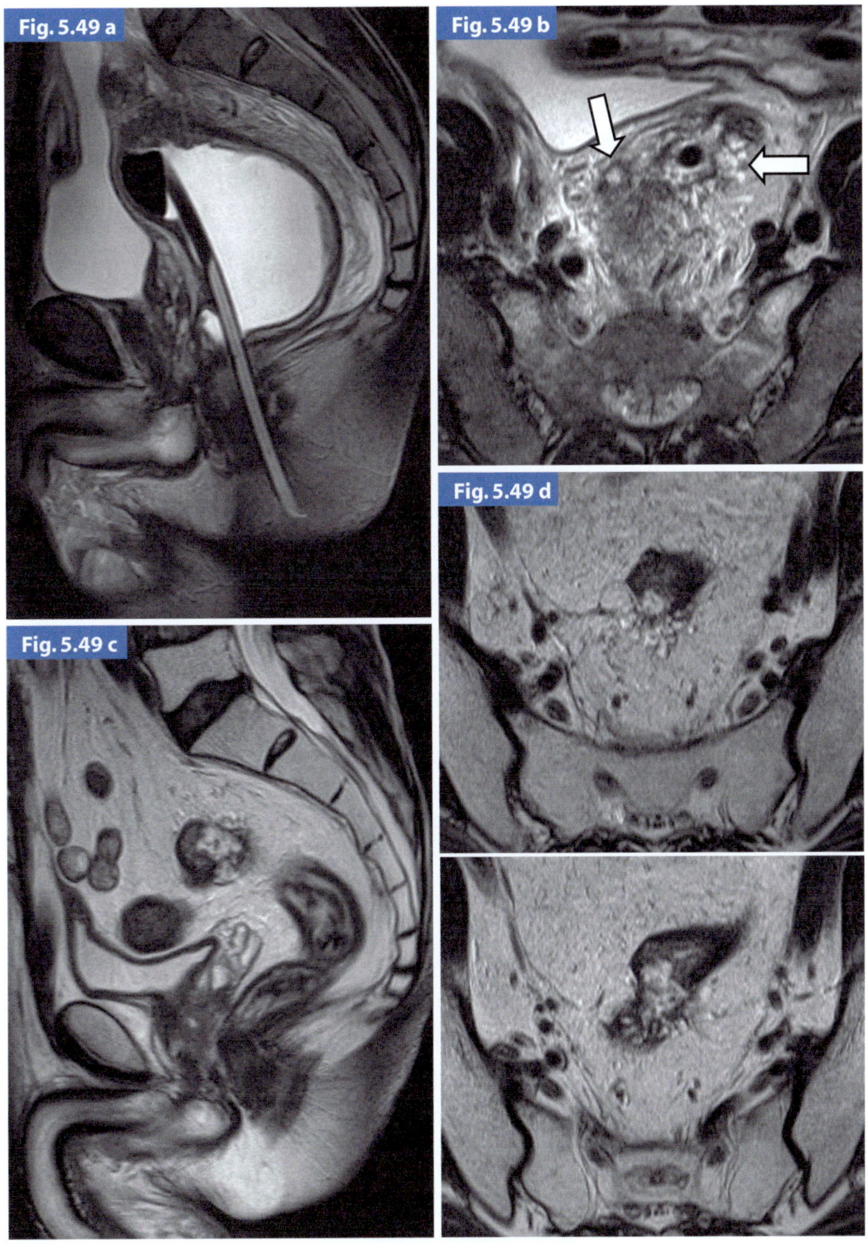

Fig. 5.49 Stage T3 rectal cancer. (**a**, **b**) Pretreatment MRI. (**a**) On the sagittal T2-TSE image, tumor stenosis of the upper rectum is treated with a decompression tube. (**b**) On the axial T2-TSE image, the wall-exceeding carcinoma forms an ill-defined mass with bright signal-intensity inclusions characteristic of mucin lakes (*arrows*). (**c**, **d**) Post-treatment MRI prior to surgery. The sagittal (**c**) and corresponding axial (**d**) T2-TSE images reveal tumor downsizing. Note the homogenously high signal of the botryoid-shaped tumor. Clinically, the tumor was staged as mucinous adenocarcinoma cT3N0 and confirmed by histopathology as ypT3N0L0V0Pn0.

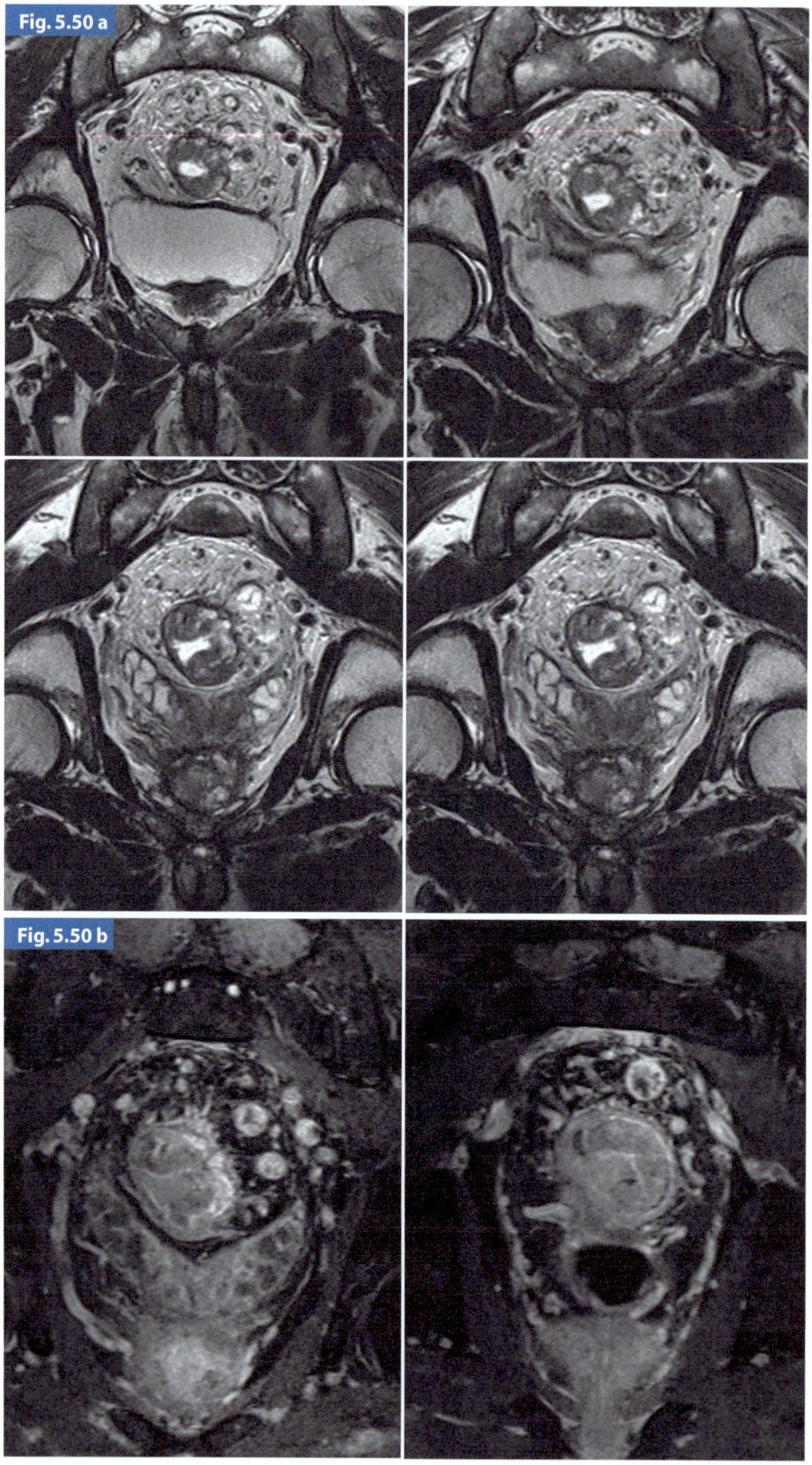

Fig. 5.50 Stage T3 rectal cancer. (**a**) Para-coronal T2-hyperTSE images at 3T reveal circular stenosing tumor of the upper rectum with perimuscular fat infiltration and extensive nodal metastases in the adjacent mesorectum. The tumor displays focal high-signal inclusions like the surrounding nodes, indicative of mucinous adenocarcinoma. (**b**) Para-coronal fat saturated CE-T1-hyperTSE images at 3T demonstrate intensive contrast enhancement of the carcinoma and the metastatic mesorectal nodes. Histopathologic diagnosis was pT3N2 G2 mucinous adenocarcinoma.

Fig. 5.51 a

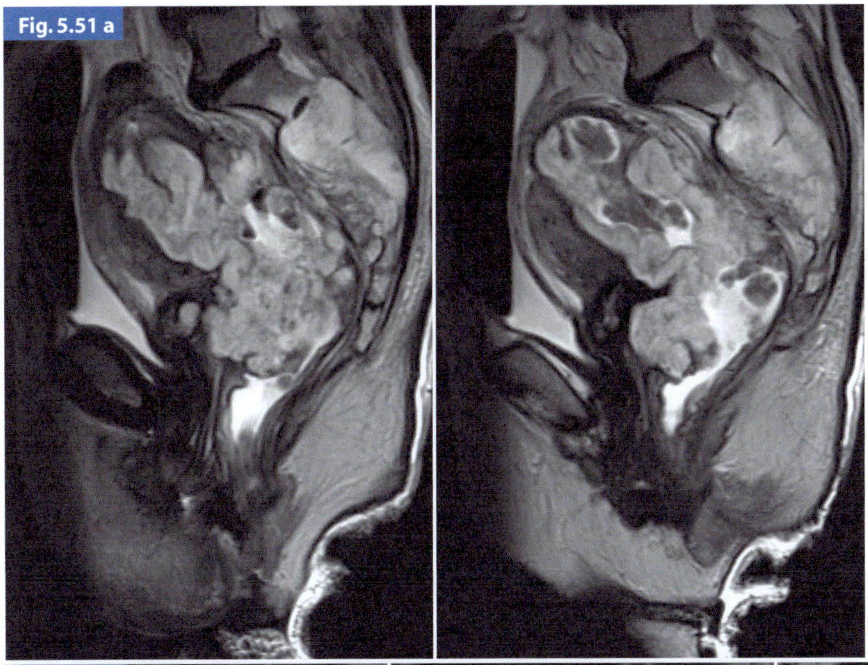

Fig. 5.51 b

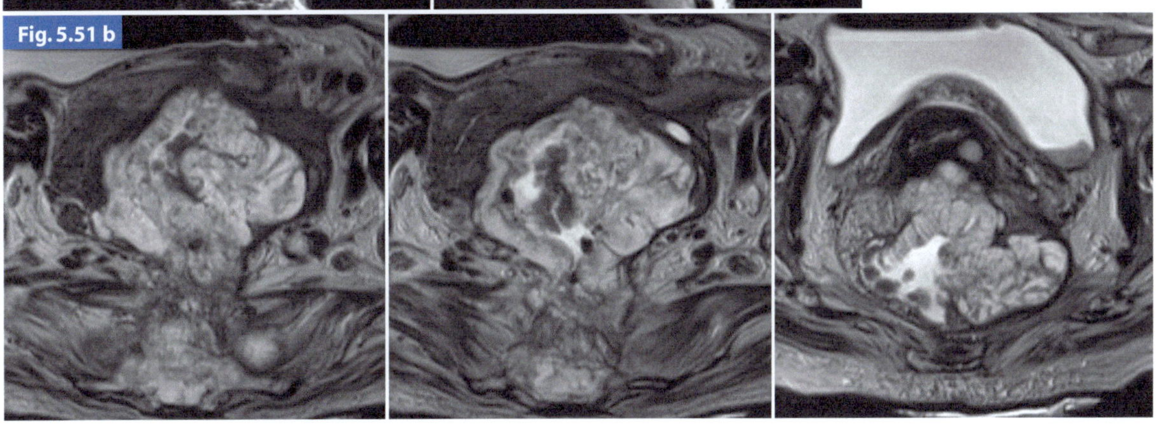

Fig. 5.51 (**a–e**) Stage T4 mucinous rectal cancer. (**a**) On the sagittal T2-TSE images, an advanced mucin containing rectal tumor is visible, which directly invades the sacral bone. Note the air-fluid level in the bladder lumen caused by a tumor fistula. (**b**) Corresponding para-axial T2-TSE images confirm the findings. Additionally, the rectal ampulla is massively widened as a result of the extensive tumor growth mimicking transmesorectal infiltration of both the uterus and vagina. (**c**) On the axial CE-VIBE 3D images, the tumor shows a papillary pattern and the mucinous parts are clearly distinguishable. The tumor fistula opens into the left bladder wall (*arrow*). DWI image (b = 750 s/mm^2) (**d**) and corresponding ADC map (**e**). The tumor is of high signal on the DWI image and also displays high signal on the ADC map, which should not be mistaken for complete necrosis. (**f**) Free-breathing axial TIRM images derived from moving-table MRI staging reveal mucinous lung metastases. The tumor was classified as a stage cT4N0M1 mucinous adenocarcinoma of the rectum.

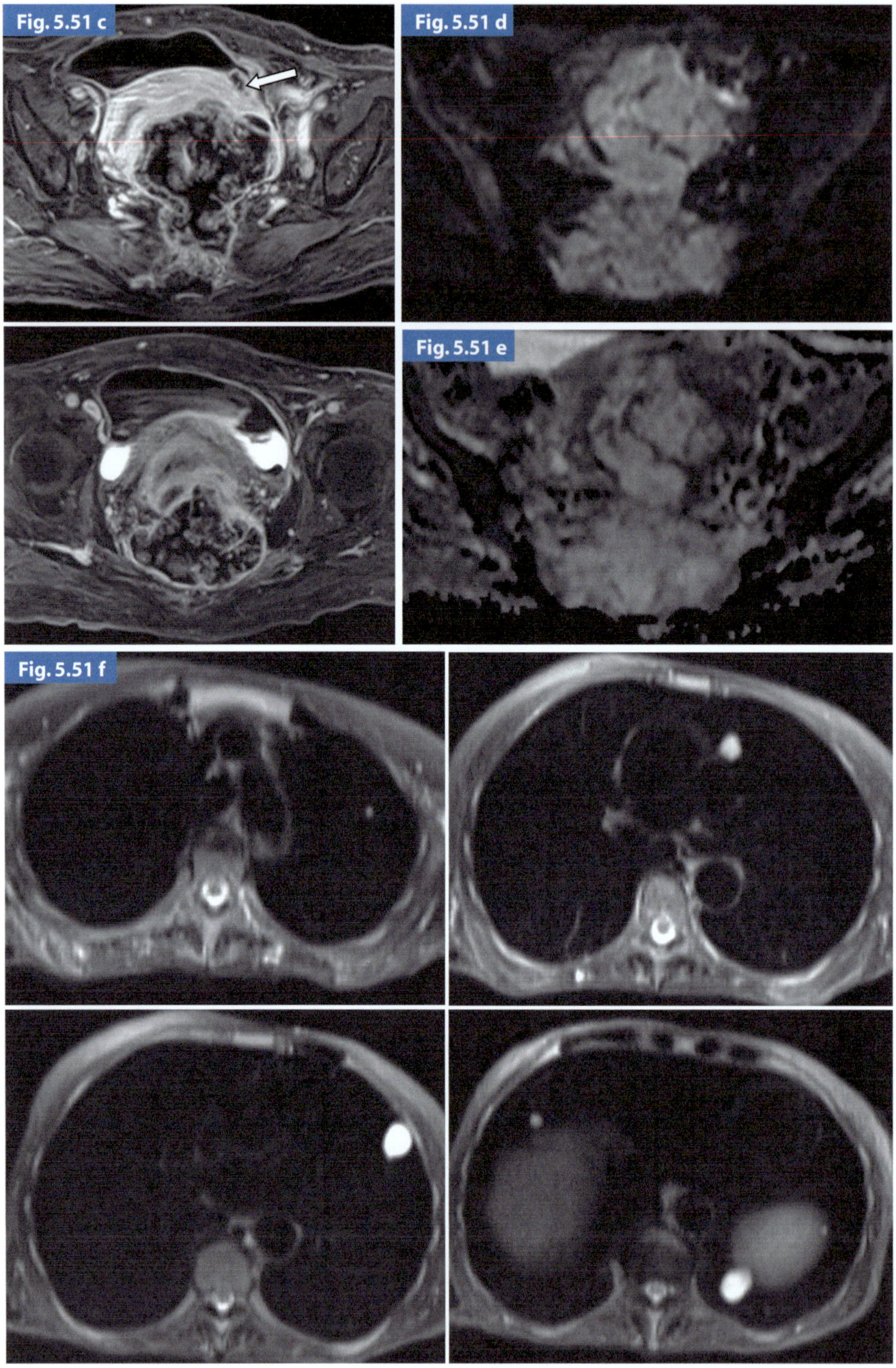
Fig. 5.51 c
Fig. 5.51 d
Fig. 5.51 e
Fig. 5.51 f

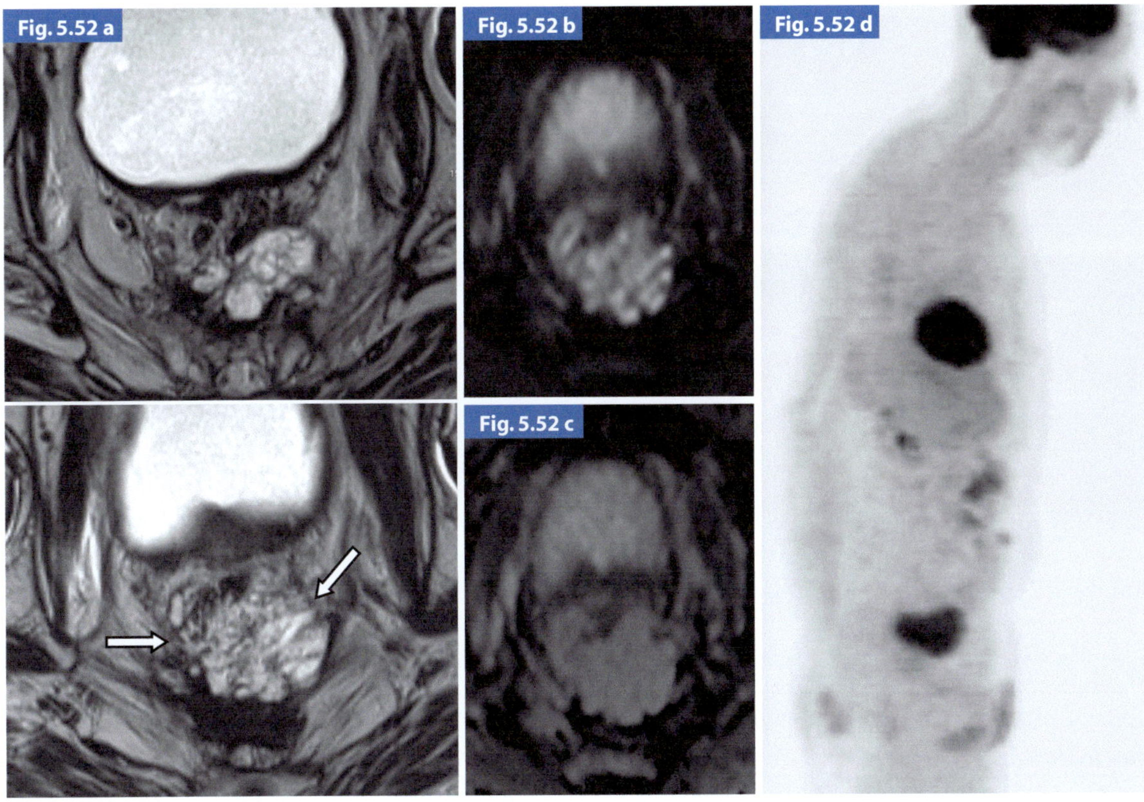

Fig. 5.52 (**a–d**) Recurrent mucinous rectal cancer. (**a**) On the para-axial T2-TSE images, a signal-rich, ill-defined mass can be identified within the low-signal presacral scar 12 years post-abdominoperineal resection of the rectum. The high signal is derived from mucin content of the lesion (*arrows*). This was confirmed by histopathology and is indicative of recurrent mucinous adenocarcinoma. Representative DWI slices ((**b**) DWI, b-value 500 s/mm^2, (**c**) ADC map) support the finding of a fluid containing tumor that was not detected by FDG-PET (**d**).

Fig. 5.53 Signet ring cell cancer of the rectum. Typical features of a signet ring cell carcinoma located in the lower rectum. (**a**) On T2-weighted sequences, the tumor normally causes diffuse thickening and signal decrease of all rectal wall layers. (**b**) On contrast agent-based sequences, the area of the tumor appears hypovascular, a finding that is contraindicative to inflammation.

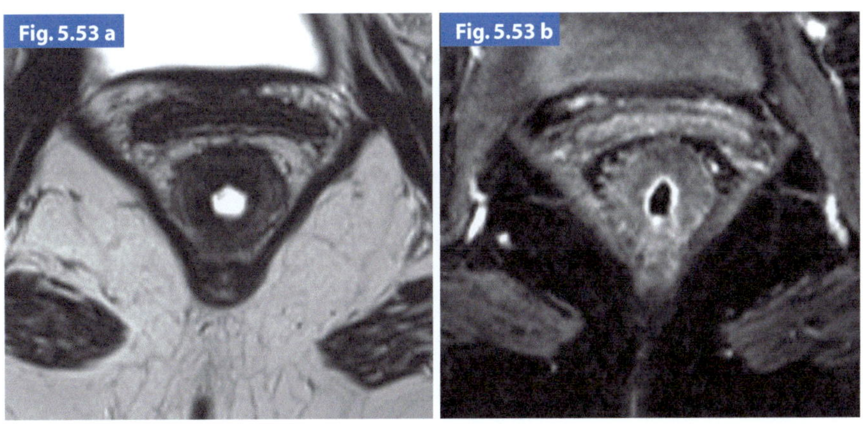

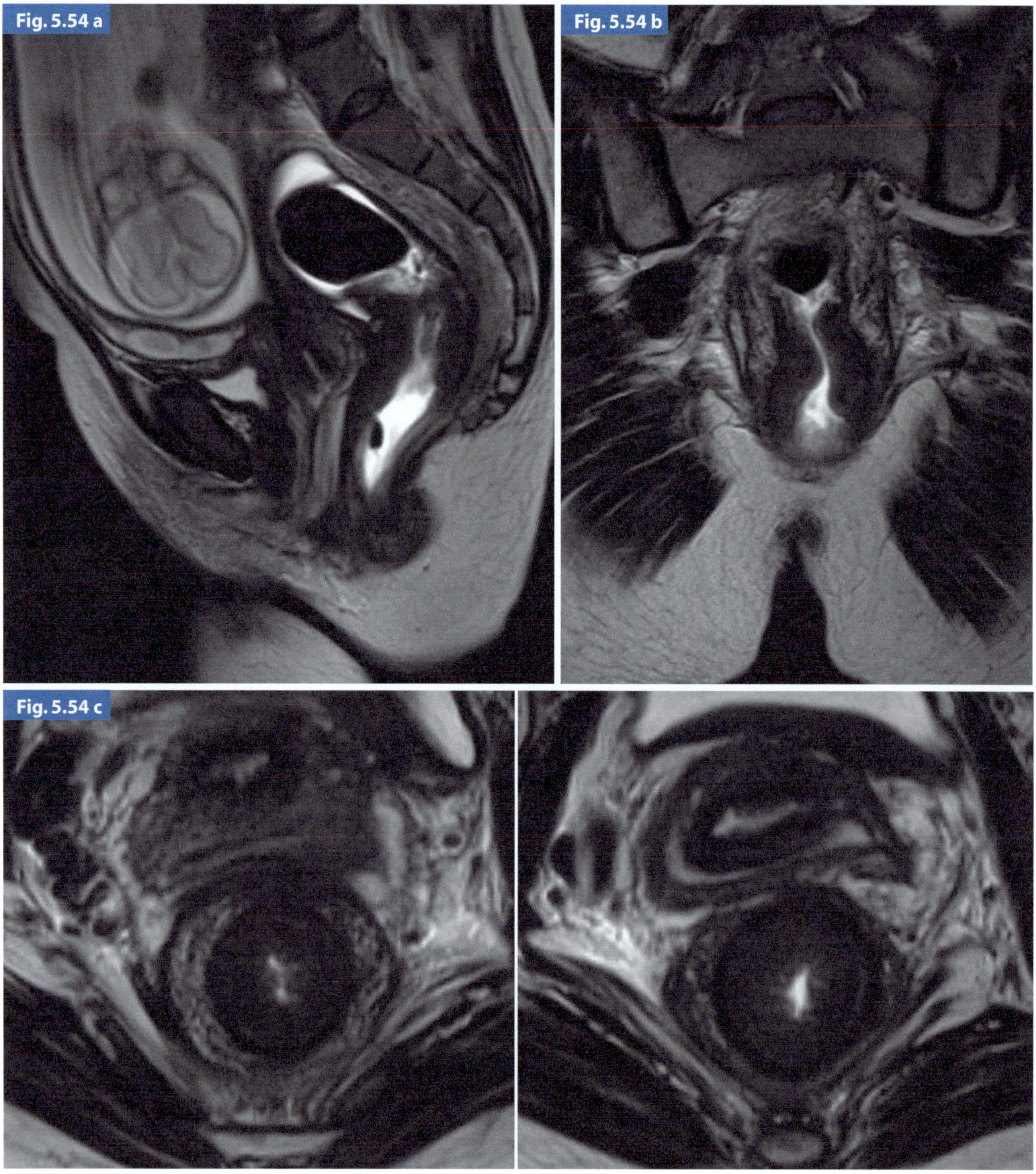

Fig. 5.54 (**a–c**) Signet ring cell cancer of the rectum. Patient history: A pregnant woman at 21 weeks gestation presented with progressive obstipation. Colonoscopy detected rectal stenosis and biopsies were taken. The sagittal (**a**) and coronal (**b**) T2-TSE images show a hypointense circular thickening of the midrectal wall. Furthermore, the normal high signal of the mesorectal fat is markedly reduced. (**c**) Representative axial T2-TSE images obtained right at the level of the high-grade rectal stenosis show the typical features of a signet ring cell carcinoma—signal drop and diffuse wall thickening. Moreover, the mesorectal fat is infiltrated mimicking fibrosis.

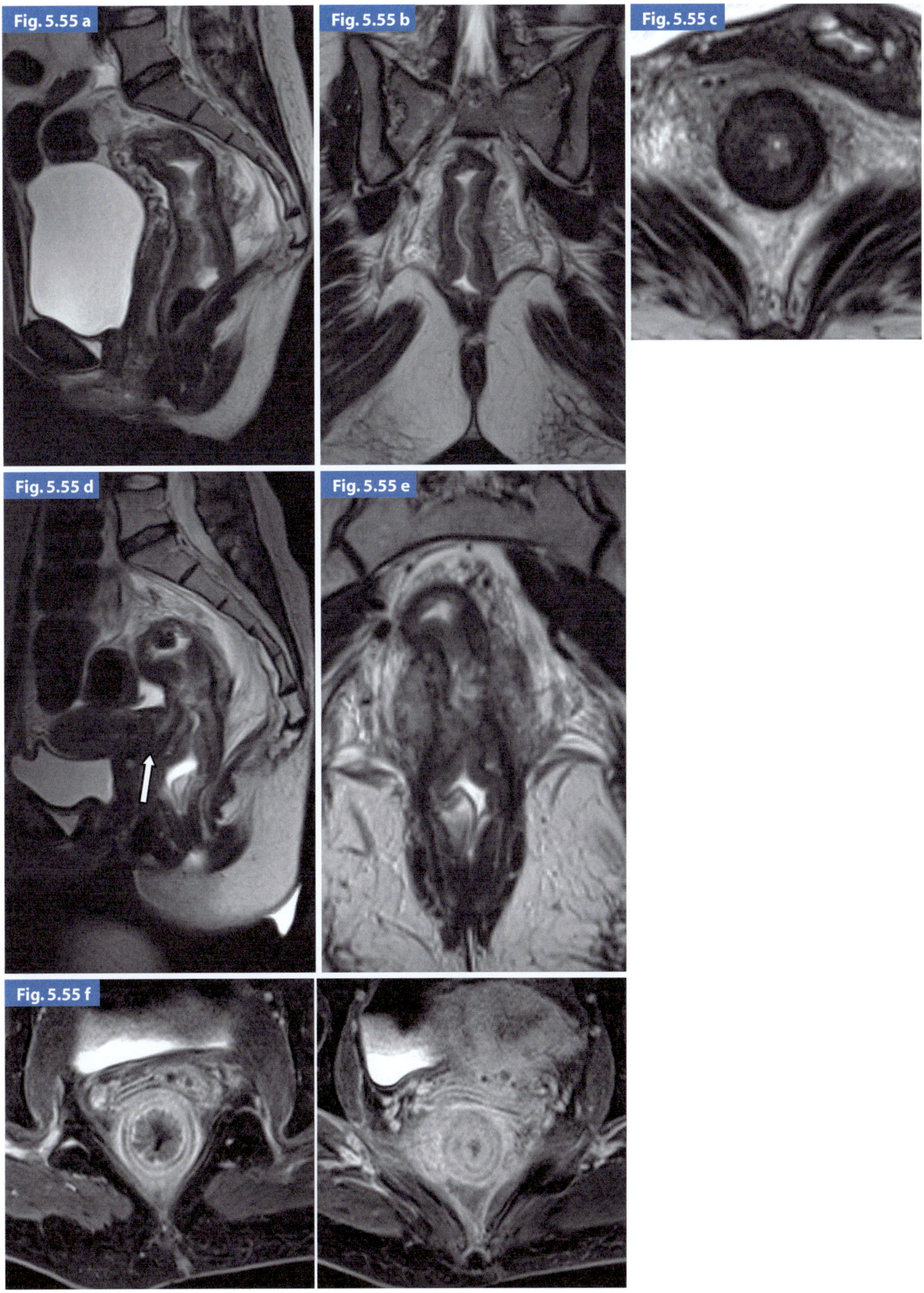
Fig. 5.55 a
Fig. 5.55 b
Fig. 5.55 c
Fig. 5.55 d
Fig. 5.55 e
Fig. 5.55 f

Fig. 5.55 g

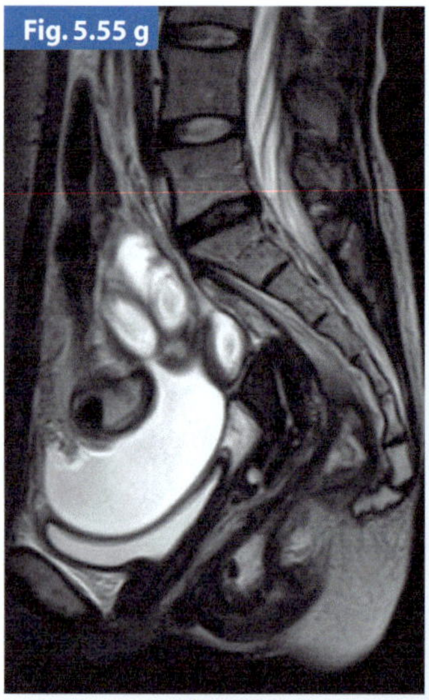

Fig. 5.55 h

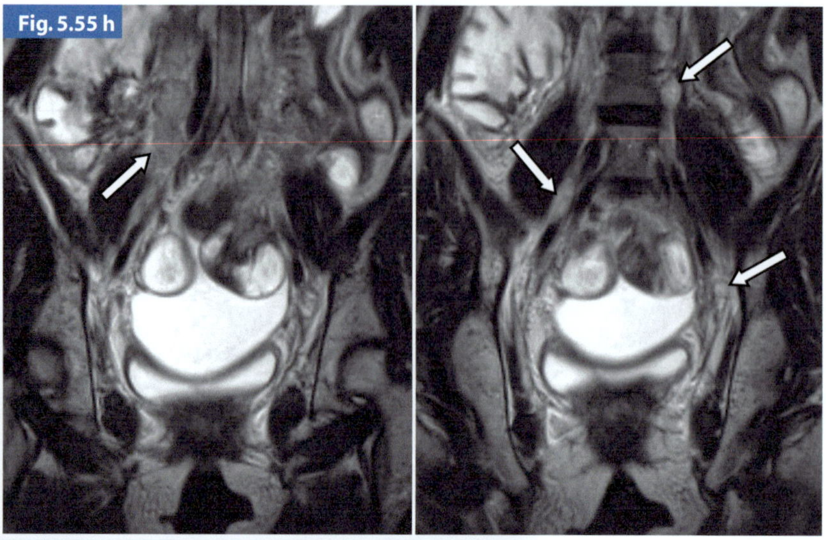

Fig. 5.55 i

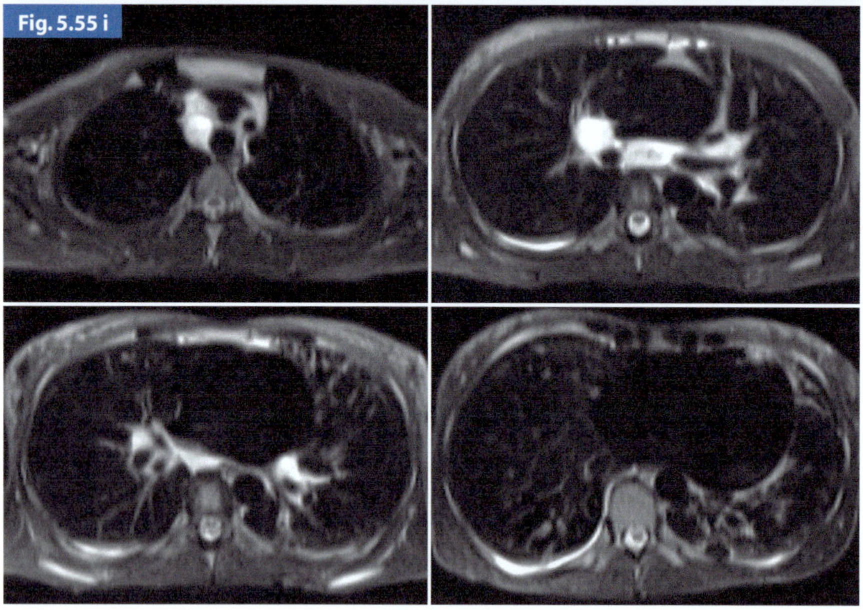

Fig. 5.55 Signet ring cell cancer of the rectum. Patient history: A 28-year-old female with progressive obstipation and anal pain. (**a–c**) Pretreatment MRI, May 2008. The sagittal (**a**), coronal (**b**), and para-axial (**c**) T2-TSE images clearly show an extensive rectal tumor with mural and extramural invasion causing rectal stenosis. The tumor provokes almost homogeneous wall thickening. Histopathologic evaluation confirmed the suspected diagnosis of a signet ring cell carcinoma. (**d–f**) Post-neoadjuvant therapy MRI, August 2008. The sagittal (**d**) and para-coronal (**e**) T2-TSE images demonstrate only partial response of the signet ring cell carcinoma to chemoradiation. In particular, the supra-anal and upper rectal portions of the tumor remained unchanged as is indicated by their low-signal intensity. In addition, tumor ingrowth into the vagina can be newly diagnosed (*arrow*). (**f**) Axial CE-VIBE 3D images obtained at the level of the lower mesorectum depict a hypovascular tumor confined to the rectal wall associated with a marked peritumorous inflammation obscuring the true extent of the disease. (**g–i**) Postoperative follow-up MRI, October 2008. Sagittal (**g**) and coronal (**h**) views show ascites, the rectal stump, and extensive nodal metastasis involving the iliac axis on both sides and the retroperitoneum (*arrows*). (**i**) The axial free-breathing TIRM images derived from the SMS moving-table staging show additional spread to the mediastinal and hilar lymph nodes. Lymphangiitis carcinomatosa is also present. Comment: Palliative abdominoperineal resection of the rectum was performed in September. During surgery, extensive peritoneal carcinosis and nodal tumor spread were found. Vaginal invasion was confirmed. The histopathologic stage was ypT4N1M1 (PER, LYM). In December 2008, the patient died of tumor-associated cachexia, only 6 months after initial diagnosis.

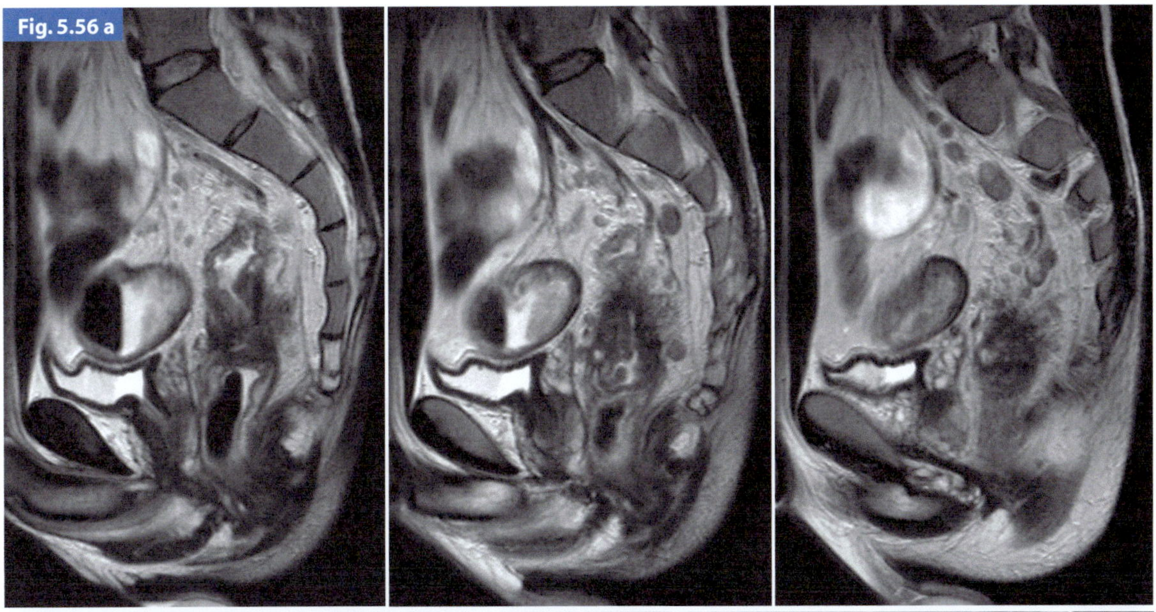
Fig. 5.56 a

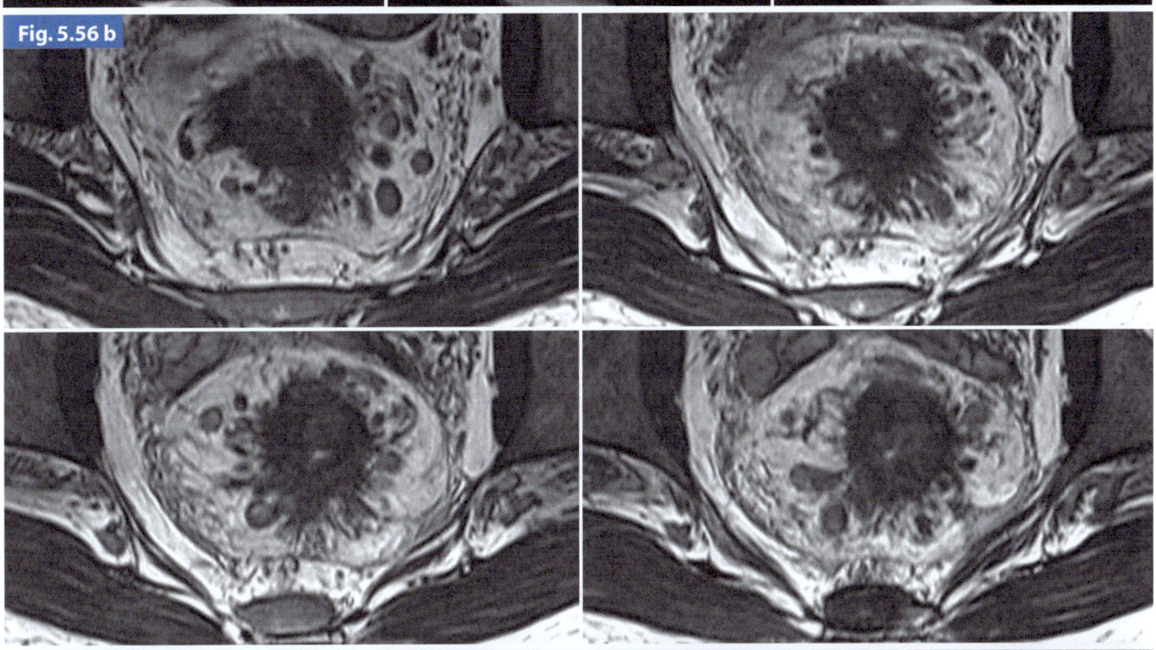
Fig. 5.56 b

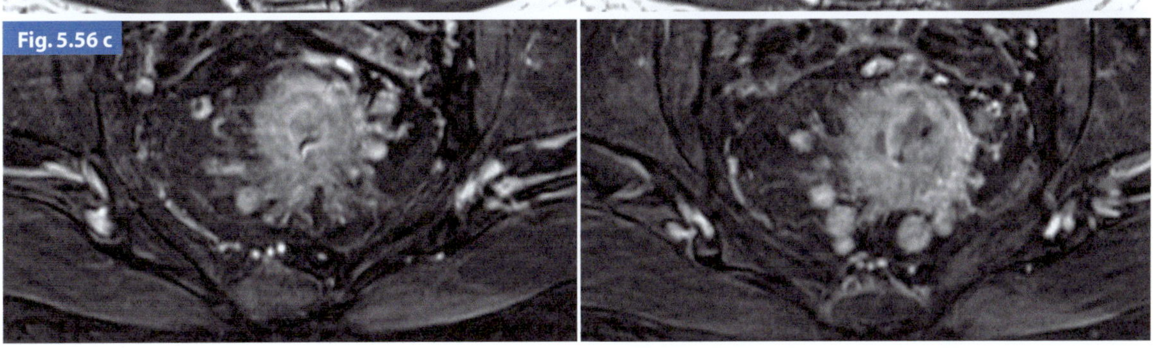
Fig. 5.56 c

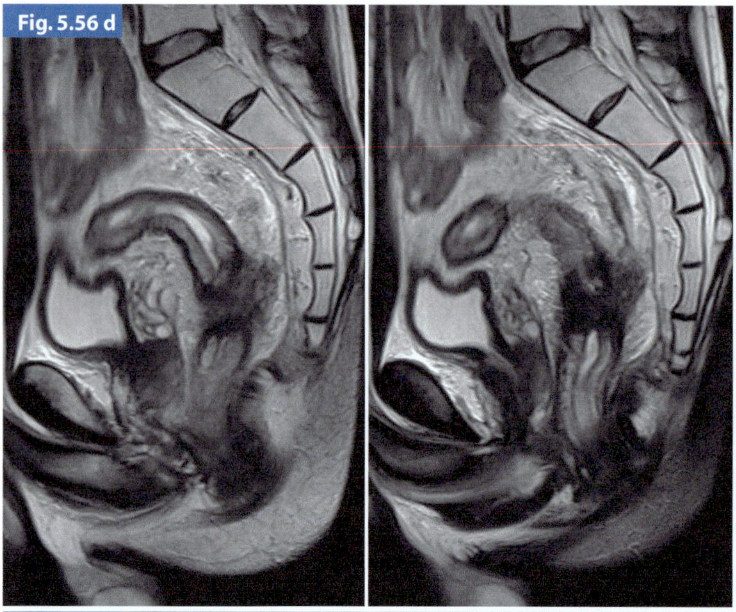
Fig. 5.56 d

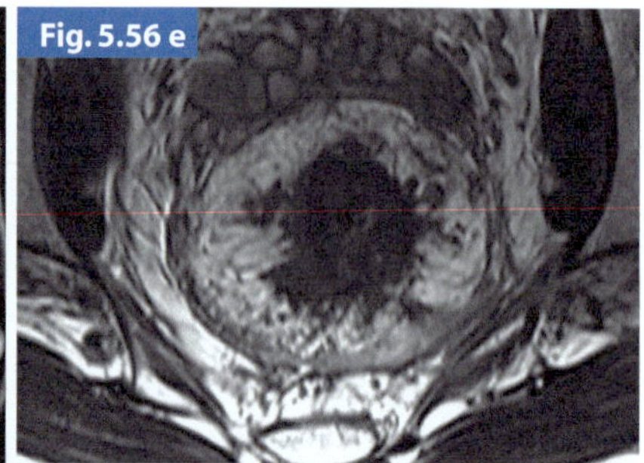
Fig. 5.56 e

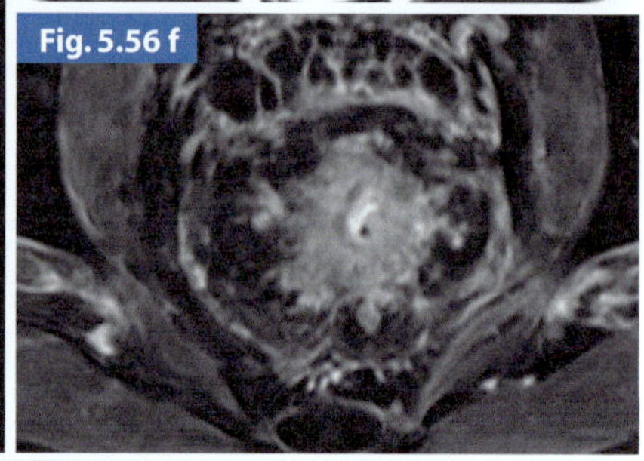
Fig. 5.56 f

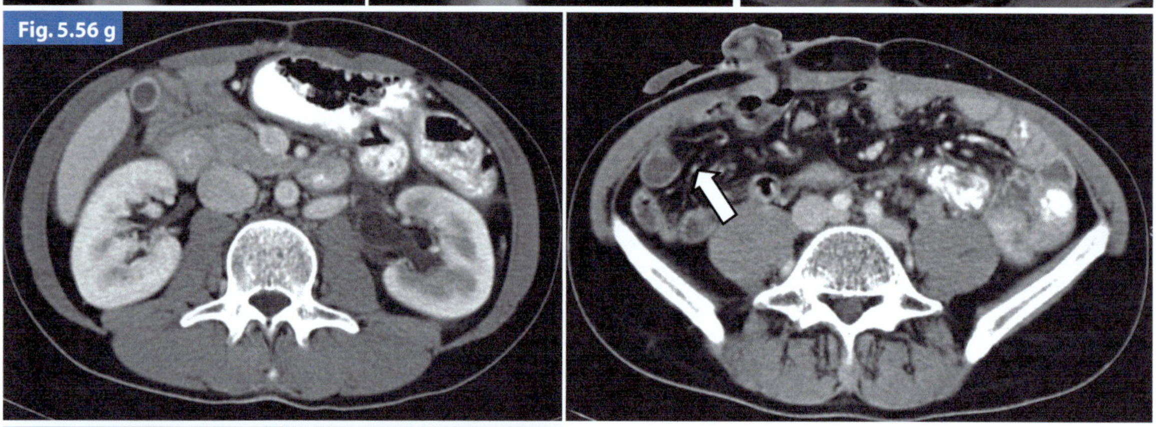
Fig. 5.56 g

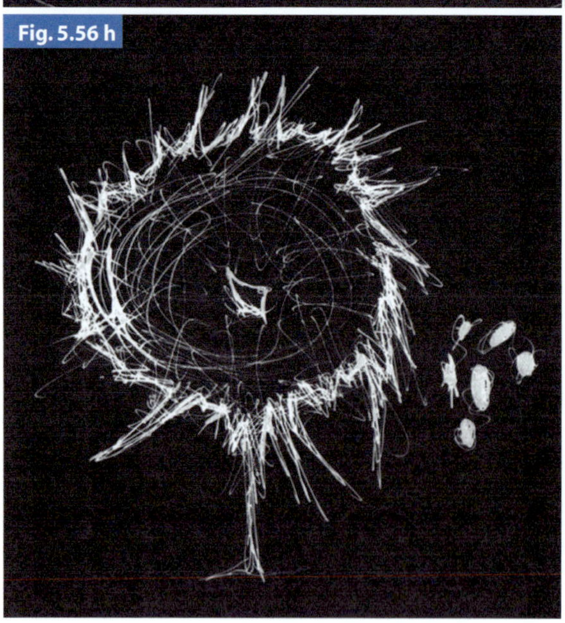
Fig. 5.56 h

Fig. 5.56 Stage T3 signet-ring cell carcinoma of the rectum. (**a–c**) Pretreatment MRI. (**a**) The sagittal T2-TSE images illustrate an advanced midrectal carcinoma with numerous metastatic nodes within the mesorectum. On the axial CISS-3D images (**b**) and corresponding axial CE-VIBE 3D images (**c**), the stenosing carcinoma has metastasized to the perimuscular fat. Parts of the pathologic nodes and the mesorectal tumor deposits are close to the circumferential resection margin. (**d–f**) Post-neoadjuvant radiochemotherapy MRI. Sagittal T2-TSE images (**d**), axial CISS-3D (**e**), and CE-VIBE 3D (**f**) images. (**g**) Follow-up MSCT scan. Therapy resulted in a slight decrease in the size of the tumor and regression of the nodal burden inside the mesorectum. However, the area exceeding the wall remained unchanged. Abdominal staging CT revealed left hydronephrosis resulting from metastasis to the ureter (*arrow*). Patient history: Longstanding ulcerative colitis. Status after subtotal colectomy and ileostomy: Following neoadjuvant therapy, an intersphincter resection with left nephrectomy was performed. Histopathology revealed stage ypT3N2M1(ureter, peritoneum) G3 signet-ring cell carcinoma. (**h**) Ink drawing: Signet-ring cell carcinoma.

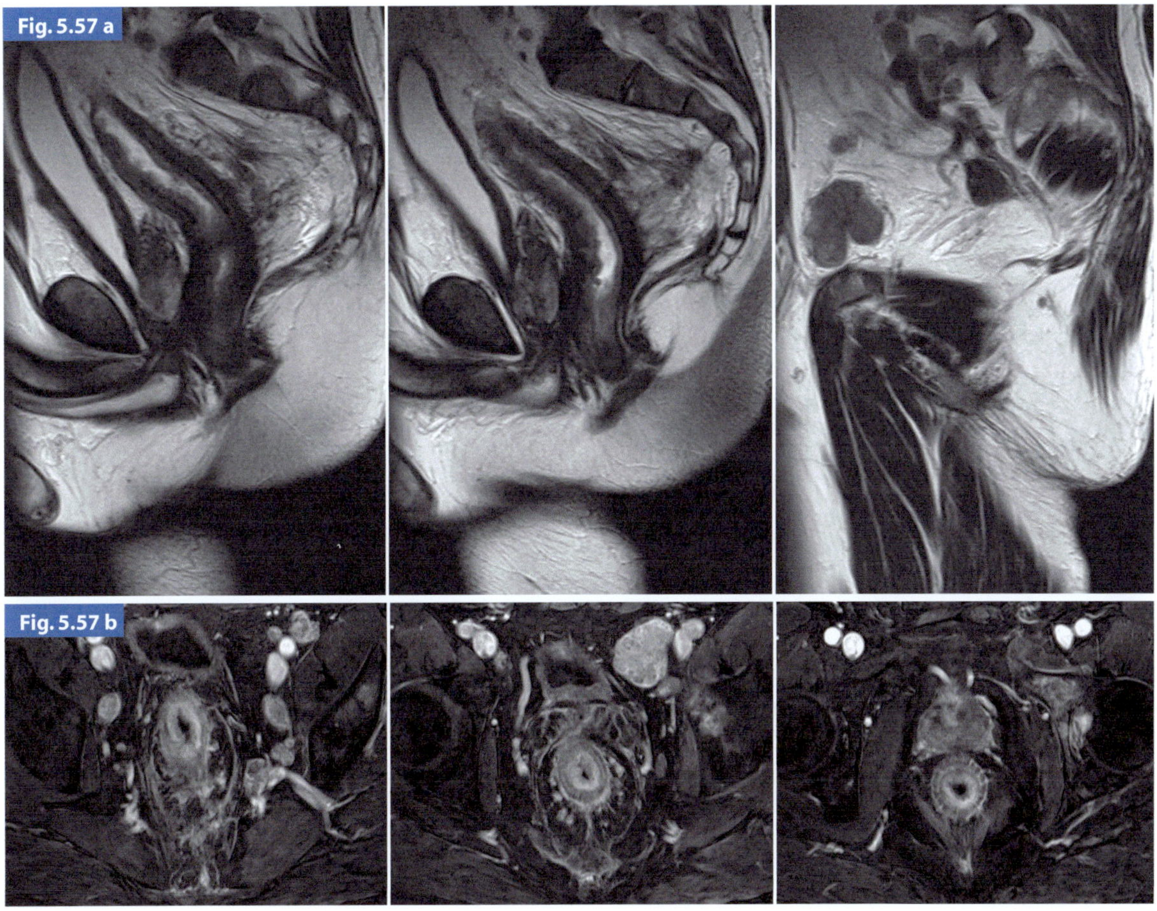

Fig. 5.57 (**a**, **b**) Stage T3 signet-ring cell carcinoma of the rectum. (**a**) Sagittal T2-TSE images show a wall-exceeding low-signal intensity tumor that involves the entire rectum, highly indicative of linitis plastica carcinoma. The tumor has spread to the left iliac nodes as is seen by the chain-like distribution of the lymph node metastases. (**b**) Axial CE-VIBE 3D images show tumor infiltration of the mesorectal fat and a thickening of the mesorectal fascia either on the basis of desmoplastic reaction or as a result of tumor invasion. In addition to the sagittal views, metastatic right iliac nodes and left acetabular bone metastasis are apparent.

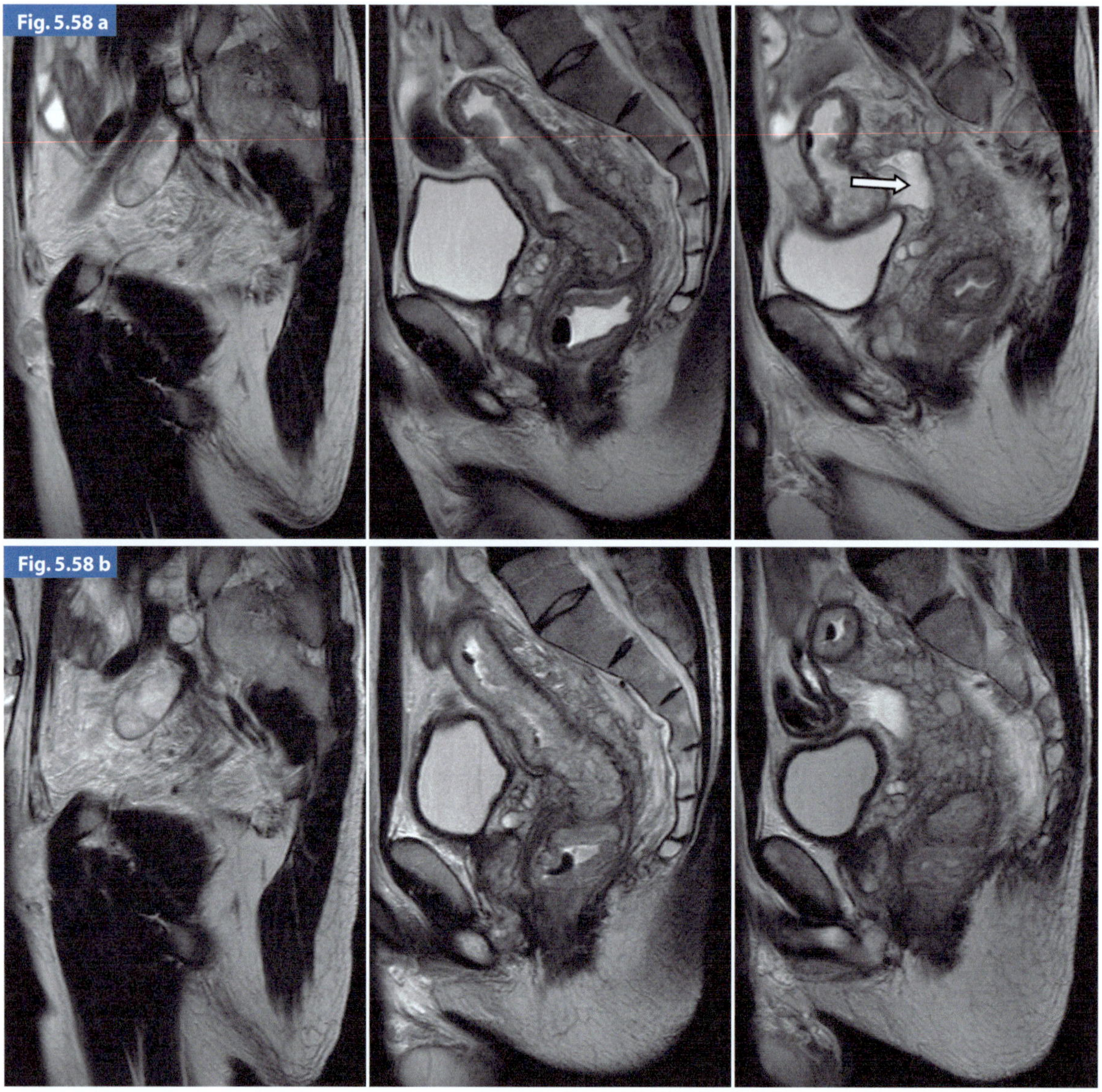

Fig. 5.58 (**a**, **b**) Stage T4 rectal cancer. (**a**) Pretreatment MRI sagittal T2-TSE images show an Advanced high-signal intensity tumor involving the whole rectum, the mesorectum, the peritoneum and the iliac axis on both sides is seen on the sagittal (**a**) T2-TSE images. The mesorectum is filled with cystic tumor masses. Ascites (*arrow*), indicative of peritoneal carcinosis (**b**) Post-neoadjuvant therapy MRI. On the sagittal (**b**) T2-TSE images tumor progress is evident. Patient history: Staging laparoscopy confirmed peritoneal carcinosis as well as hepatic metastases. Biopsy revealed a poorly differentiated signet ring cell carcinoma. Protective ileostomy and a sigmoid mucous fistula were created. The combination of the wall-exceeding tumor, peritoneal infiltration, iliac and retroperitoneal lymph node metastases, and hepatic metastases led to the clinical stage cT4N2M1. Comment: At first appearance, the histopathologic diagnosis of a signet ring cell carcinoma contradicts the signal characteristics of the tumor and its metastases on MRI. However, the extent of rectal wall infiltration and mesorectal tumor load, the shape of the involved rectum resembling linitis plastica, and the concomitant peritoneal seeding are features of signet ring cell cancer. The dedifferentiation of the carcinoma may have contributed to a modification of the MR signal.

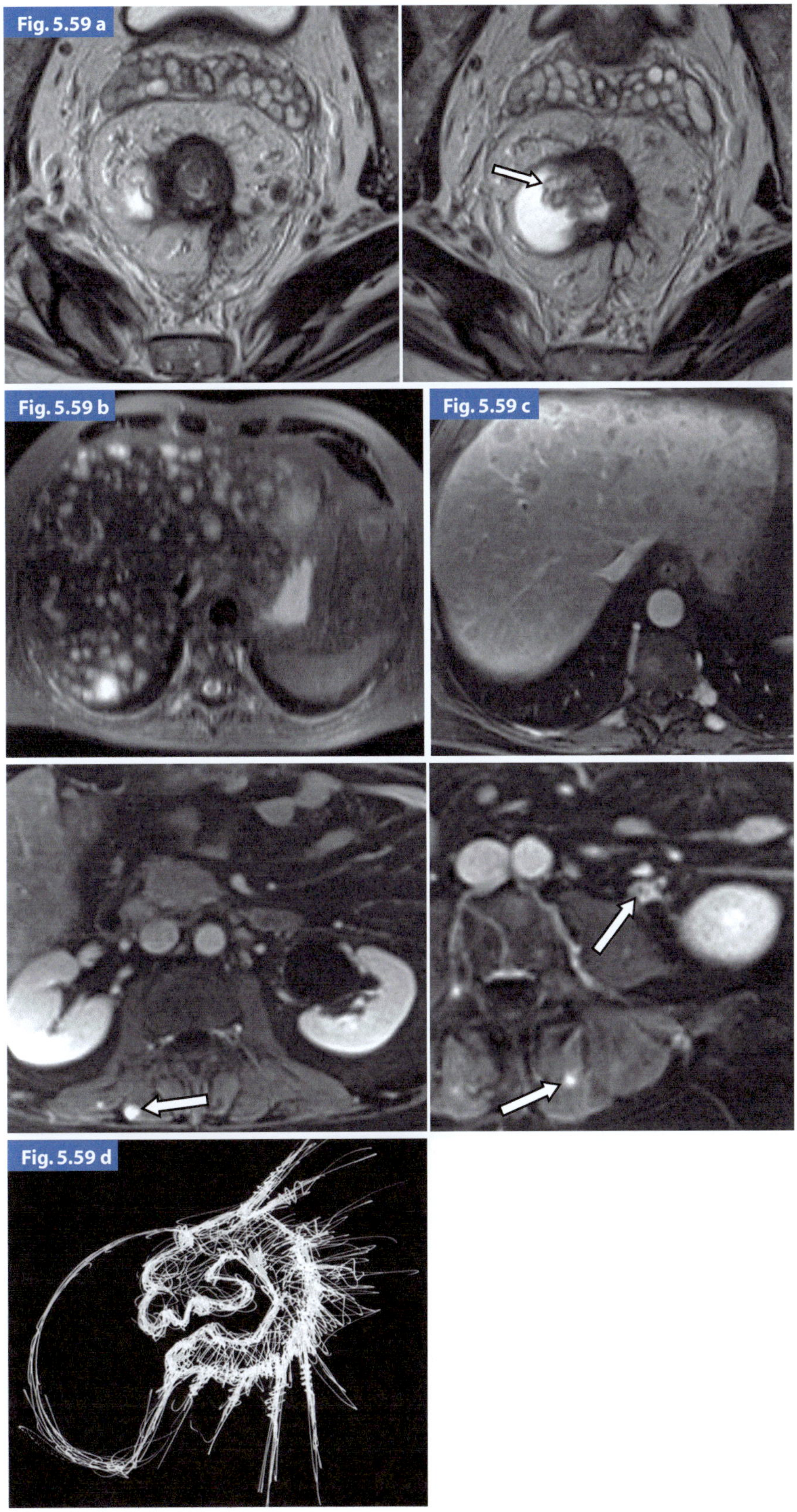

Fig. 5.59 Small cell neuroendocrine cancer of the rectum. (**a**) Para-axial T2-TSE images reveal advanced rectal cancer with invasion of the mesorectal fat and mesorectal nodal spread. The tumor contains a signal-rich luminal portion that resembles tubulovillous adenoma (*arrow*) as well as a wall-exceeding part with intermediate signal intensity. Axial TIRM image (**b**) and corresponding axial CE-FLASH-2D images (**c**) derived from moving-table M-staging show extensive liver metastasis, concomitant bone metastases, soft tissue metastasis (*arrows*), and an infiltration of the left ureter (*arrow*) causing hydronephrosis at initial presentation. (**d**) Ink drawing: Wall-exceeding neuroendocrine carcinoma.

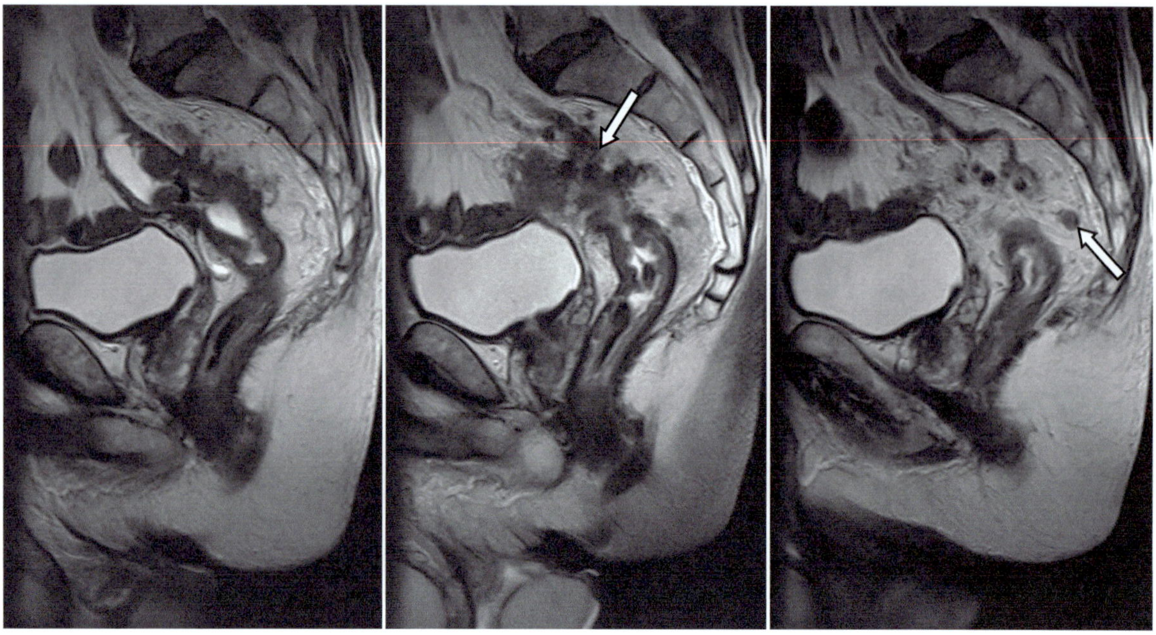

Fig. 5.60 Stage T3 rectal cancer. Sagittal T2-TSE images reveal negative prognostic features of rectal cancer such as extramural venous invasion and more than three mesorectal lymph node metastases (*arrows*), which are associated with clinical stage V2N2. Histopathology diagnosed stage pT3N2M1 (liver) L1V1 rectal cancer.

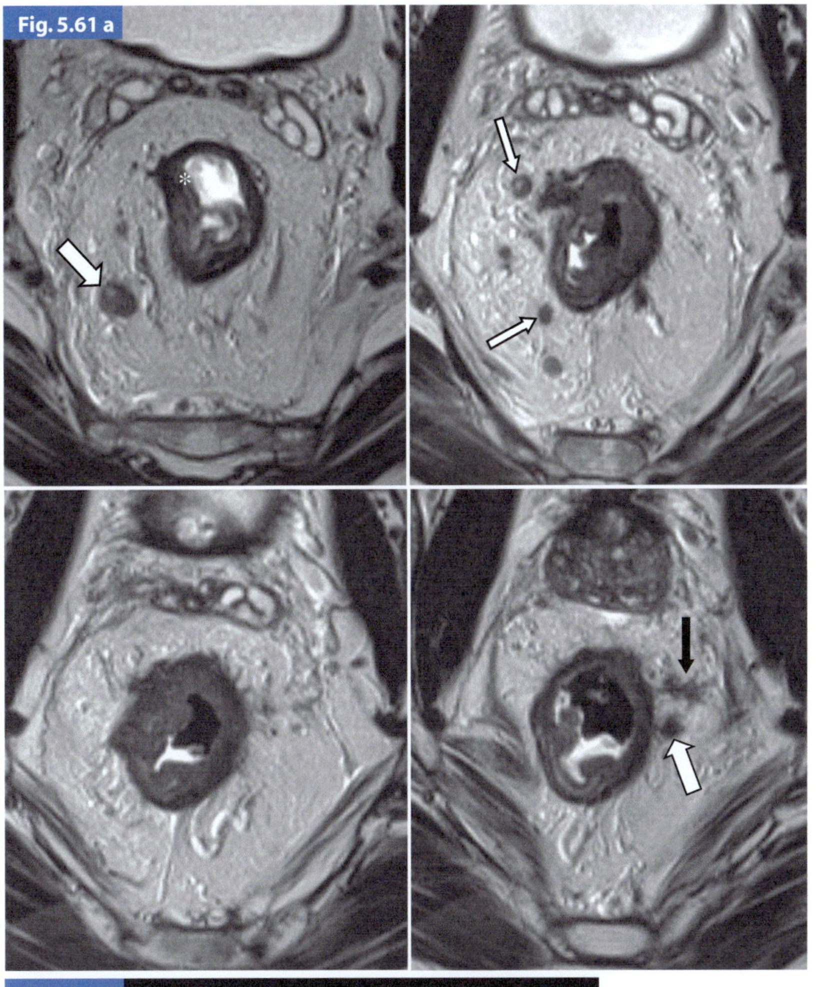

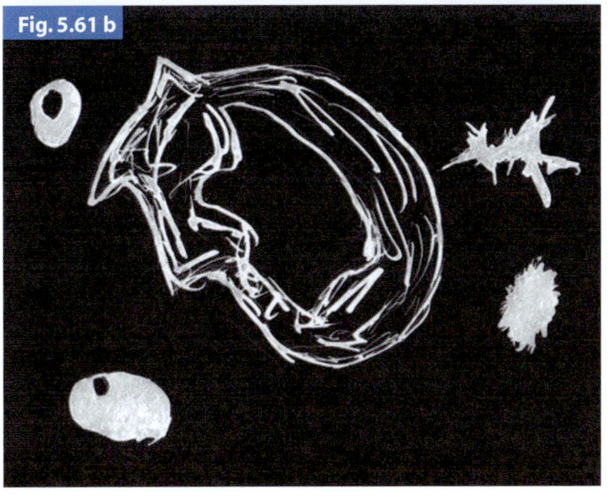

Fig. 5.61 Stage T3 rectal cancer. (**a**) Preoperative MRI, axial (A) T2-TSE images show a stenosing carcinoma with circular growth, tumor exulceration, and wall penetration. The irregular shape and signal inhomogeneities of the surrounding mesorectal nodes are signs of metastatic involvement (*white arrows*). Additionally, a typical mesorectal tumor deposit is demonstrated with irregular shape and low-signal intensity (*black arrow*). The histopathologic stage was diagnosed as pT3N2M1 (liver) G2. (**b**) Ink drawing: Features of metastatic lymph nodes and tumor deposit.

Fig. 5.62 a

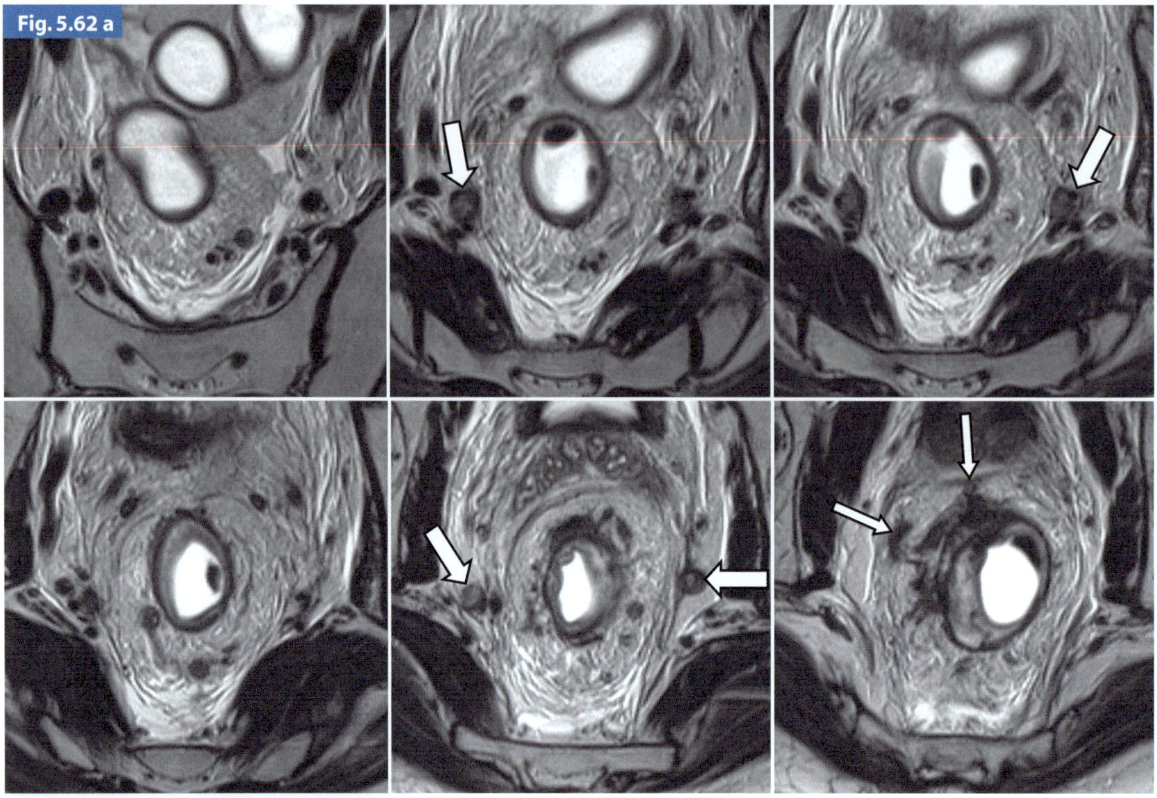

Fig. 5.62 b

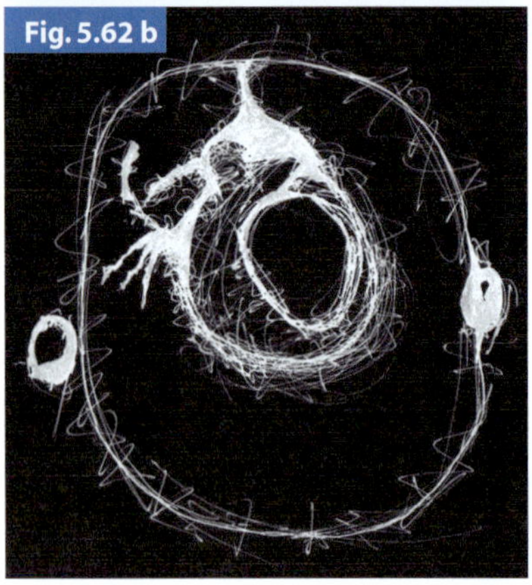

Fig. 5.62 Stage T3 rectal cancer. (**a**) Para-axial T2-TSE images display status post-neoadjuvant radiochemotherapy and show the presence of nodal metastases within the mesorectum and along the internal iliac vessels on both sides (*arrows*). Additionally, venous infiltration and involvement of the Denonvilliers' fascia is visible (*small arrows*). (**b**) Ink drawing: Perimesorectal nodal disease, extramural venous invasion.

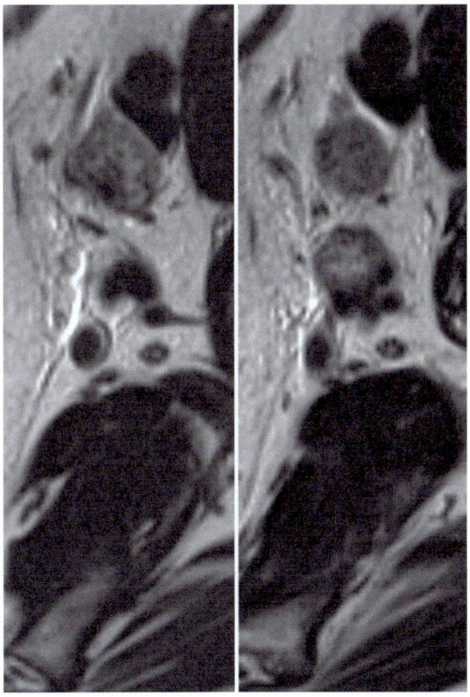

Fig. 5.63 Pelvic sidewall nodes. The axial T2-TSE images display left iliac lymph node metastases presenting with inhomogenous signal intensity and irregular borders.

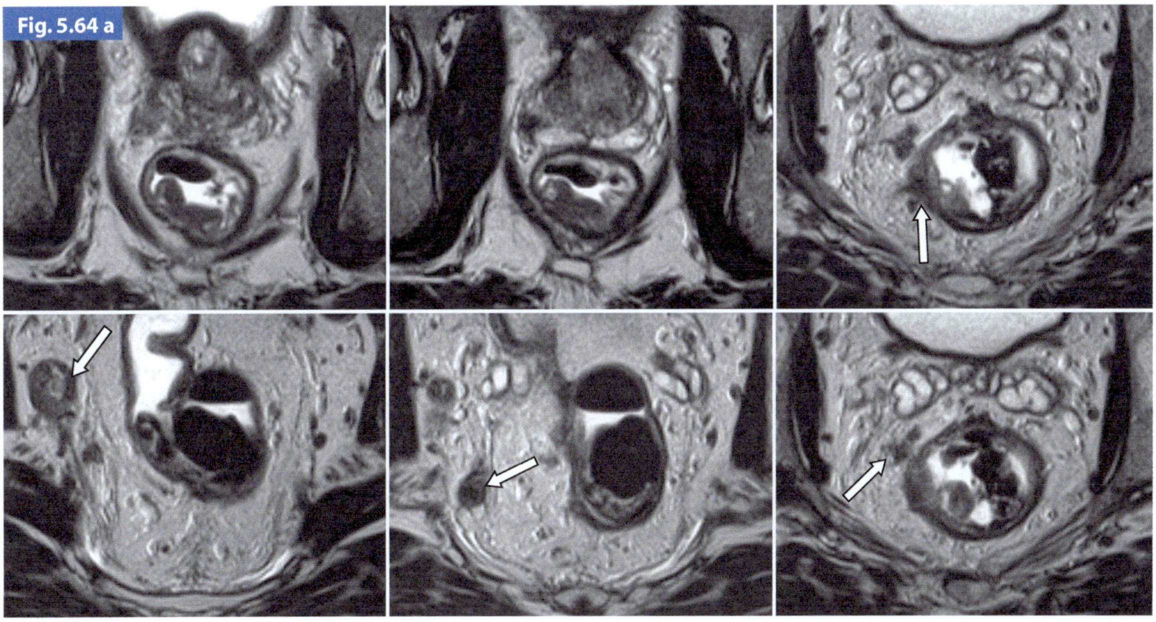

Fig. 5.64 Stage pT1 rectal cancer. Course of the disease. (**a**) pretreatment MRI, September 2007. Rectal cancer with intramural spread. Two different locations of the cancer can be seen on the para-axial (**a**) T2-TSE images, a clinical stage T2 tumor arising from the lower rectum and a second tumor originating from the wall of the midrectum. The upper focus is infiltrating the perimuscular fat and was therefore clinically staged as T3 (*arrow*). Additionally, the axial T2-TSE images reveal negative prognostic patterns associated with rectal cancer: first, suspicious right pelvic sidewall lymph nodes due to their size, signal inhomogeneity, and irregular borders (*arrows*), second, extramural venous invasion at 10 o'clock lithotomy position (*arrow*).

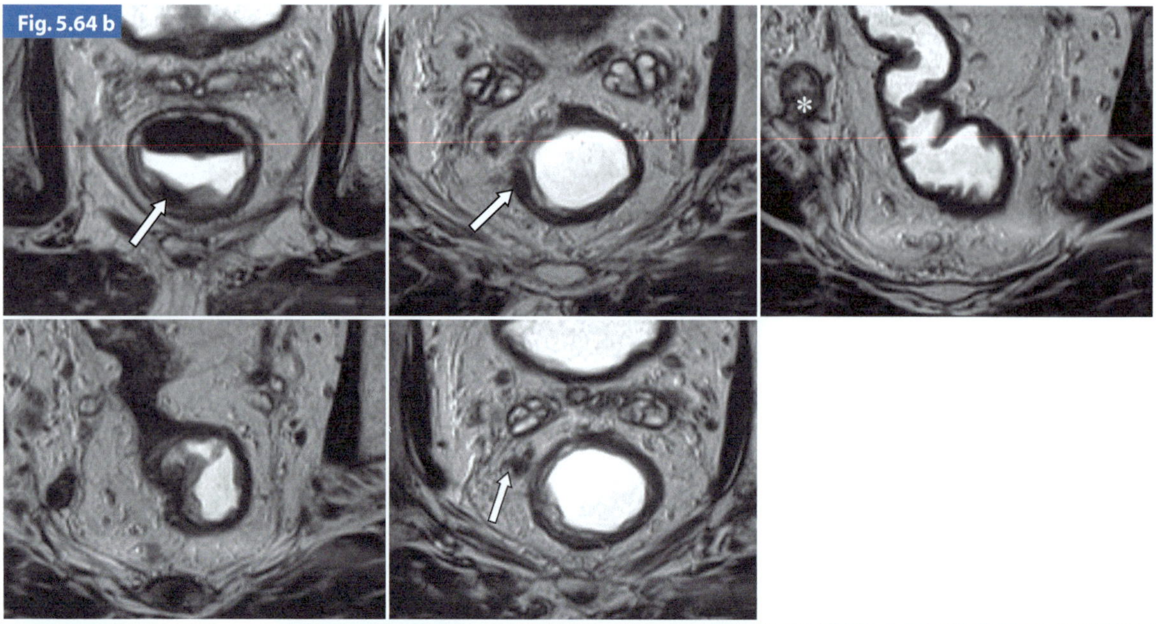

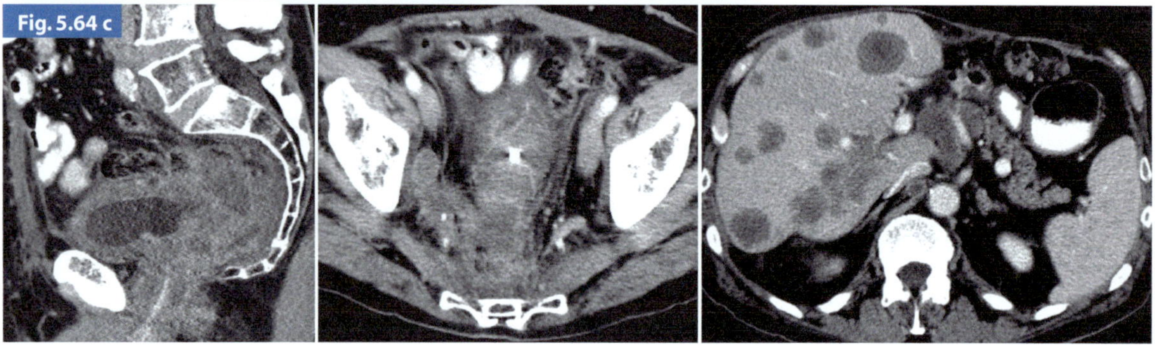

Fig. 5.64 (**b**) post-neoadjuvant therapy MRI, November 2007. Compared to the initial MRI, tumor shrinkage and fibrosis is evident on the para-axial (**b**) T2-TSE images as a result of chemoradiation (*arrows*). In contrast, the pelvic sidewall nodes and the venous invasion remain unchanged (*asterisk*, *arrow*). The initial MRI in September identified more than three mesorectal lymph node metastases and the control MRI in November also revealed liver metastasis, (not illustrated). Patient history: In December 2007 abdominoperineal resection without right pelvic lymphadenectomy was performed. In February 2008 additional anatomical resections of the liver segments 2 and 3 and an atypical resection of the segment 4 was done. At histopathologic examination, the rectal cancer was classified as ypT1N2L1V1M1 (liver) R0. (**c**) Follow-up CT, June 2008. During follow-up CT detects tumor dissemination. The local tumor relapse involves the entire sacral hollow down to the perineal scar seen on the sagittal reformatted image. The tumor recurrence directly invades the urinary bladder, the prostate, the seminal vesicles and the right pelvic sidewall at the level of the lymph nodes described in the initial MRI. In addition, nodal metastases around the celiac trunk and an extensive liver metastasis are present.

5.7 Recurrent Rectal Cancer

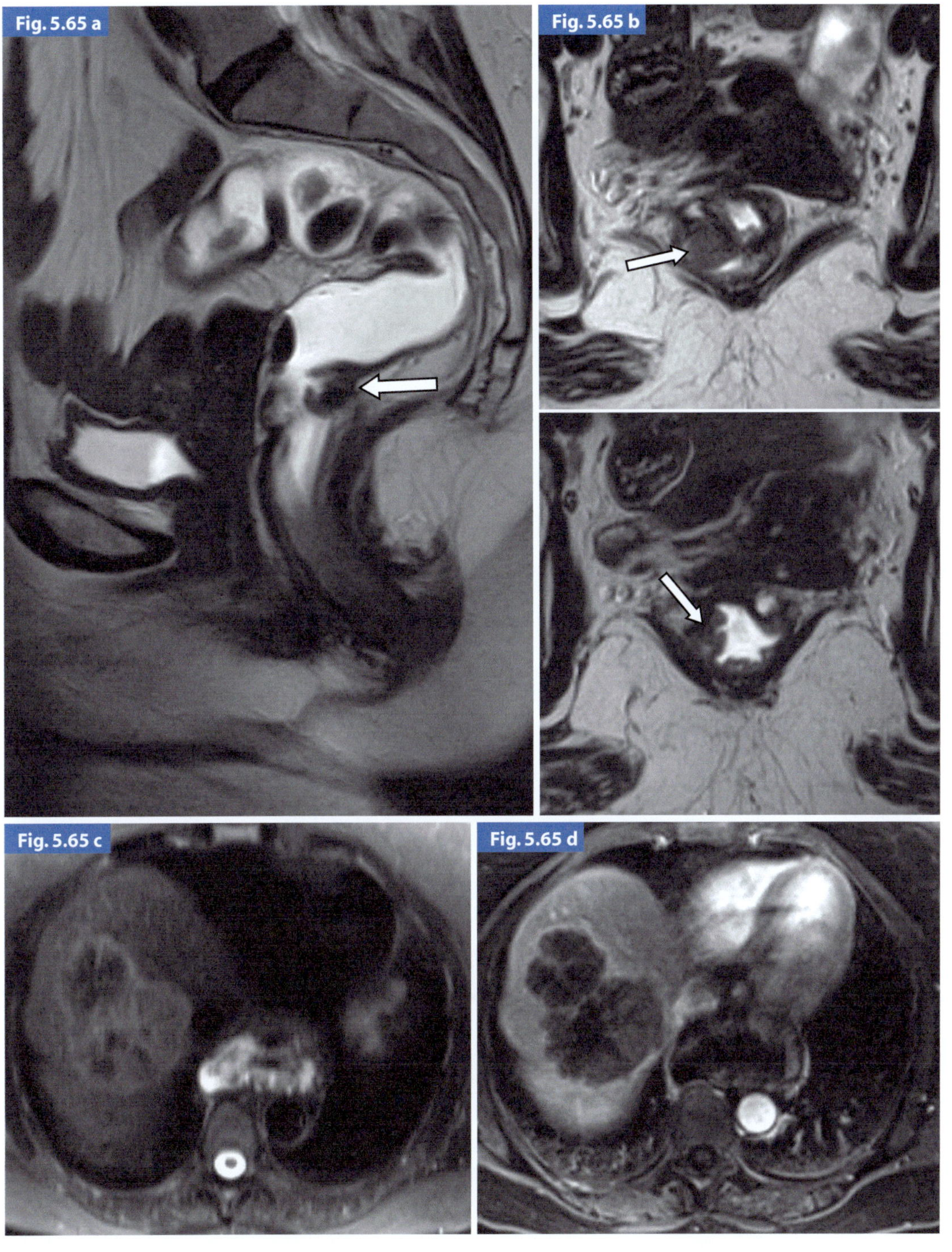

Fig. 5.65 Course of the disease. Sagittal (**a**) and para-axial (**b**) T2-TSE images show polypoid luminal recurrence with central ulceration at the site of the anastomosis after rectal cancer resection (*arrows*). Axial free-breathing TIRM images (**c**) and corresponding axial CE-FLASH 2D images (**d**) from the moving-table M-staging reveal extensive liver metastasis as well as axial hernia.

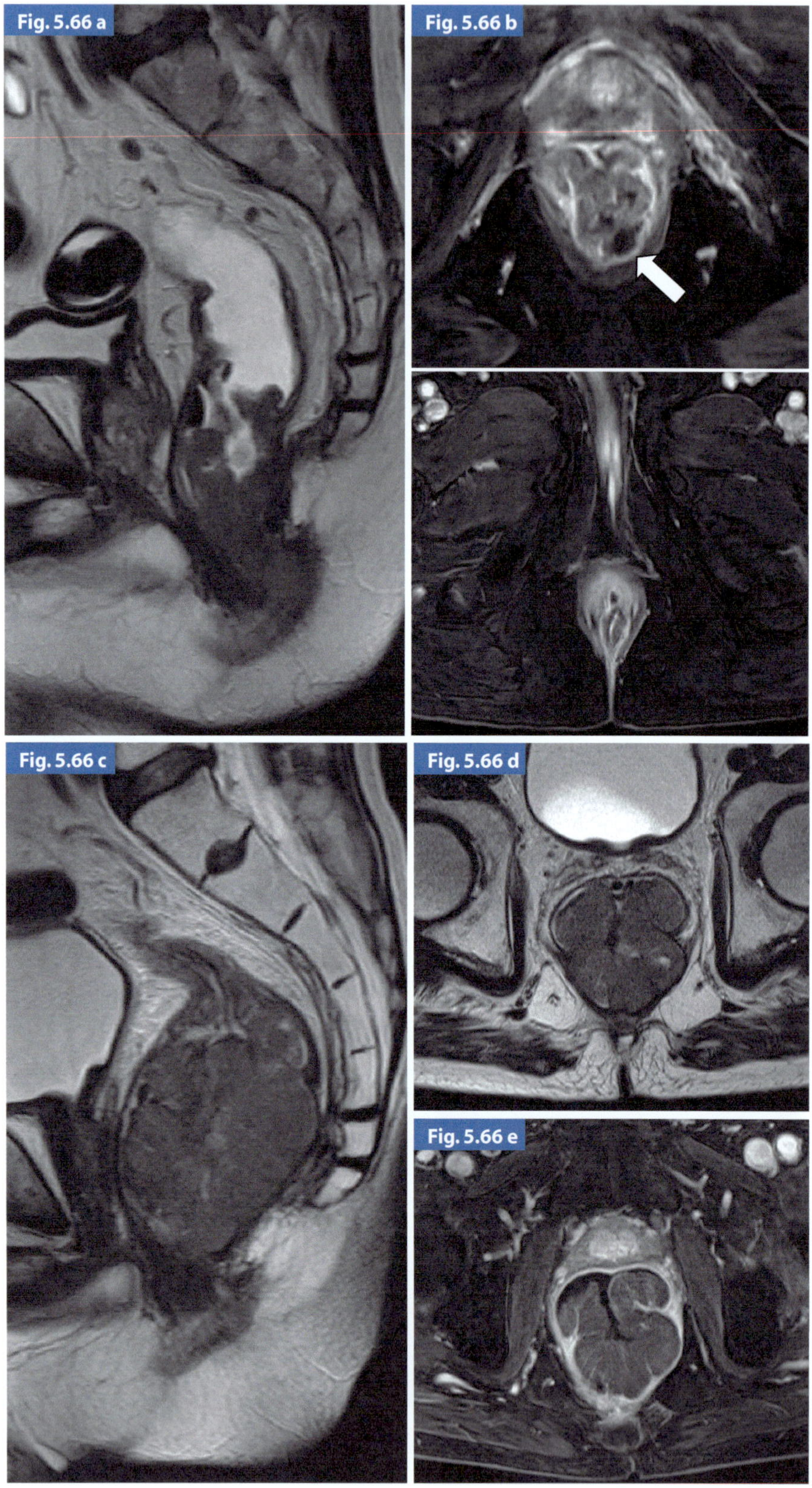

Fig. 5.66 Course of the disease. Patient history: Carcinoma of the lower rectum with infiltration of the anal channel diagnosed in 2004 and clinically staged as cT3N1. Neoadjuvant radiochemotherapy was performed. The patient refused abdominoperineal resection and only agreed to TEM, which was carried out in April 2005. In November 2005, the patient was readmitted with transanal bleeding resulting from local recurrence. Extensive hepatic metastasis was coexistent and a palliative sigmoidostomy was created. (**a**, **b**) Pretreatment MRI: October 2004. On the sagittal T2-TSE image (**a**) and the corresponding axial CE-VIBE 3D images (**b**), a stenosing tumor of the lower rectum can be seen invading the anal channel. At the level of the anorectal junction, the tumor shows wall-exceeding growth (*arrow*). (**c**–**e**) Posttreatment MRI: November 2005. The sagittal (**c**) and axial (**d**) T2-TSE images and the corresponding axial CE-VIBE 3D image (**e**) reveal subtotally stenosing local tumor recurrence with extensive involvement of the mesorectum.

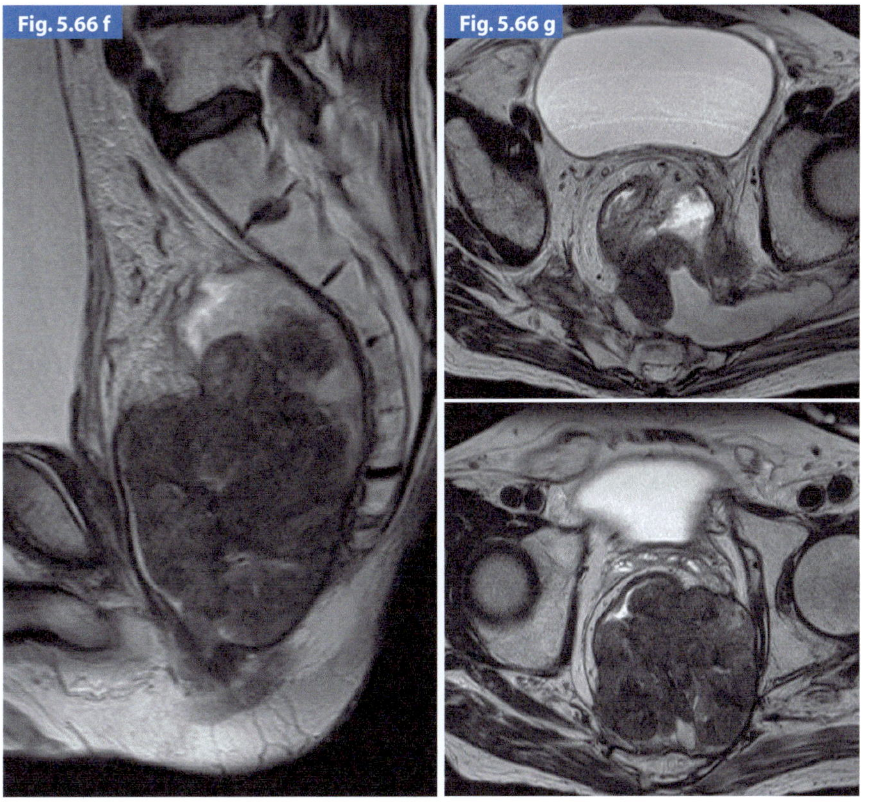

Fig. 5.66 (**f**, **g**) Control MRI: June 2006. The sagittal (**f**) and axial (**g**) T2-TSE images expose tumor perforation with abscess development in the left sciadic foramen. The mesorectum is also completely occupied by tumor masses.

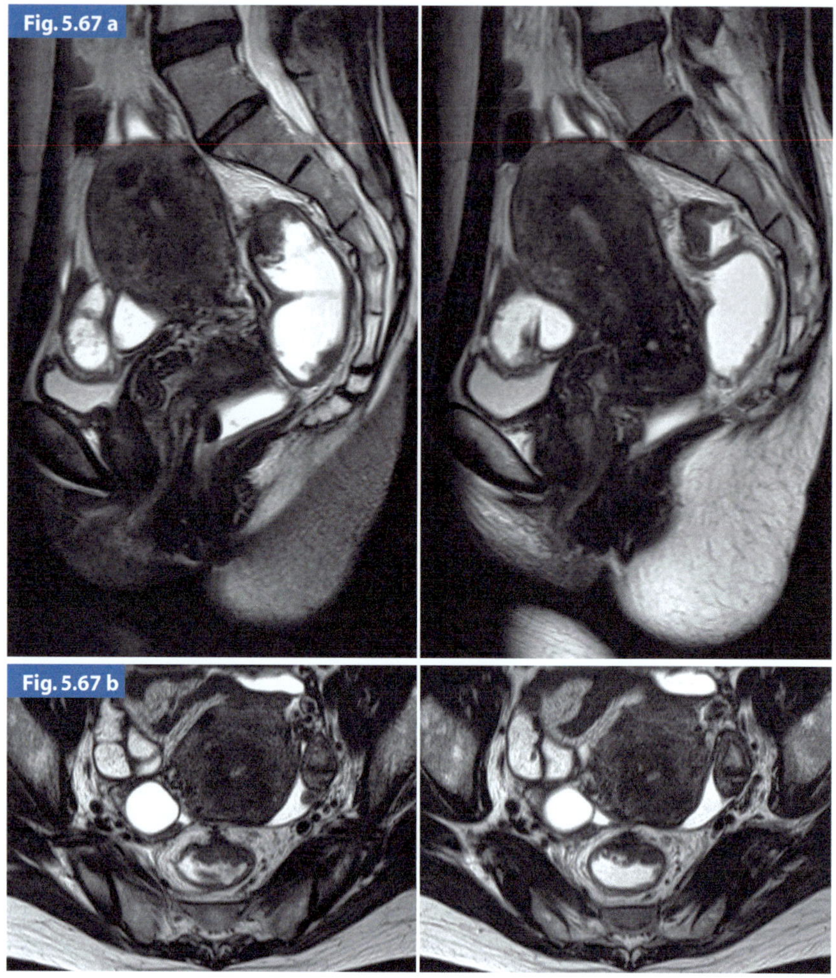

Fig. 5.67 Course of the disease. Patient history: Status after discontinuity resection resulting from perforated rectal cancer. (**a**) The sagittal T2-TSE images display tumor recurrence arising from the roof of the rectal stump. (**b**) Corresponding axial T2-TSE images additionally depict wall exceedance at 12-o'clock into a scar formation. Deep anterior resection of the rectum was performed. Histopathology diagnosed rpT3N0L0V0 local recurrence.

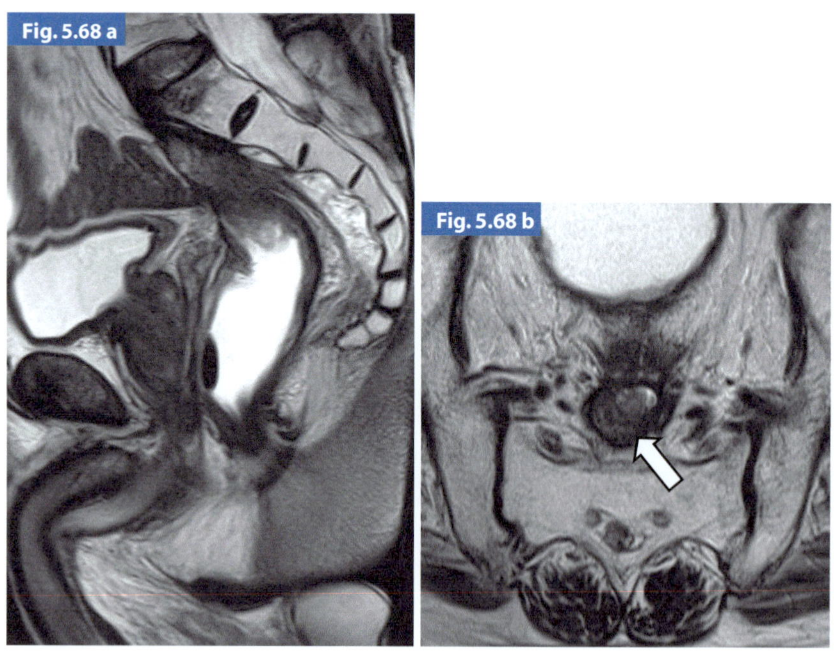

Fig. 5.68 Course of the disease. Two years following deep anterior rectum resection, the patient developed endoscopically nonpassable luminal and extraluminal anastomotic tumor recurrence shown on the sagittal (**a**) and axial (**b**) T2-TSE image (*arrow*). Additional bone metastasis confined to the body of the first sacral vertebra is outlined on the sagittal image.

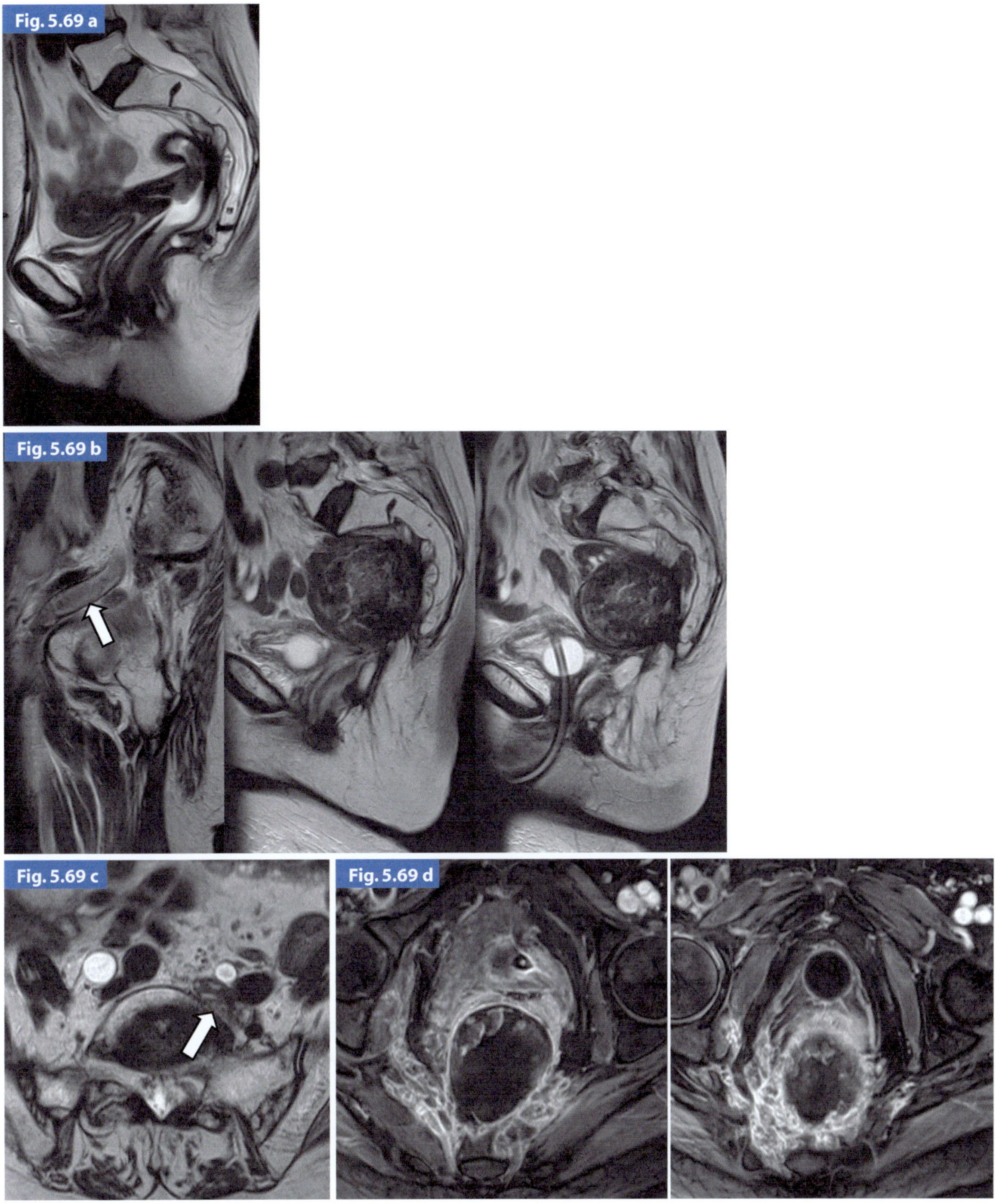

Fig. 5.69 a

Fig. 5.69 b

Fig. 5.69 c

Fig. 5.69 d

Fig. 5.69 Course of the disease. Patient history: 2002 deep anterior resection resulting from pT4N1M0 G2 midrectal adenocarcinoma. (**a**) Initial follow-up pelvic MRI of the year 2003 at our institution. The sagittal (**a**) T2-TSE image shows luminal anastomotic recurrence immediately above a broad rectovaginal fistula. Salvage surgery consisting of abdominoperineal resection and en bloc hysterectomy was carried out. Histopathology revealed stage rpT4N0 recurrent rectal cancer. (**b**–**d**) 2005 control MRI. (**b**) On the sagittal T2-TSE images, an extensive local tumor recurrence is detectable causing right deep vein thrombosis (*arrow*). (**c**) Additionally, axial T2-TSE image shows ureteral infiltration with hydronephrosis on both sides and a thrombus in the left common iliac vein (*arrow*). (**d**) The corresponding axial CE-VIBE 3D images reveal a centrally necrotic local recurrence with tumor deposits along the sacral nerves, the scar, and right pelvic sidewall.

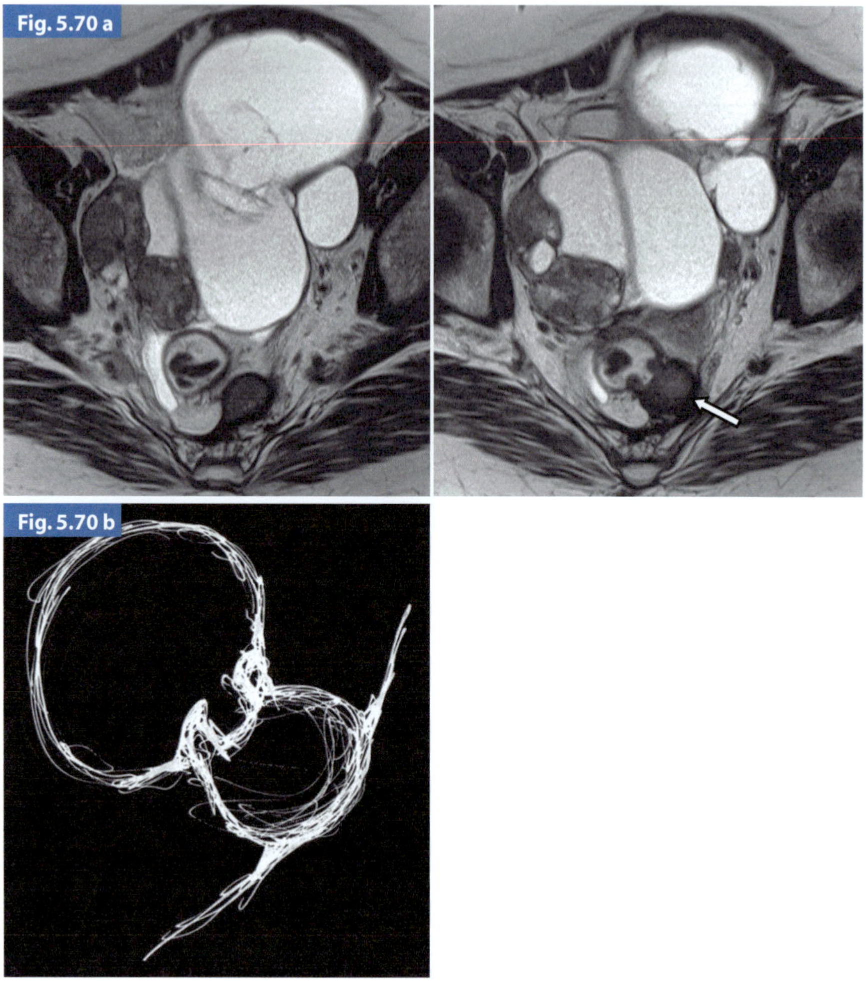

Fig. 5.70 (**a**) Recurrent rectal cancer and ovarian cancer. Para-axial T2-TSE images reveal combined luminal and extraluminal local tumor recurrence at the site of the anastomosis with central ulceration (*arrow*). Ovarian cancer comprised of solid and cystic components is also present. Histopathology diagnosed pT3b G3 carcinoma involving both ovaries and rpT3N0 recurrent rectal cancer. (**b**) Ink drawing: Combined luminal and extraluminal recurrence.

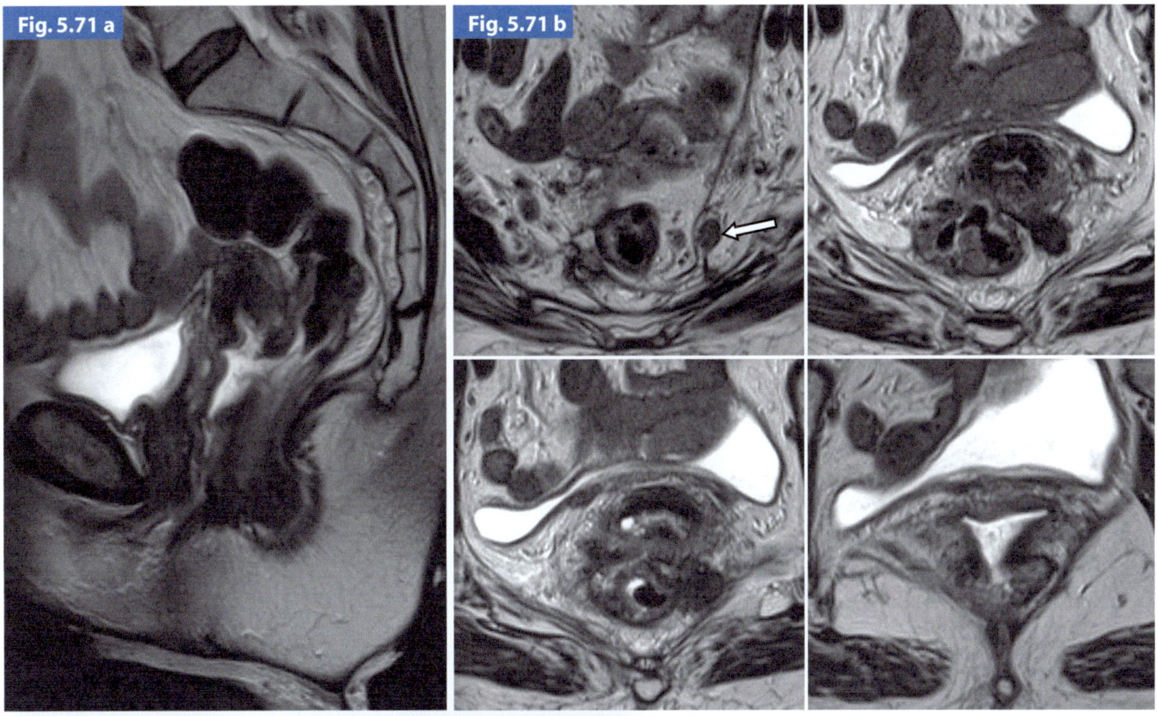

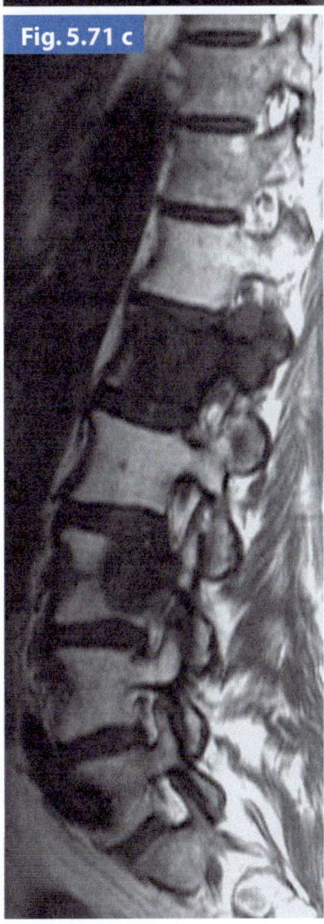

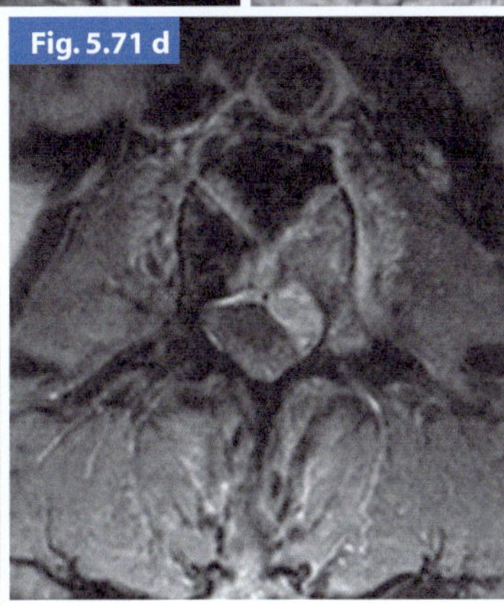

Fig. 5.71 Patient history: Status after deep anterior rectal resection including the posterior vaginal wall resulting from pT4N0 rectal carcinoma. The development of a neorectal-vaginal fistula and metastatic spread to the liver, lungs, and bone are noted. (**a**) On the sagittal T2-TSE image, a broad fistula track is seen with rectally administered water passing into the vaginal cavity. (**b**) Axial T2-TSE images reveal luminal and extraluminal recurrent rectal cancer at the level and above the anastomosis. Tumor deposit is seen outside the descending mesocolon (*arrow*). Sagittal T1-TSE (**c**) and corresponding axial CE-FLASH 2D (**d**) images exemplify metastatic spread to the first and third lumbar segment with epidural tumor involvement.

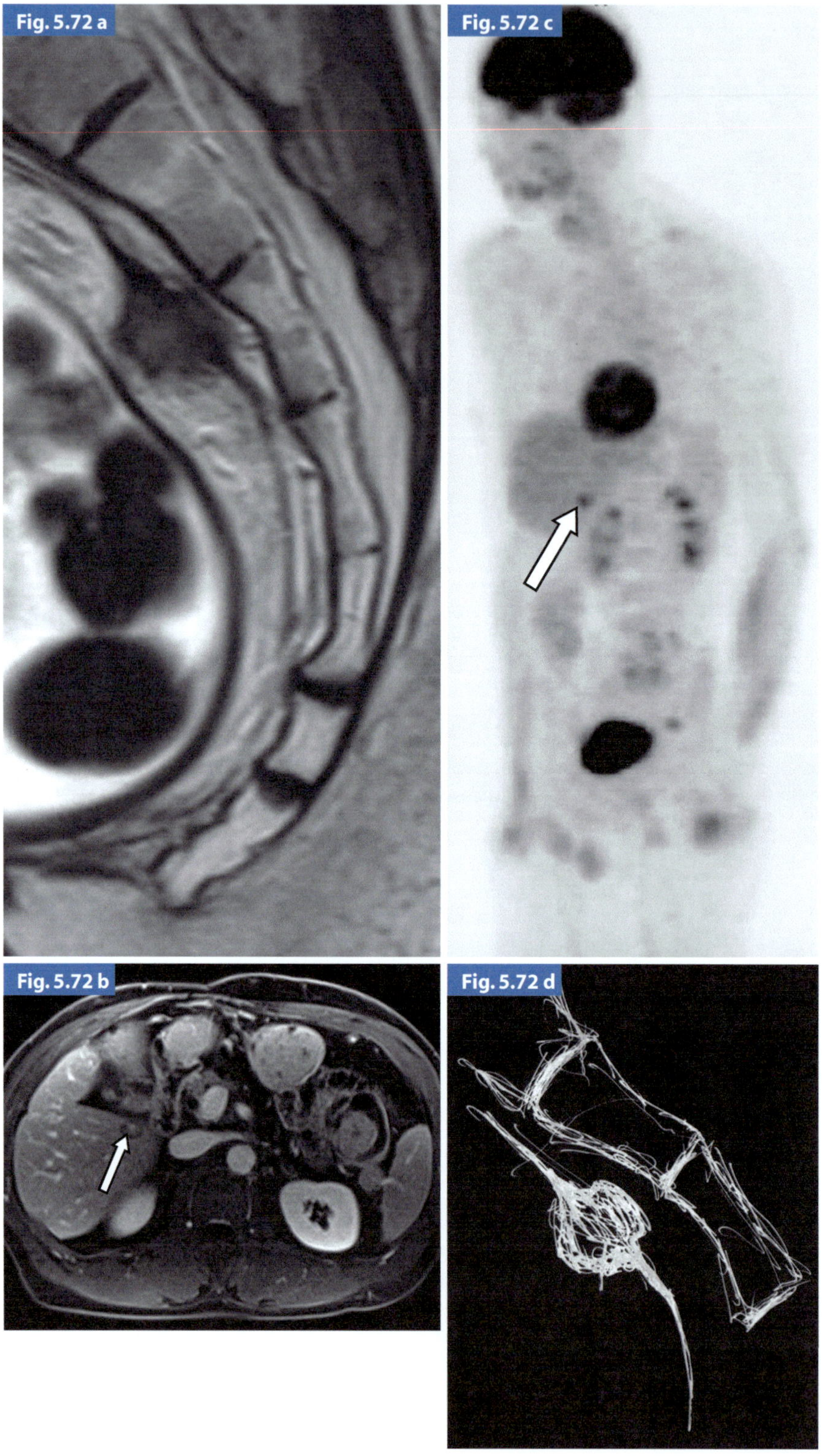

Fig. 5.72 (**a**) Sagittal T2-TSE image demonstrates extraluminal local recurrence invading the presacral fascia. (**b**) Axial CE-FLASH 2D image derived from the SMS moving-table examination reveals liver metastasis (*arrow*) confirmed by PET (**c**, *arrow*). (**d**) Ink drawing: Extraluminal local recurrence.

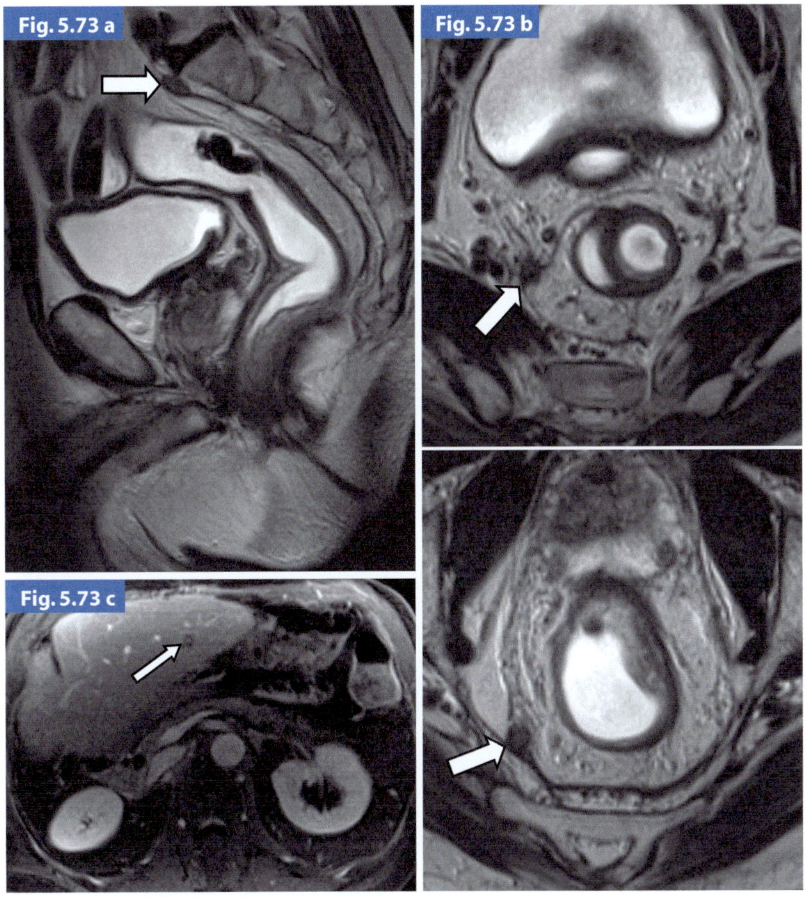

Fig. 5.73 Lateral residual disease. Patient history: Status after pT2N0M0 G2 adenocarcinoma of the rectosigmoid, extended right hemihepatectomy due to metachronous liver metastases, and salvage surgery of locally recurrent rectal cancer. Follow-up MRI, increasing CEA-values. Sagittal (**a**) T2-TSE image shows a normal anastomosis without signs of recurrence. At the level of the promontory delineation of a small nodular mass (*arrow*). Para-axial (**b**) T2-TSE images reveal additional nodes at the level and below the colonic anastomosis (*arrows*) suggestive of lateral residual disease. SMS-FLASH-2D image (**c**) shows a hypovascular liver metastasis in the remaining left liver (*arrow*).

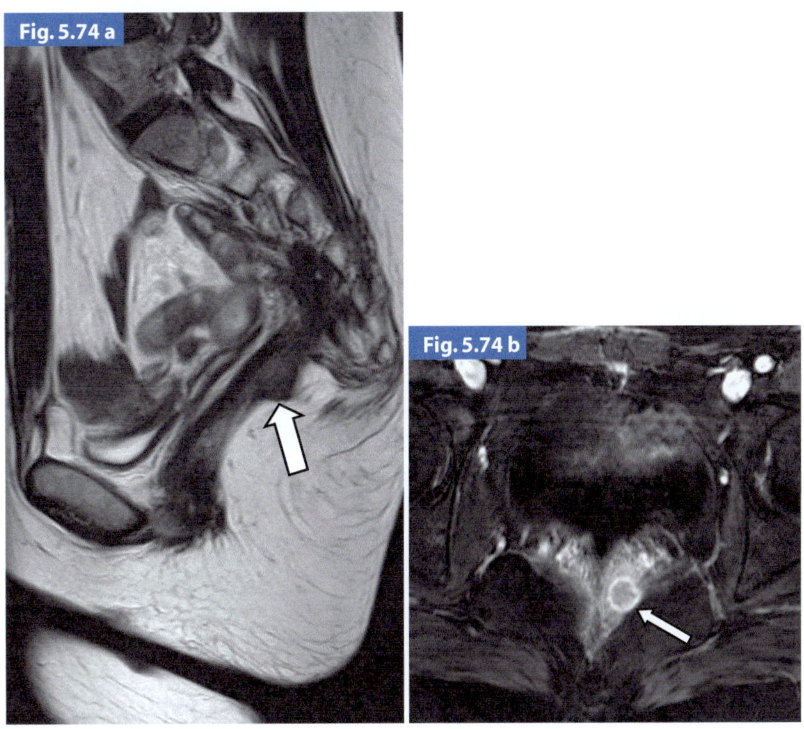

Fig. 5.74 On the sagittal T2-TSE (**a**) and axial CE-FLASH (**b**) three-dimensional images, a nodular tumor recurrence is seen within the pelvic scar 2 years after abdomino-perineal resection.

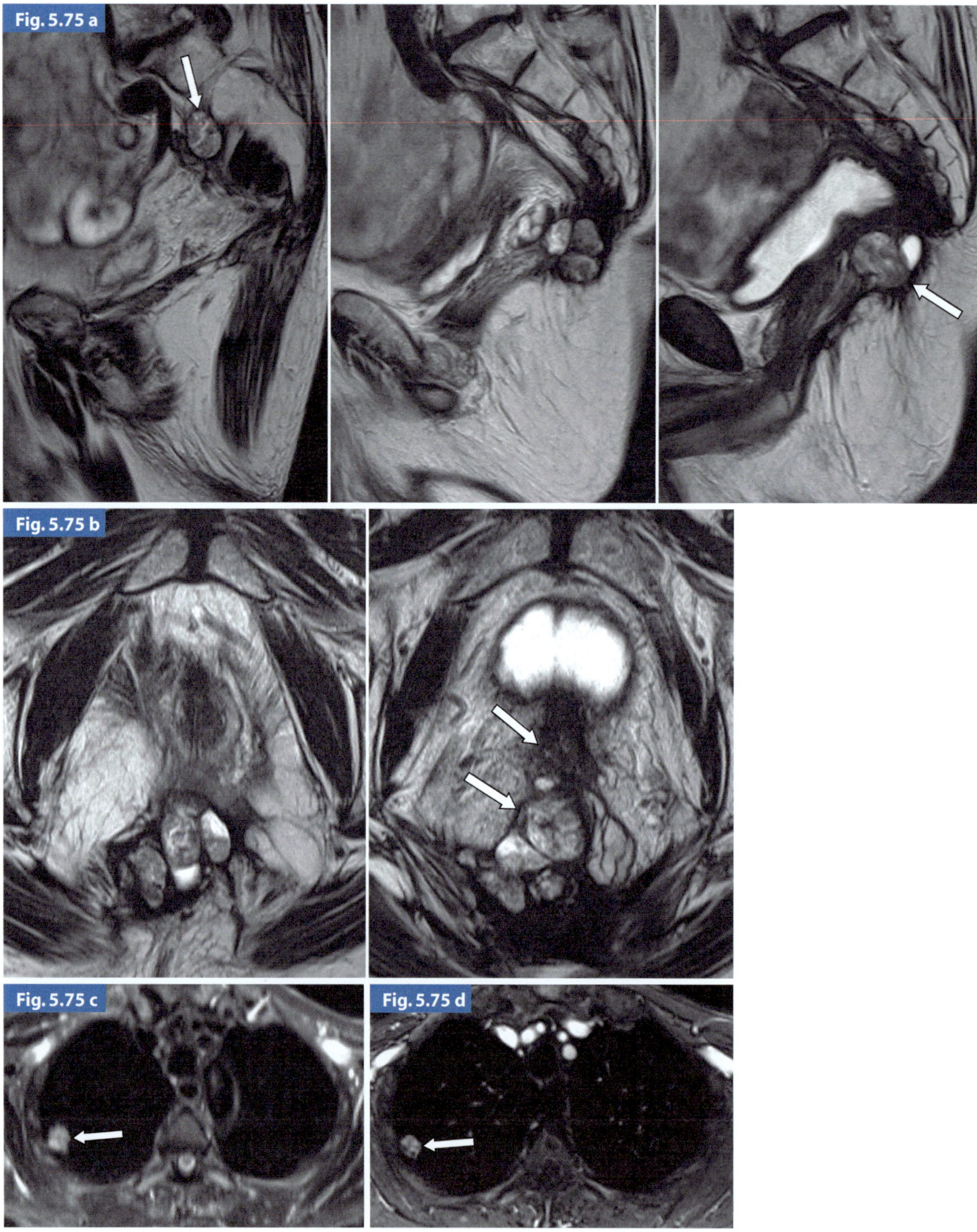

Fig. 5.75 Recurrent metastasizing rectal cancer. (**a**) Sagittal T2-TSE images display a second local tumor recurrence within the pelvic scar after abdominoperineal resection of the rectum and salvage surgery including distal sacrectomy for locally recurrent cancer (*arrow*). Additionally, a right iliac lymph node metastasis can be observed (*arrow*). (**b**) The inhomogenously high-signal intensity of the extraluminal second tumor recurrence shown on the para-axial T2-TSE images corresponds to mucinous adenocarcinoma. The seminal vesicles and the prostate are already infiltrated (*arrows*). Axial free-breathing TIRM (**c**) and corresponding axial breath-hold CE-FLASH 2D (**d**) images derived from SMS moving-table staging reveal solitary metastasis in the upper lobe of the right lung (*arrows*).

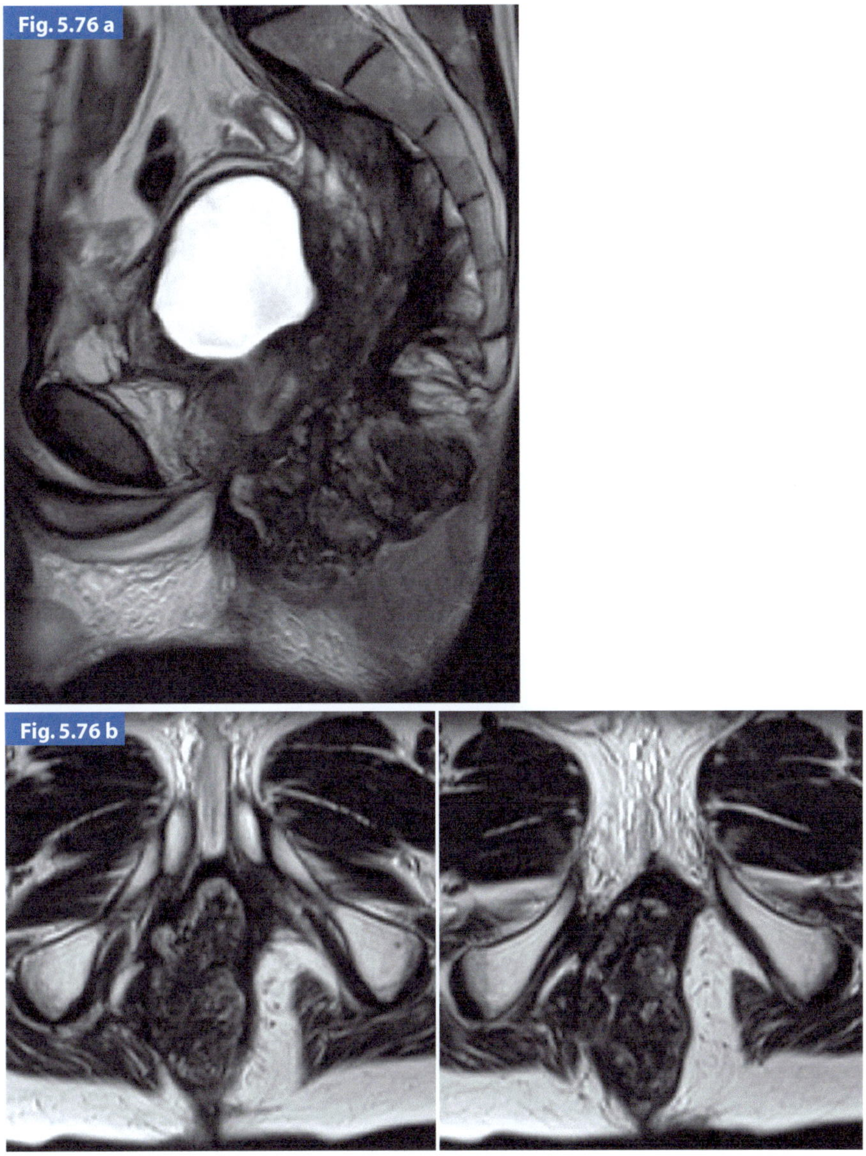

Fig. 5.76 Sagittal (**a**) and axial (**b**) T2-TSE images with typical findings in a patient with a second local recurrence of rectal cancer after abdominoperineal resection and exenteration. Also present, extensive low-signal tumor formation within the perineal scar, reaching to the penile root.

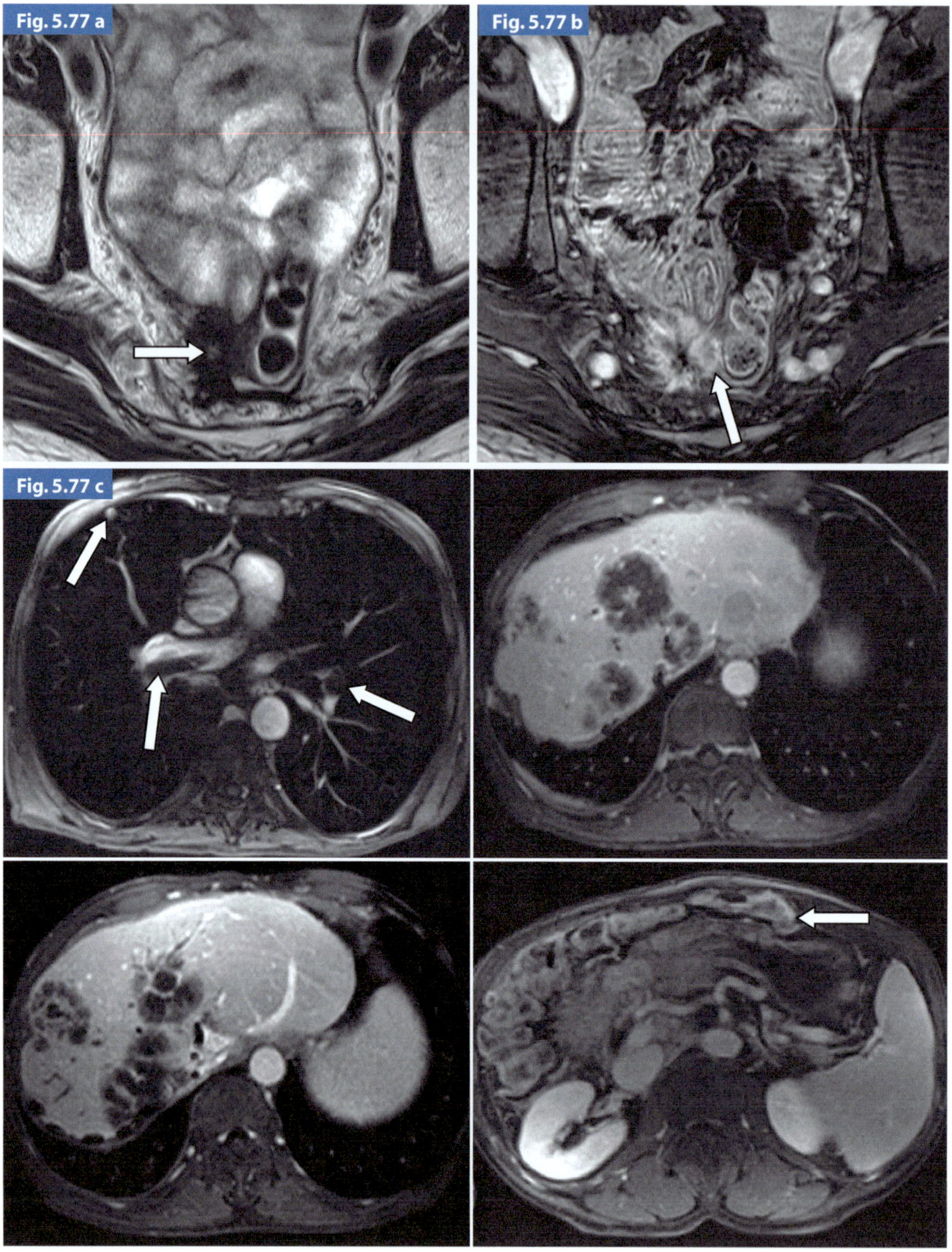
Fig. 5.77 a
Fig. 5.77 b
Fig. 5.77 c

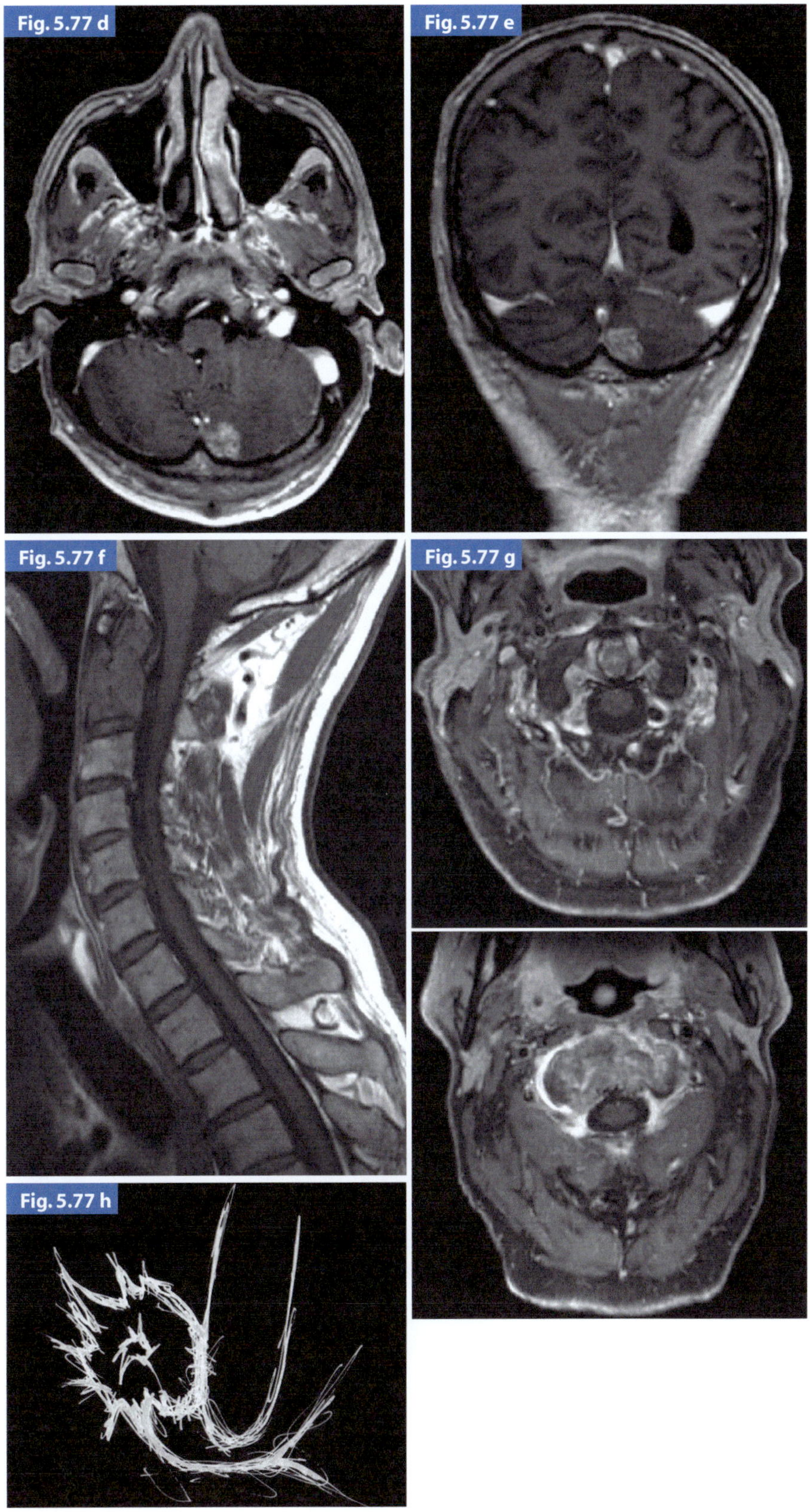

Fig. 5.77 Metastasizing recurrent rectal cancer. On the axial T2-TSE (**a**) and corresponding axial CE-VIBE (**b**) three-dimensional images, extraluminal local tumor recurrence is seen within a scar following deep anterior rectum resection. Note the signal-rich center of the hypointense scar indicative of tumor regrowth (*arrow*). The tumor recurrence involves the wall of the adjacent neorectum (*arrow*). (**c**) On the axial CE-FLASH 2D images derived from concomitantly performed SMS moving-table examination, a pulmonary metastasis in the right lung is visible. Paraneoplastic pulmonary embolism is also apparent (*arrows*). Typical colorectal liver metastases resembling a cockade are seen following right hemihepatectomy and abdominal wall metastasis (*arrow*). Axial (**d**) and coronal (**e**) CE-MPRAGE images reveal left cerebellar metastasis. Concomittant bone metastasis in the axis with epidural component is shown on the sagittal T1-TSE (**f**) and the axial CE-FLASH 2D (**g**) images. (**h**) Ink drawing: Extraluminal recurrence within a scar.

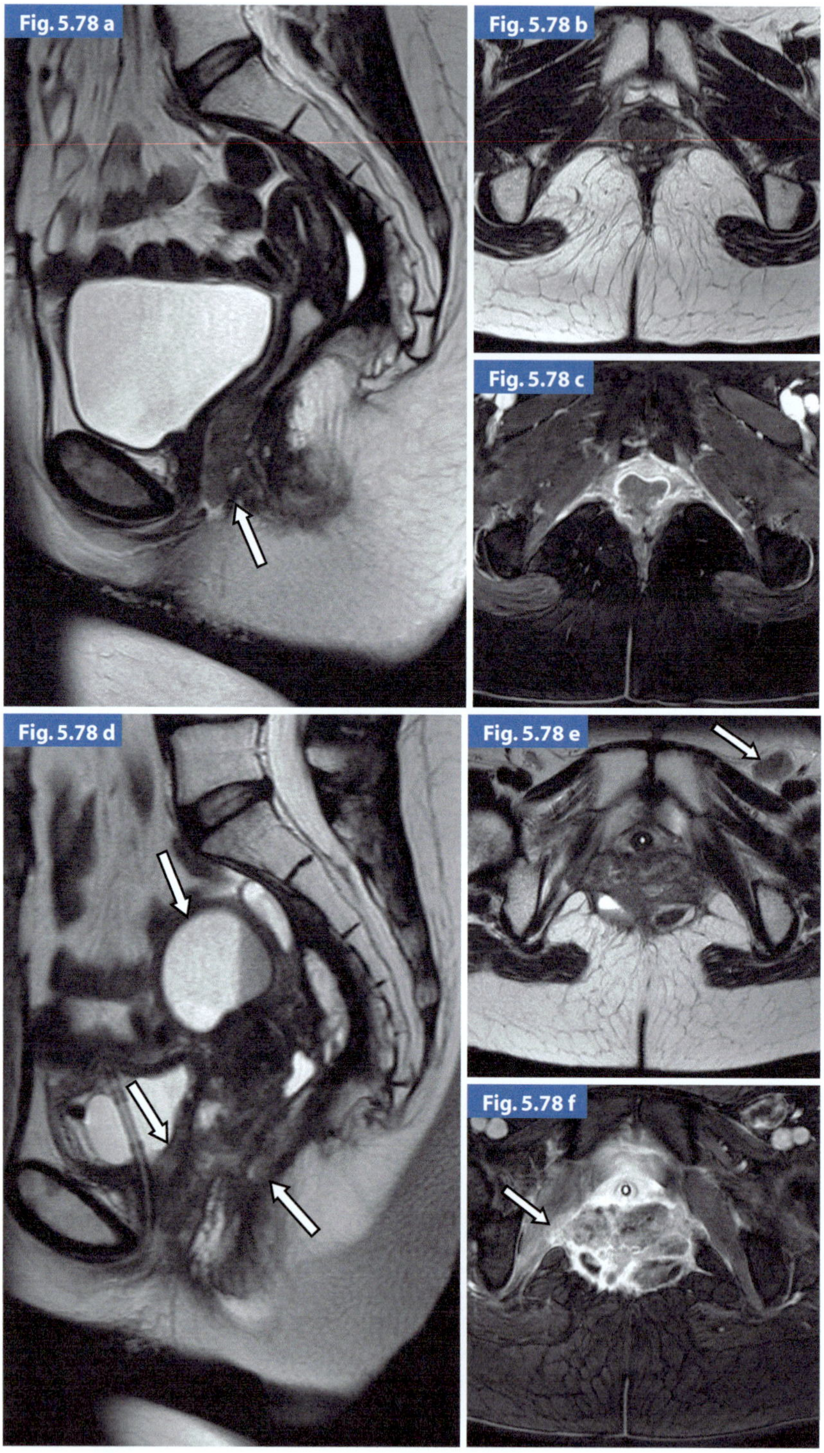

Fig. 5.78 Recurrent rectal cancer, course of the disease. Patient history: Status after radiochemotherapy and abdominosacral amputation of the rectum with resection of the posterior vaginal wall in 2004 resulting from pT4N2M0 rectal cancer. In 2005 the patient was readmitted with elevated CEA-levels and a palpable vaginal tumor. (**a–c**) First follow-up MRI, November 2005. On the sagittal T2-TSE image (**a**) and the axial T2-TSE (**b**) and CE-VIBE 3D (**c**) images, local tumor recurrence is seen with infiltration of the pelvic scar and the vagina producing an exophytic intravaginal mass (*arrow*). (**d–f**) Control MRI, June 2006. The sagittal (**d**) and axial (**e**) T2-TSE and (**f**) CE-VIBE 3D images reveal notable tumor progression with infiltration of the vagina, uterus, bladder, urethra, scar, and right pelvic sidewall. Additionally, lymph node metastasis occurred in the left groin. Uterine bleeding is demonstrated (*arrows*). Note the signal increase of the pelvic scar in T2 with tumor invasion. The tumor recurrence was treated with multiorgan resection and gracilis-flap. Histopathology diagnosed stage rpT4 R1 recurrent rectal cancer and a stage pTis high-grade bladder cancer.

Fig. 5.78 (**g–i**) Final control MRI, October 2006. Demonstration of the third local tumor recurrence on the sagittal (**g**) and axial (**h**) T2-TSE images and the corresponding axial (**i**) CE-VIBE 3D images. Rapidly growing tumor nodules along the gracilis-flap to the inside of the left thigh (*arrows*). In addition, the pelvic scar is completely interspersed by tumor nests. The right internal obturator muscle is invaded. Tumor nodules can be seen around the pudendum (*arrows*).

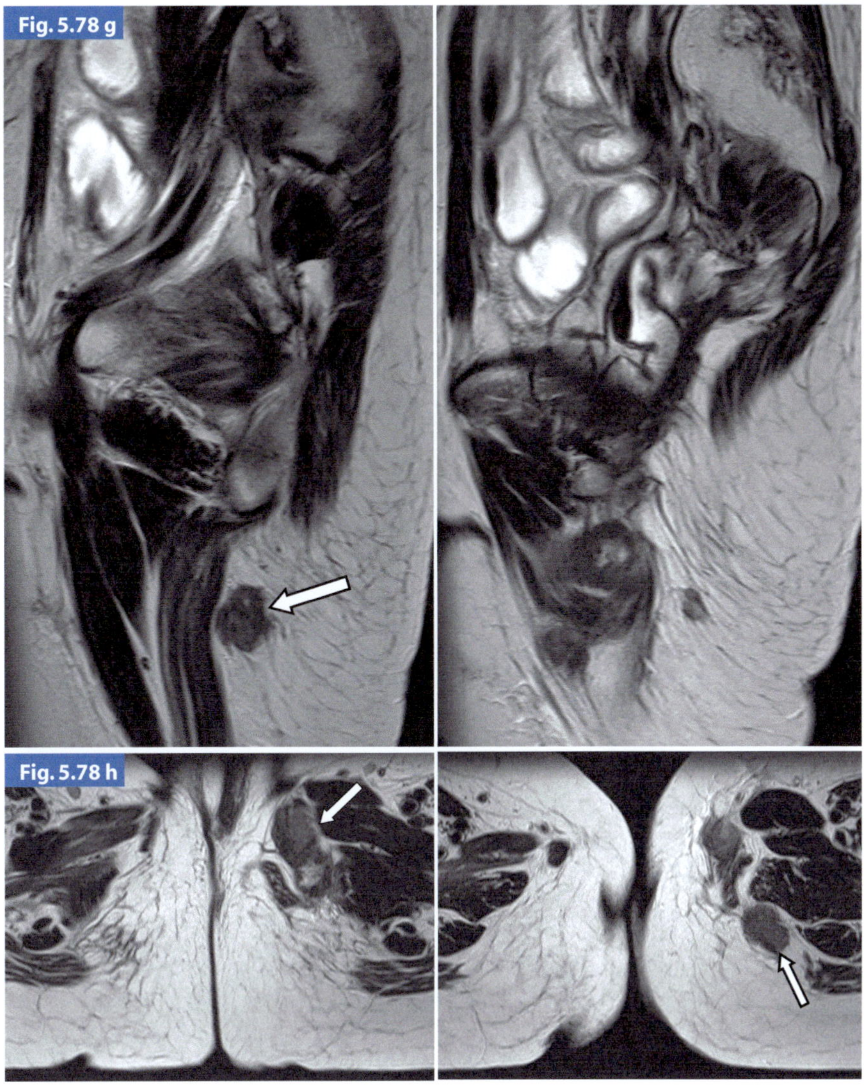

Fig. 5.78 i

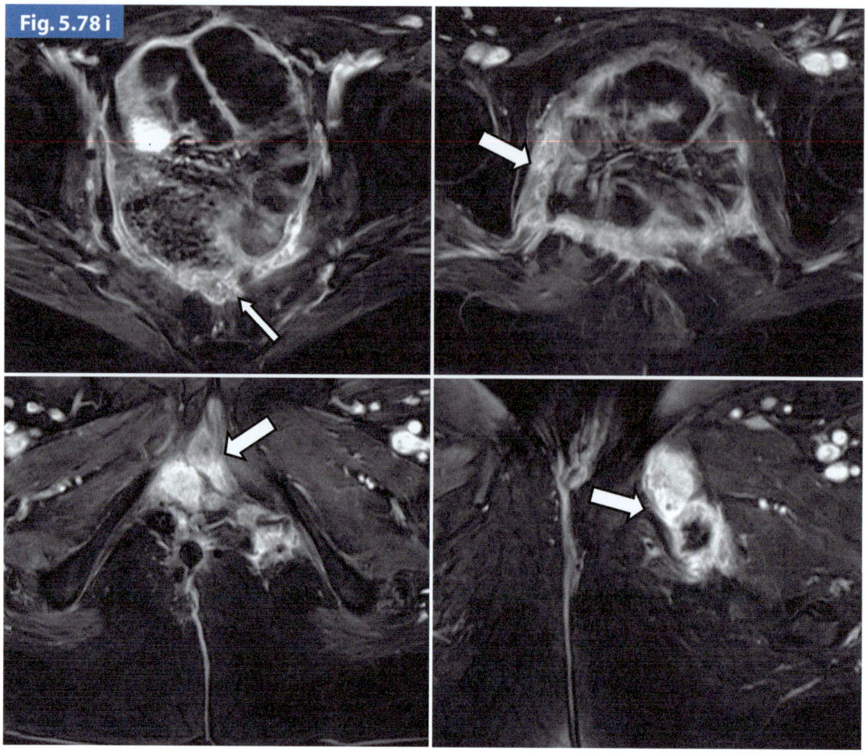

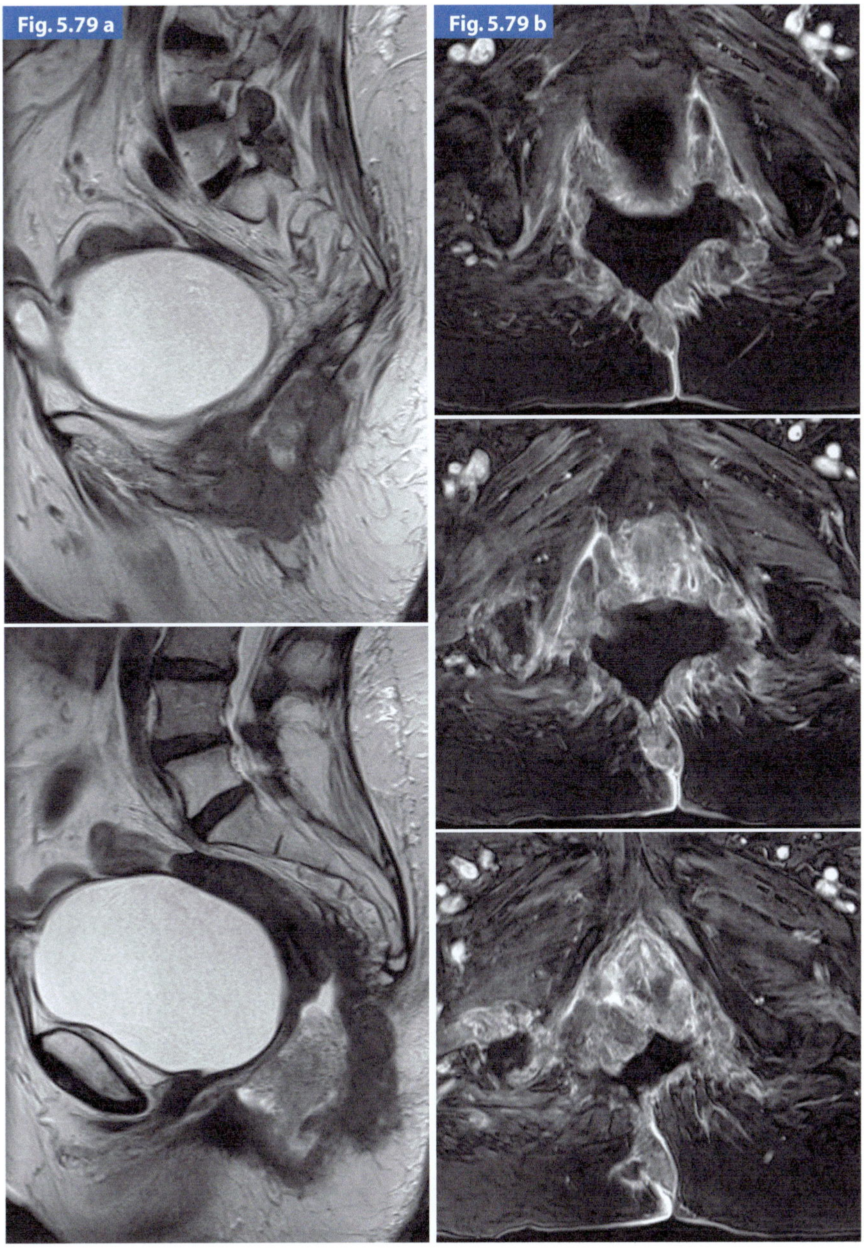

Fig. 5.79 Patient with rectal cancer on the basis of ulcerative coilitis was treated with abdominoperineal resection. In the course, she developed wound healing deficit. (**a**) Sagittal T2-TSE images reveal a thick-walled abscess formation and nodular masses affecting the pelvic floor and the vagina. (**b**) Axial contrast-enhanced VIBE 3D images show a fluid-filled wound cavity that forms a common channel with the vagina and is surrounded by a rim of tumor tissue extending to the pelvic sidewalls, the vesical outlet, the rima ani, and the right quadratus femoris muscle.

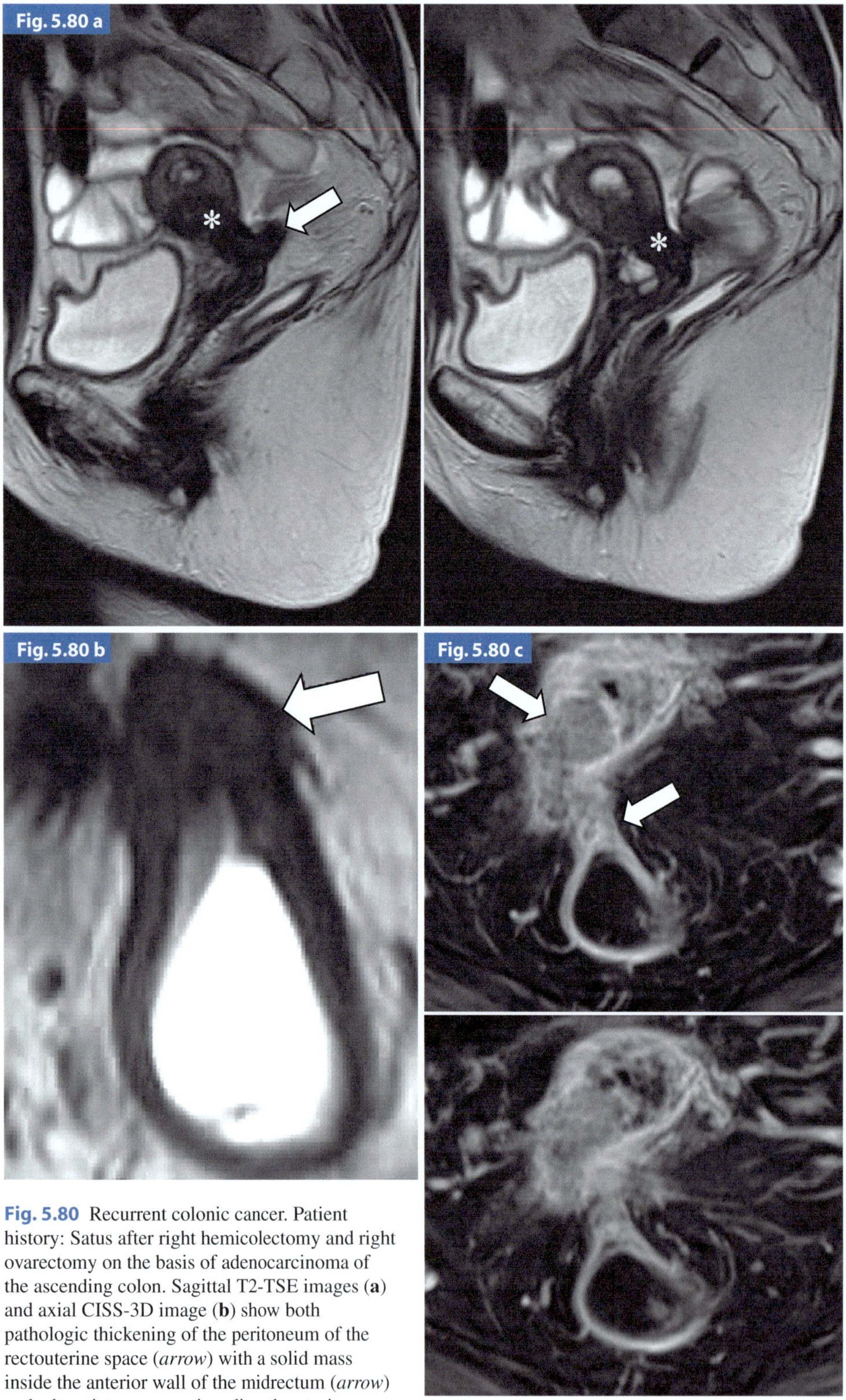

Fig. 5.80 Recurrent colonic cancer. Patient history: Satus after right hemicolectomy and right ovarectomy on the basis of adenocarcinoma of the ascending colon. Sagittal T2-TSE images (**a**) and axial CISS-3D image (**b**) show both pathologic thickening of the peritoneum of the rectouterine space (*arrow*) with a solid mass inside the anterior wall of the midrectum (*arrow*) and a hypointense mass invading the uterine cervix and neck (*asterisks*). (**c**) Axial CE-VIBE 3D images show local recurrence with unterine invasion as well as involvement of the peritoneal reflection and midrectum (*arrows*).

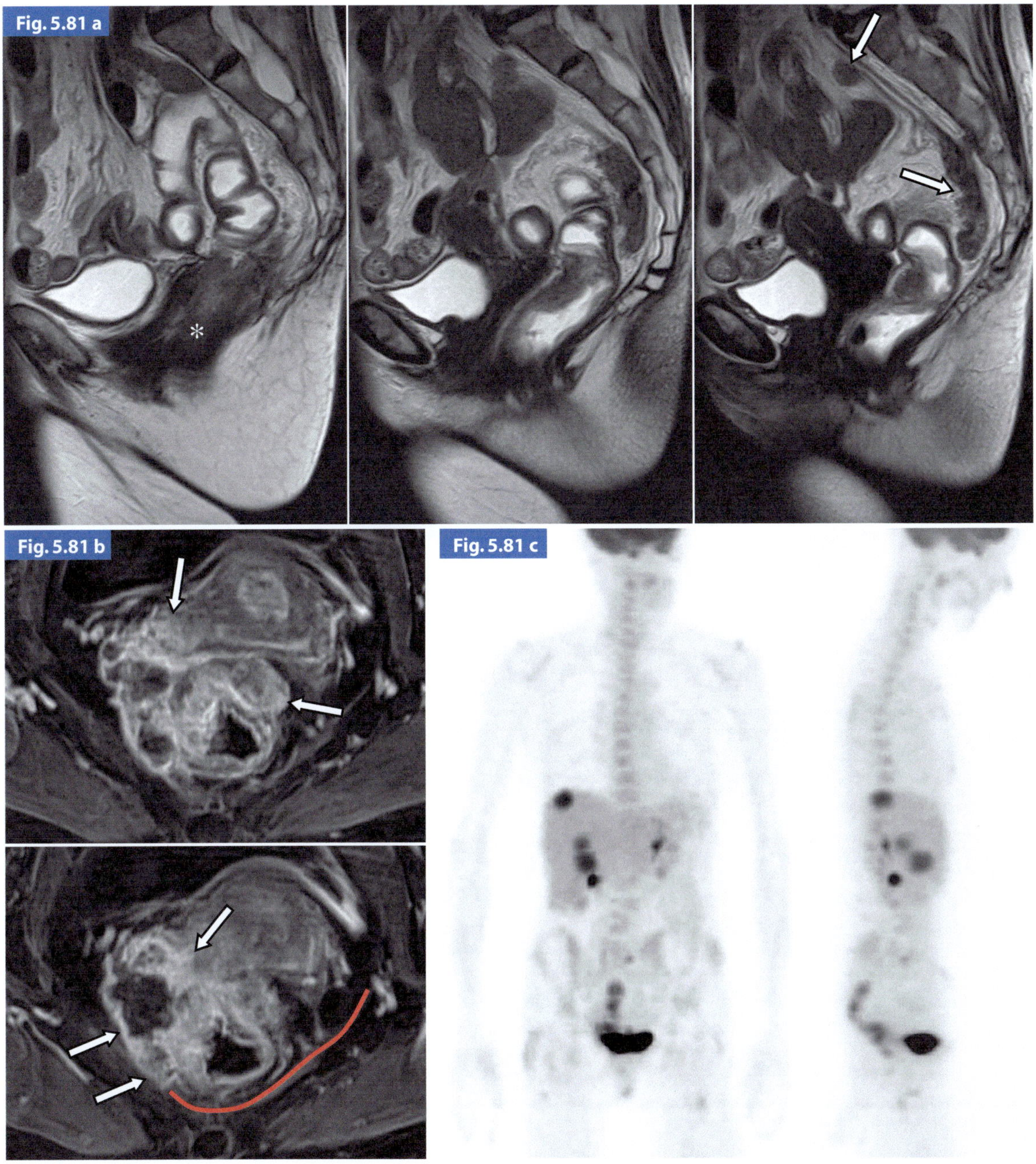

Fig. 5.81 Patient history: Status after TEM resulting from stage pT1N0M0 G1 rectal cancer. (**a**) Sagittal T2-TSE images reveal advanced luminal and extraluminal local tumor recurrence of the midrectum (*asterisk*) with an elongated mesorectal tumor deposit and a lymph node metastasis along the superior rectal artery (*arrows*). (**b**) Axial CE-VIBE 3D images demonstrate the luminal and extraluminal component of the recurrence between 7- and 3-o'clock lithotomy position involving the mesorectum, the right levator ani muscle, and the right posterior vaginal wall (*arrows*, *red line* indicates the normal course of the levator muscle), associated with stage rcT4. The findings were confirmed by FGD-PET (**c**) and additional hepatic metastasis was detected.

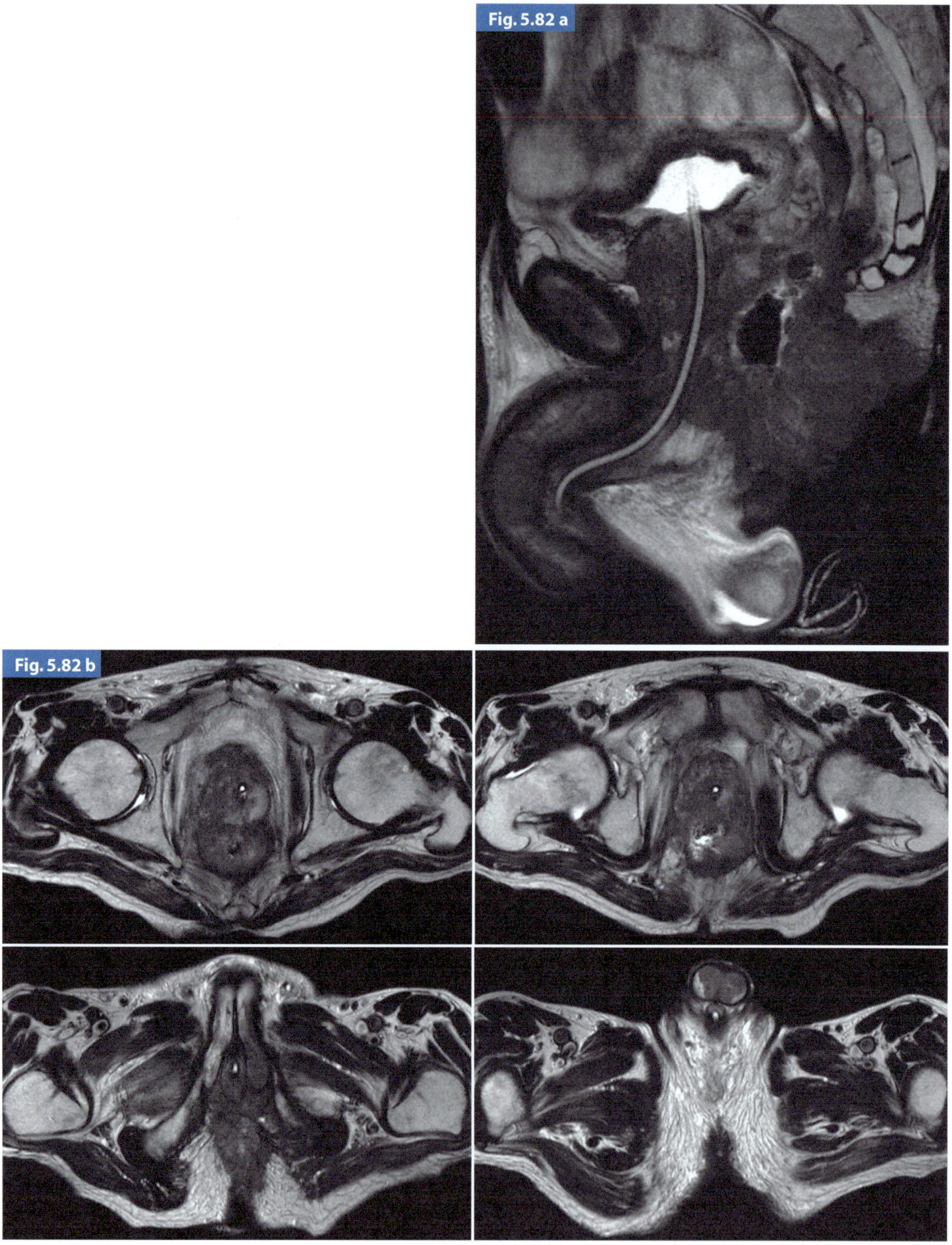

Fig. 5.82 Sagittal (**a**) and axial (**b**) T2-TSE images reveal advanced centrally necrotic local rectal cancer recurrence invading the perineal scar, the prostate, the penile root, the cavernous bodies, and the urethra.

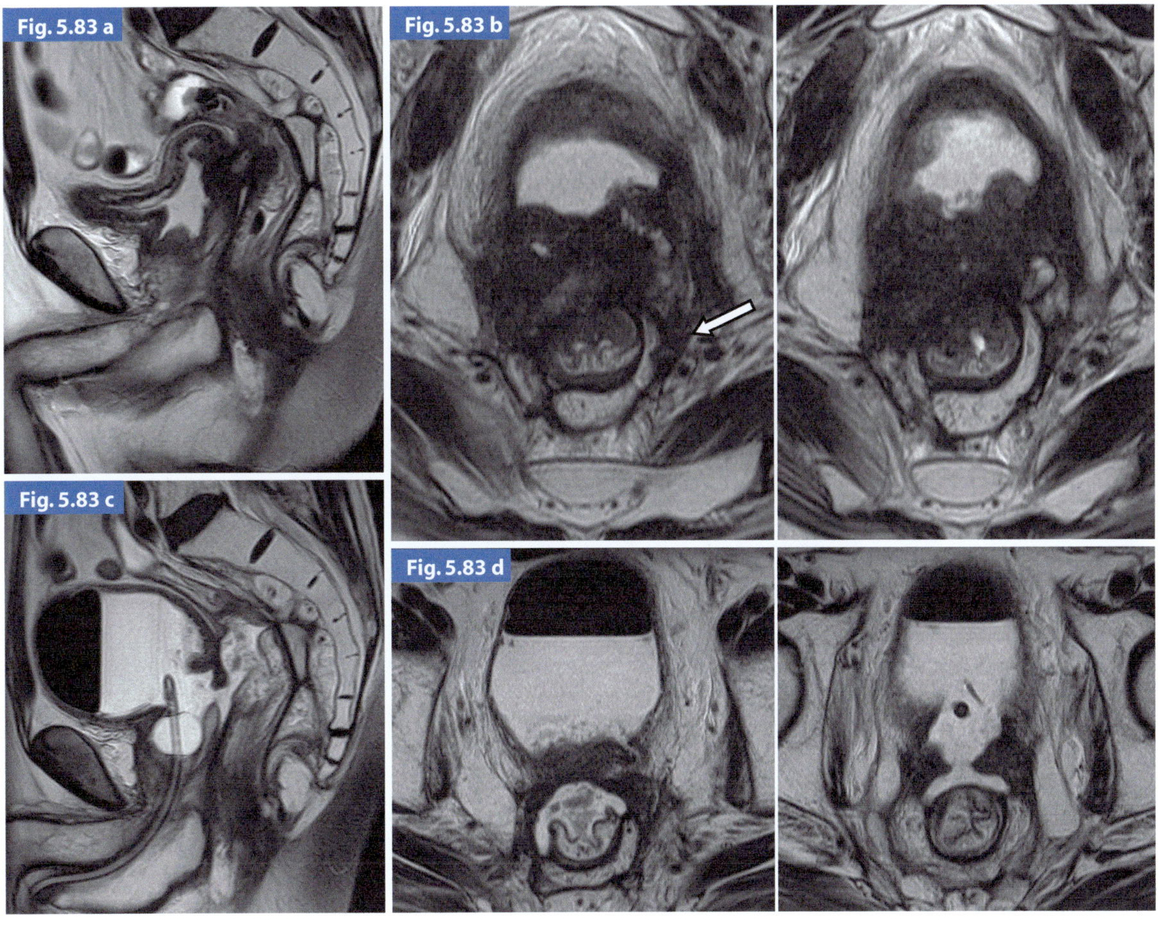

Fig. 5.83 (**a**, **b**) Initial follow-up MRI. Advanced luminal and extraluminal anastomotic recurrence is present on the sagittal (**a**) and para-axial (**b**) T2-TSE images. The tumor extends per continuitatem to the seminal vesicles and urinary bladder and involves the perianastomotic scar (*arrow*). (**c**, **d**) Control MRI during adjuvant radiochemotherapy. Downsizing of the recurrent tumor could be achieved visible on the sagittal (**c**) and para-axial (**d**) T2-TSE images. As a treatment-related complication, tumor fistula occurred and established communication between the neorectum and the urinary bladder. Note the air in the bladder lumen.

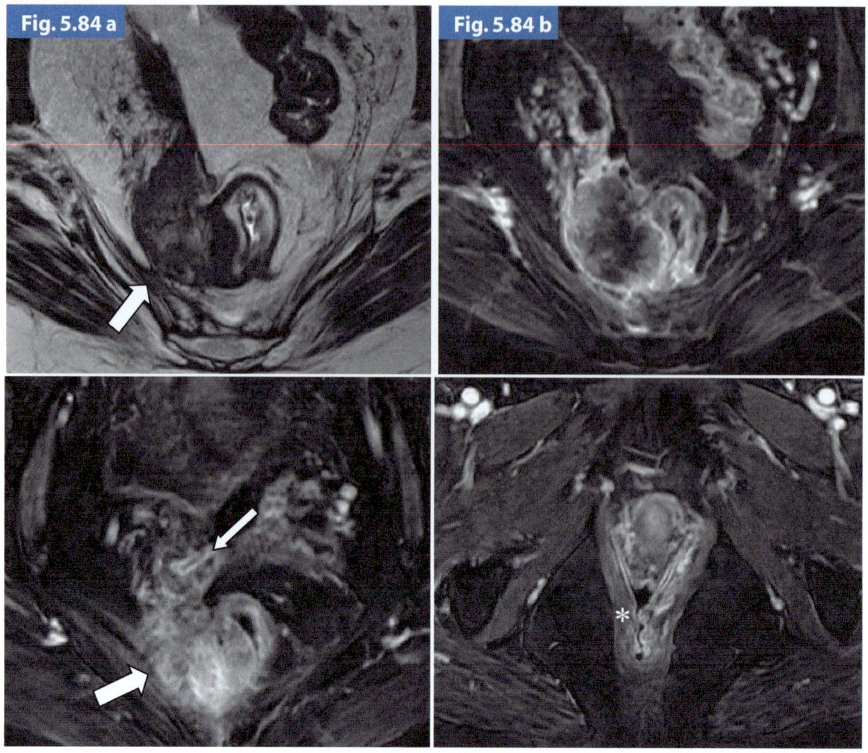

Fig. 5.84 Local recurrence of rectal cancer. Patient history: Status after supraanal TEM surgery for low-lying rectal cancer, development of a rectovaginal fistula and known liver and lung metastases. On the axial T2-SPACE (**a**) and axial CE-VIBE (**b**) three-dimensional images, extensive local recurrence is seen with infiltration of the rectal wall, the mesorectal fat and fascia, the right levator muscle (*arrow*), and the posterior wall of the vagina (*small arrow*). Additionally, persistent rectovaginal fistula can be detected (*asterisk*).

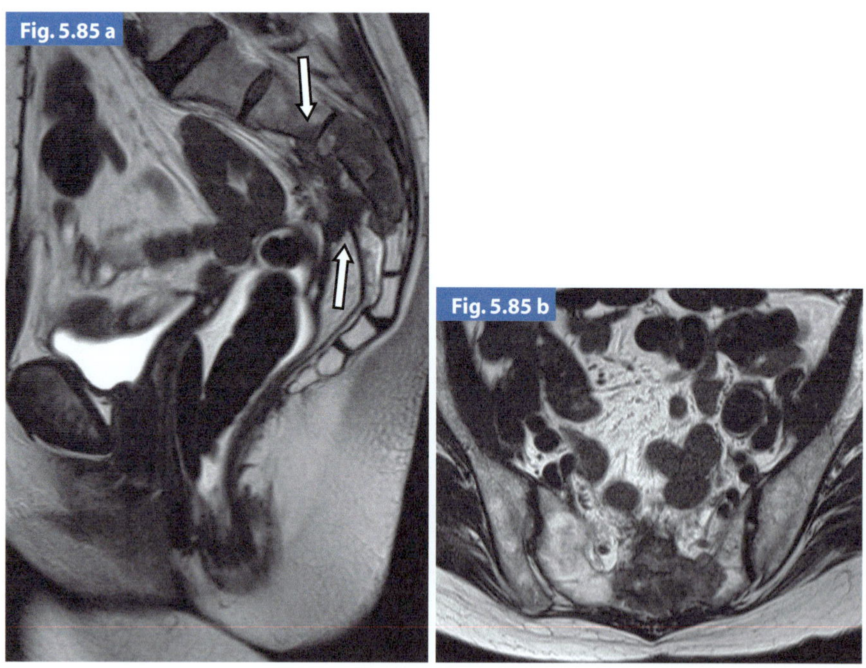

Fig. 5.85 The sagittal (**a**) and axial (**b**) T2-TSE images reveal extraluminal local tumor recurrence involving the presacral scar and the sacral bone between S2 and S4 (*arrows*).

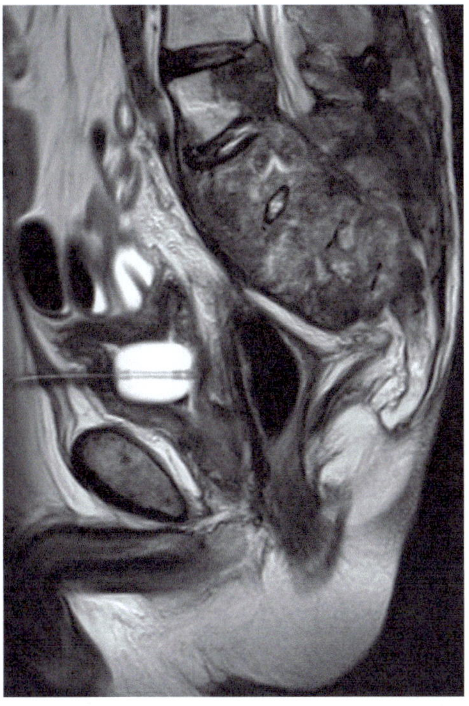

Fig. 5.86 Broad extraluminal recurrence of rectal cancer. On the sagittal T2-TSE image, a massive tumor infiltration of the sacral and fifth lumbar vertebral bone is seen occupying the sacral spinal channel.

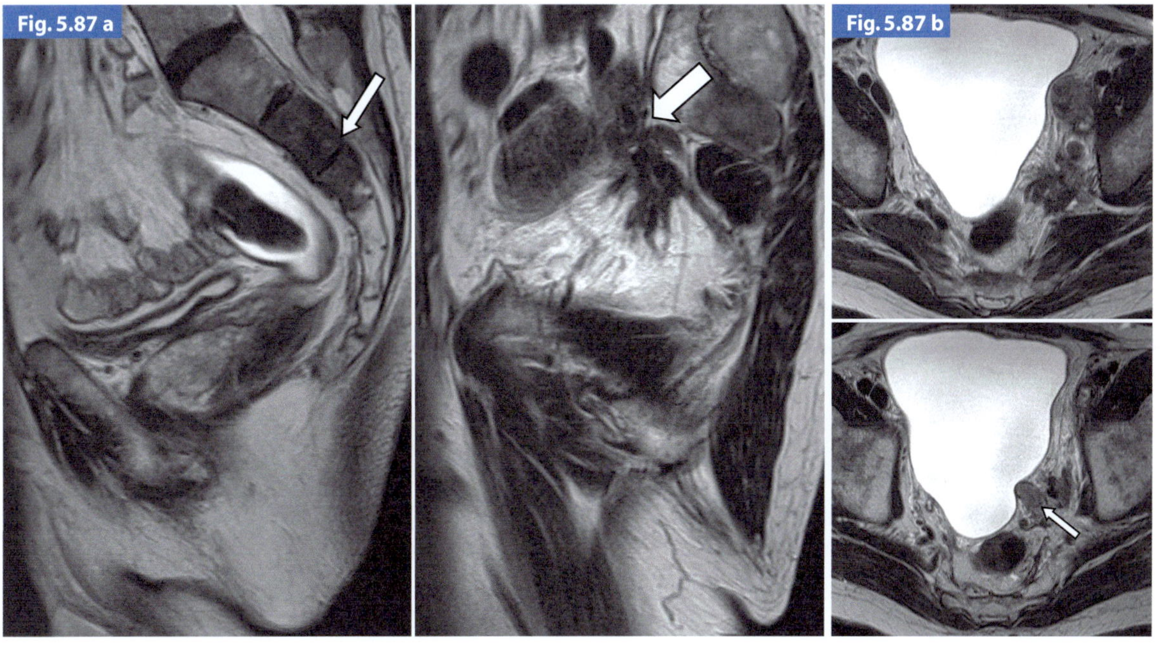

Fig. 5.87 (**a**) The sagittal T2-TSE images demonstrate involvement of the sacral bone at the level of the S2 and S3 segment. Additionally, left pelvic sidewall recurrence with adjacent lymph node metastases is evident (*arrows*). (**b**) Aggravatingly, the axial T2-TSE images depict infiltration of the left ureter (*arrow*).

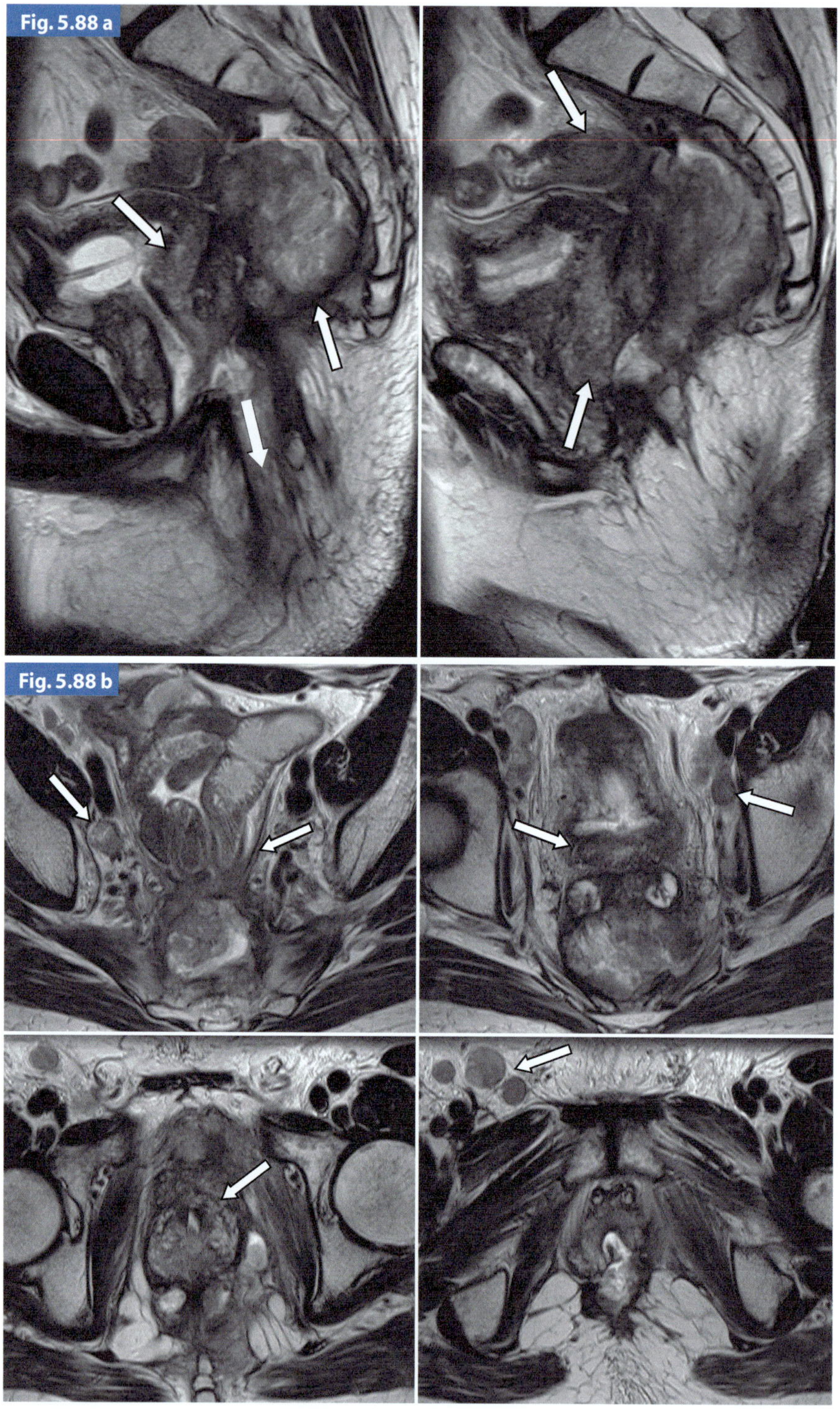

Fig. 5.88 Example of an extensive local tumor recurrence with infiltration of the pelvic scar after abdominoperineal resection of the rectum: Sagittal (**a**) and para-axial (**b**) T2-TSE images, and corresponding axial (**c**) CE-VIBE 3D images. The partially necrotic recurrence involves the prostate, seminal vesicles, bladder, urethra, peritoneum, ileum, pelvic sidewall, and sacral bone. Iliac and inguinal lymph node metastases are also present. Tumor fistula to the urethra and the perineum (*arrows*).

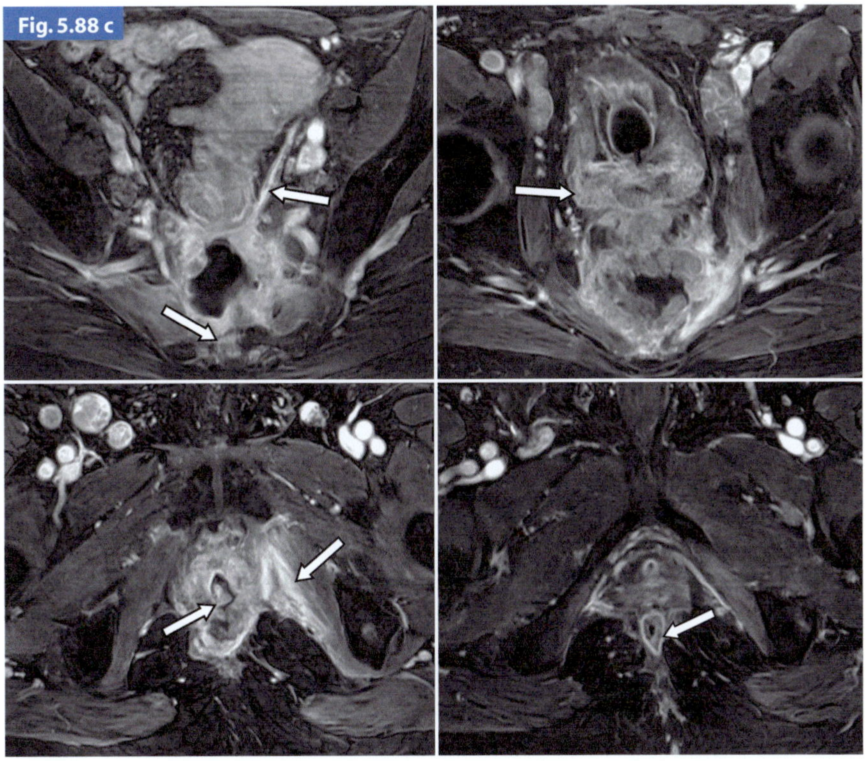

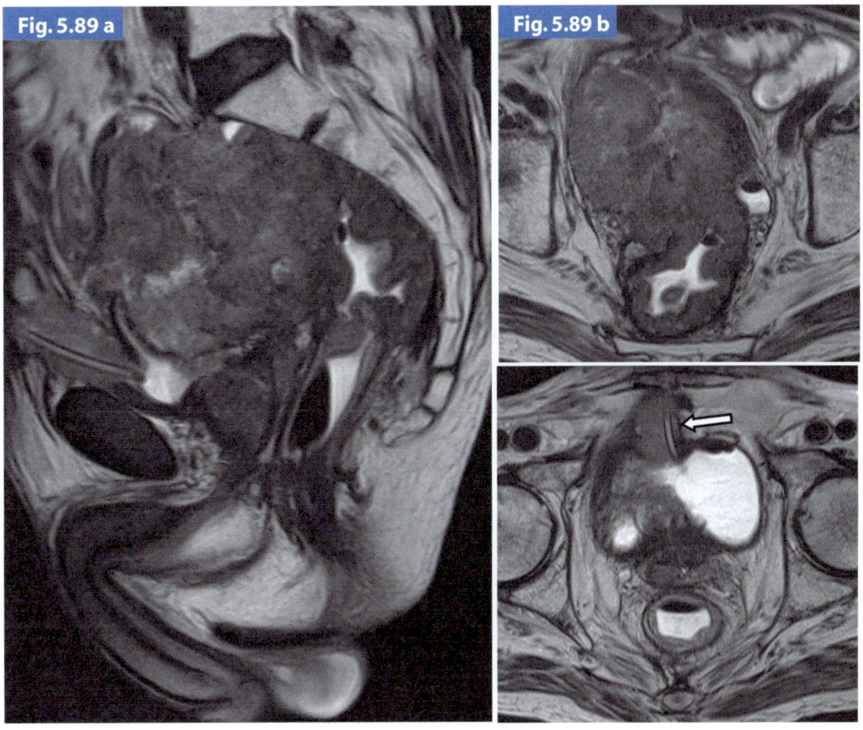

Fig. 5.89 The sagittal (**a**) and axial (**b**) T2-TSE images expose a large local tumor recurrence invading the anastomosis, the descending colon, the bladder, the seminal vesicles and prostate, the parietal pelvic fascia, and the tissue around the suprapubic catheter (*arrow*).

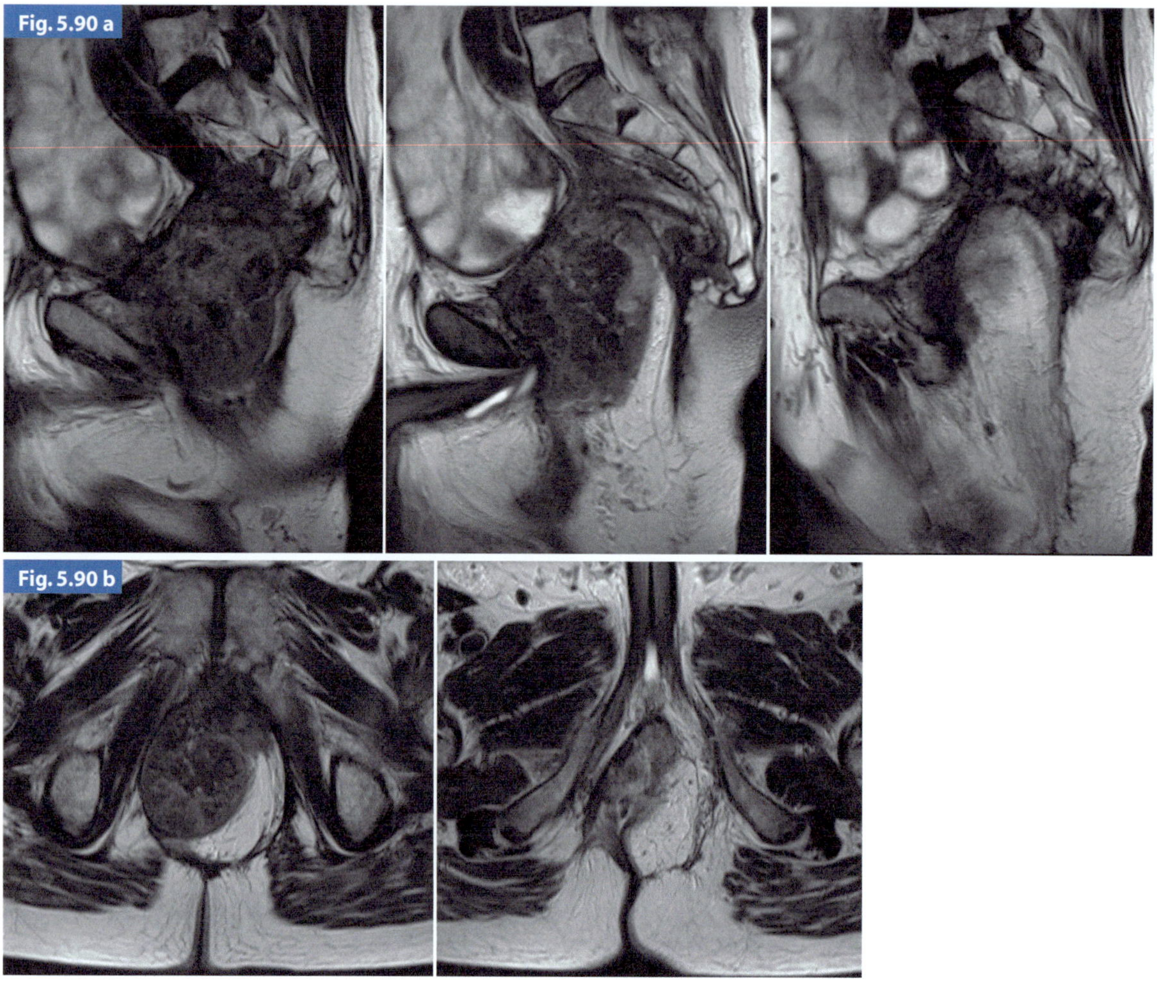

Fig. 5.90 Patient history: Status after pelvic exenteration and perineal reconstruction, second recurrence. Sagittal (**a**) and axial (**b**) T2-TSE images show an extensive second local recurrence of rectal carcinoma occupying the pelvic scar and infiltrating the flap reconstruction.

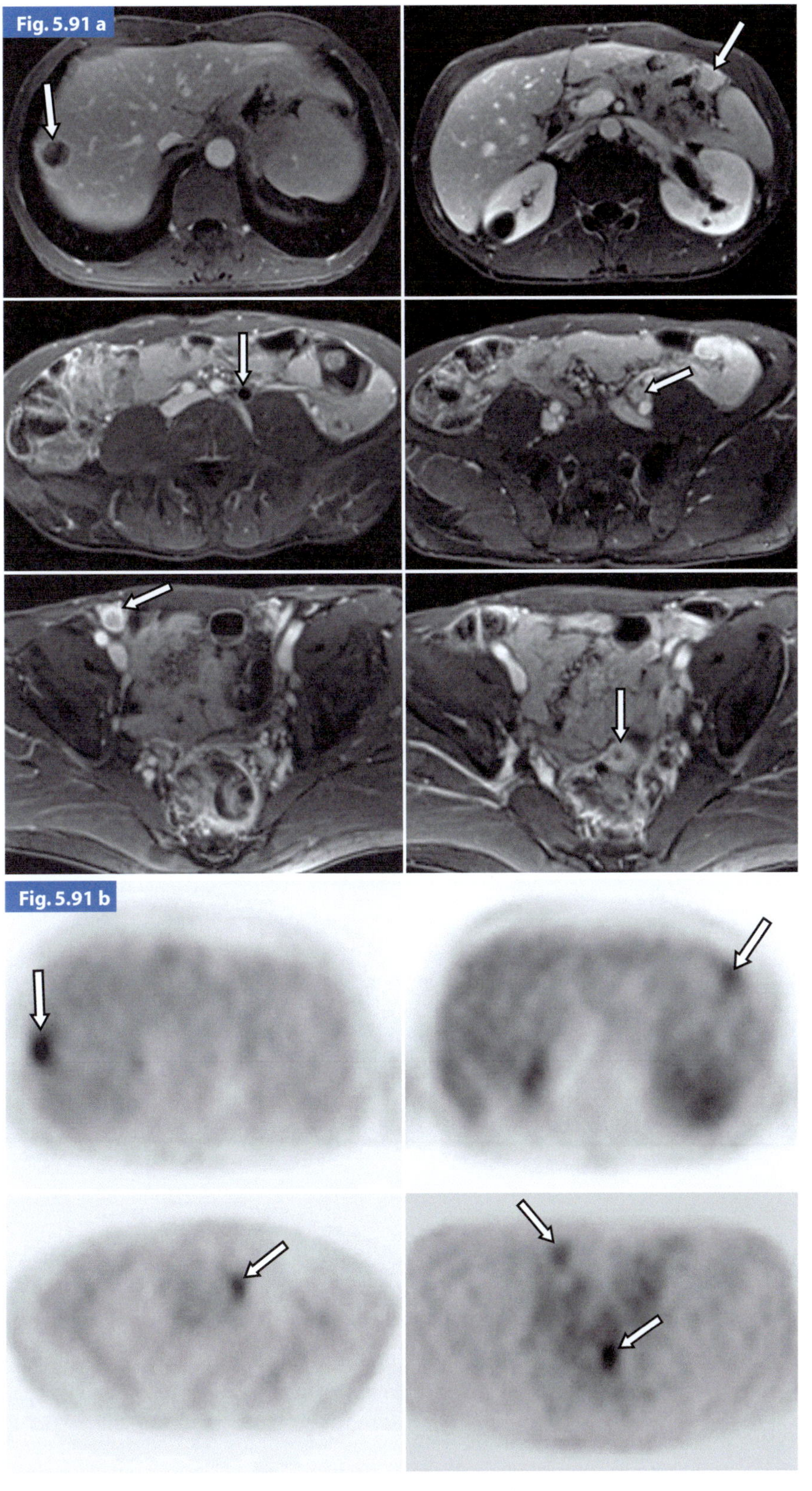

Fig. 5.91 Patient history: Status after rectosigmoid resection, PME, and pelvic peritonectomy in 2005 resulting from rectosigmoid cancer, stage pT4N1M1 (peritoneal) L1 G3, R1. Status after 12 cycles of FOLFIRI + Avastin until 2006. Restaging in 2007 with initial diagnosis of a liver metastasis. Axial breath-hold CE-FLASH 2D images from the SMS moving-table staging (**a**) and corresponding axial FDG-PET data (**b**) reveal a solitary superficial metastasis in the liver segment 7 (*arrows*), a peritoneal nodule (*arrows*), hydronephrosis and left ureteral stenosis resulting from tumor infiltration (*arrows*), a mesorectal lymph node metastasis (*arrows*), and a peritoneal node adjacent to the cecal colon (*arrows*). Subsequent atypical and anatomic resection of the liver segments 8 and 7, partial resection of the right diaphragm, deep anterior resection of the rectum, left ureteral resection, partial resection of the transverse colon and Sugarbaker procedure with hyperthermic intraperitoneal chemotherapy (HIPEC) were carried out. Histopathology described left ureteral metastasis, extensive peritoneal carcinosis, infiltration of the right diaphragm resulting from liver metastasis, omental metastases, and mesorectal lymph node metastases.

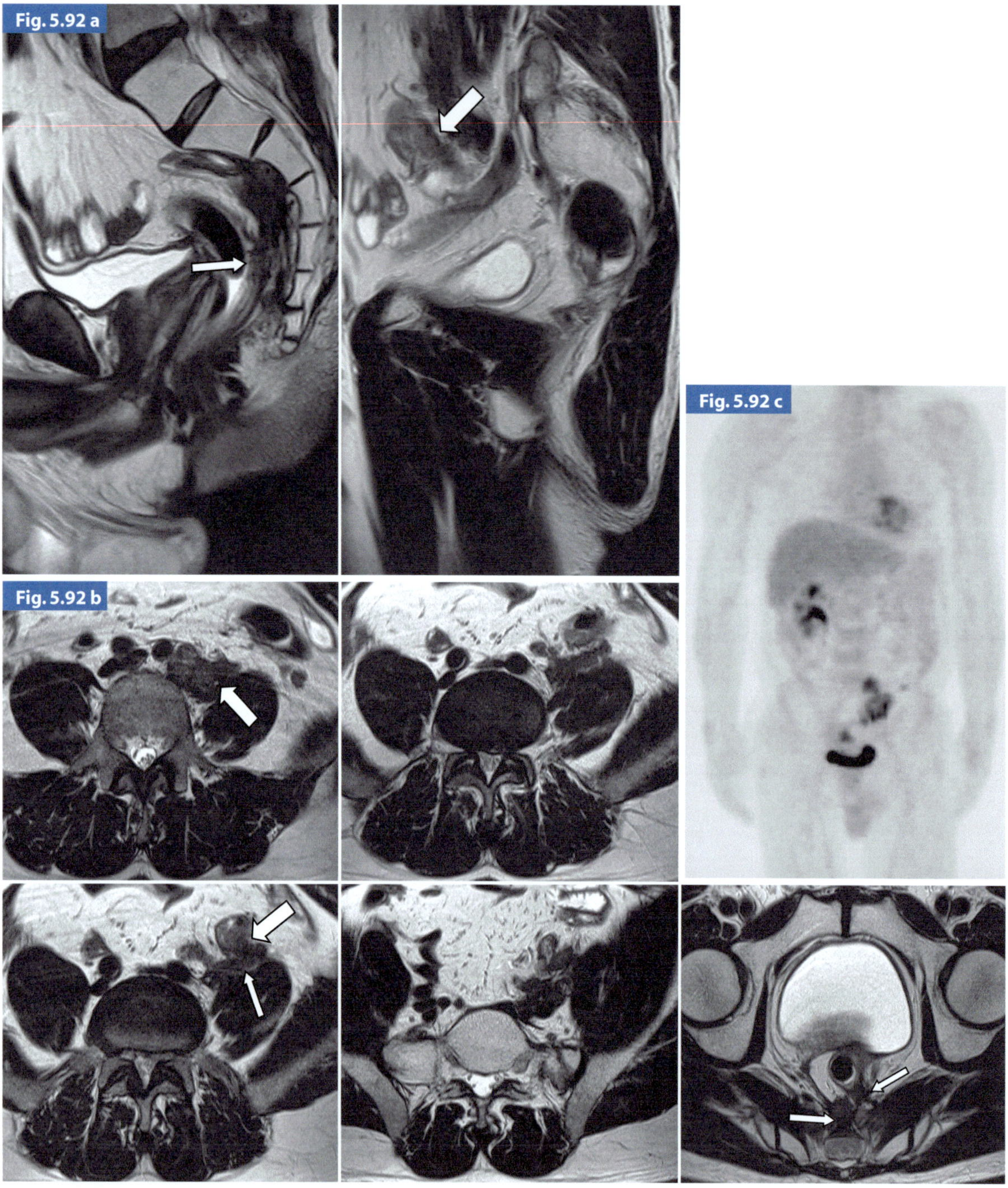

Fig. 5.92 Recurrent rectal cancer and metachronous carcinoma of the descending colon. Patient history: in 2002 rectal cancer was diagnosed and laparoscopic anterior resection of the rectum was performed. Histopathology revealed stage pT3N1 rectal cancer. In 2005, elevated CEA levels gave rise to the displayed MRI and PET examinations. (**a**) The sagittal T2-TSE images exhibit presacral local tumor recurrence at the level of the S2 and S3 segments with involvement of the rectal anastomosis (*small arrow*). A metachronous carcinoma in the descending colon can also be seen (*arrow*). (**b**) Axial T2-TSE images reveal left iliac lymph node metastases (*arrow*) and wall-exceeding tumor of the descending colon (*arrow*) with adhesion to the left psoas muscle (*arrow*). The local tumor reccurence infiltrates the presacral fascia and the rectal anastomosis between 4- and 5-o'clock lithotomy positions (*arrows*). The findings were corroborated by FDG-PET (**c**).

5.8 Unusual Metastatic Spread of Colorectal Cancer

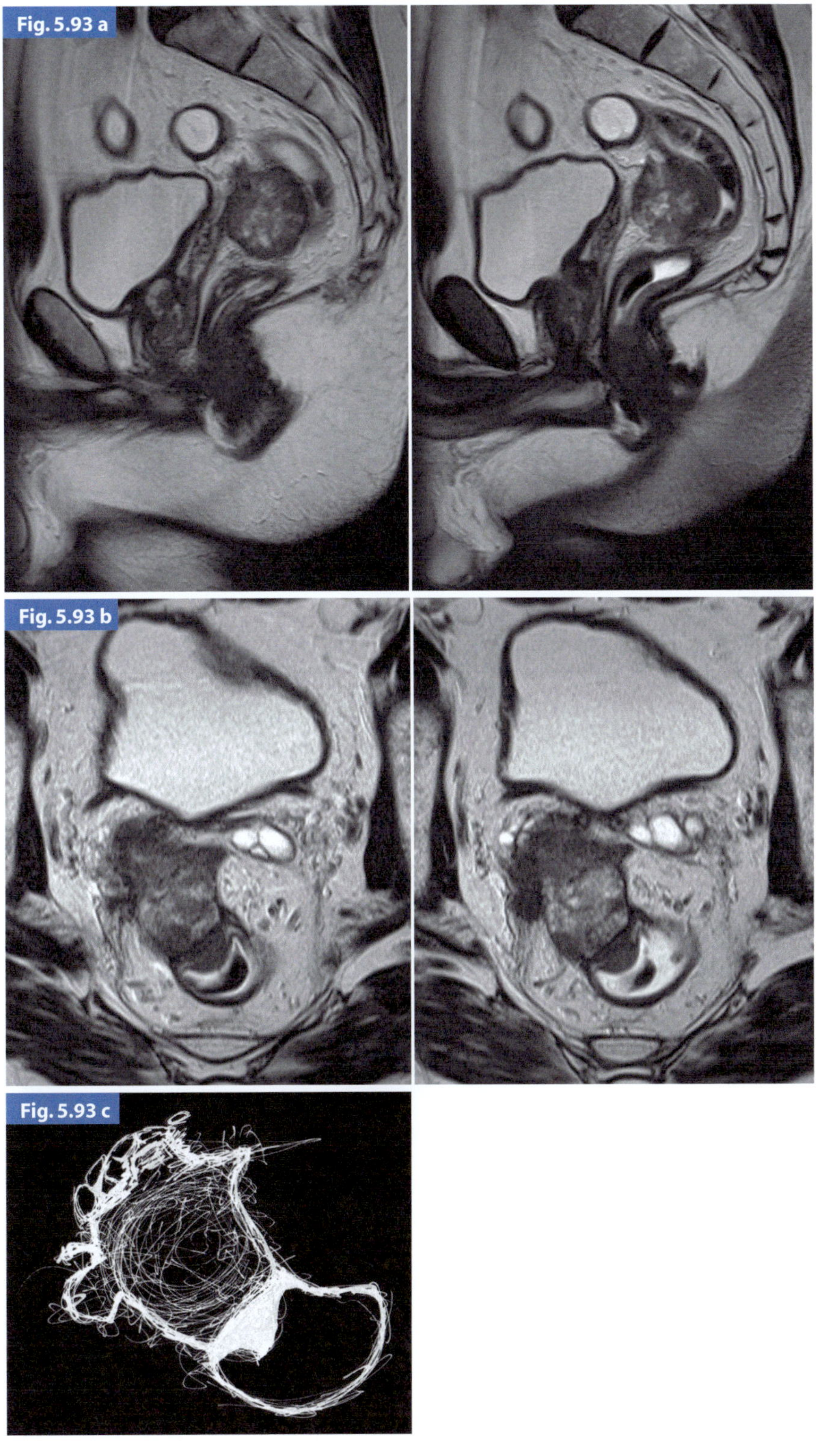

Fig. 5.93 Recurrent cecal cancer. Patient history: Status after right hemicolectomy for cecal cancer. Continuously rising CEA-levels during follow-up. Sagittal (**a**) and axial (**b**) T2-TSE images reveal a metastasis in the rectovesical pouch with invasion of the right seminal vesicles, the mesorectal fat and all layers of the adjacent midrectum, confirmed by histopathology. (**c**) Ink drawing: peritoneal metastasis

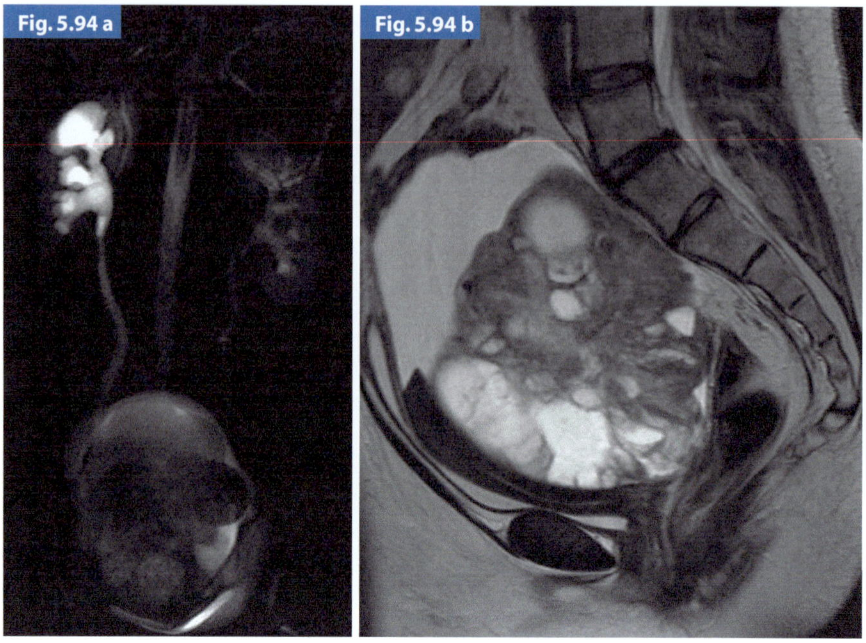

Fig. 5.94 Ovarian metastasis of sigmoid cancer. On the coronal RARE image (**a**), hydronephrosis resulting from ureteral compression is seen. Extensive tumor with cystic and solid components that cause ascites is detectable on the sagittal (**b**) T2-TSE image displacing urinary bladder, uterus, and neorectosigmoid. The tumor seems to originate from the right ovary which could not be differentiated. Patient history: Right ovariectomy was performed and histopathology diagnosed a colon cancer metastasis.

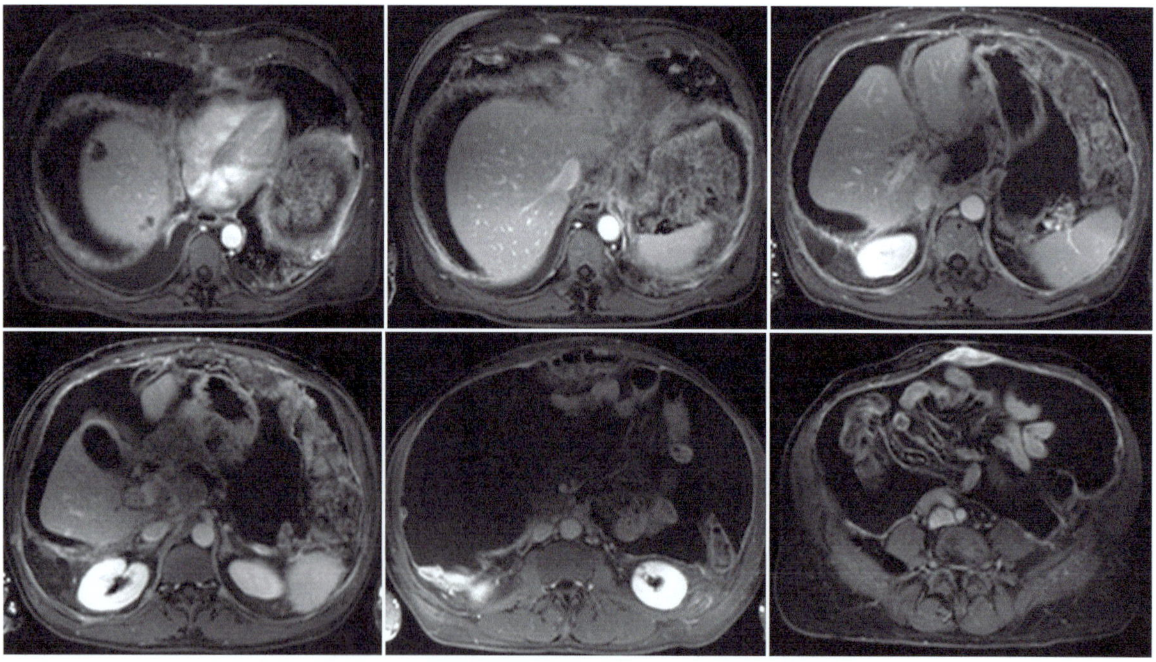

Fig. 5.95 Peritoneal carcinosis resulting from stage T4 mucinous adenocarcinoma of the rectum. The axial CE-FLASH 2D images reveal characteristics of an advanced peritoneal spread including large ascites, involvement of the greater and lesser omentum, and the liver parenchyma.

Fig. 5.96 Stomach metastasis of a moderately differentiated tubular adenocarcinoma of the rectum. (**a**) Coronal HASTE image, (**b**) axial T1-FLASH 2D, and (**c**) corresponding axial CE-FLASH 2D images show an intra-/extraluminal stomach metastasis (*arrow* in **a**) causing antral stenosis (*arrow* in **c**). The metastasis infiltrates the duodenum (*arrow* in **b**) and the left anterior chest wall (*arrow* in **b**).

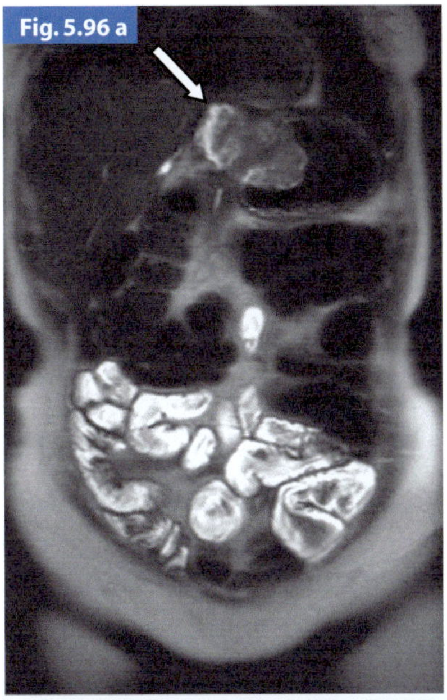

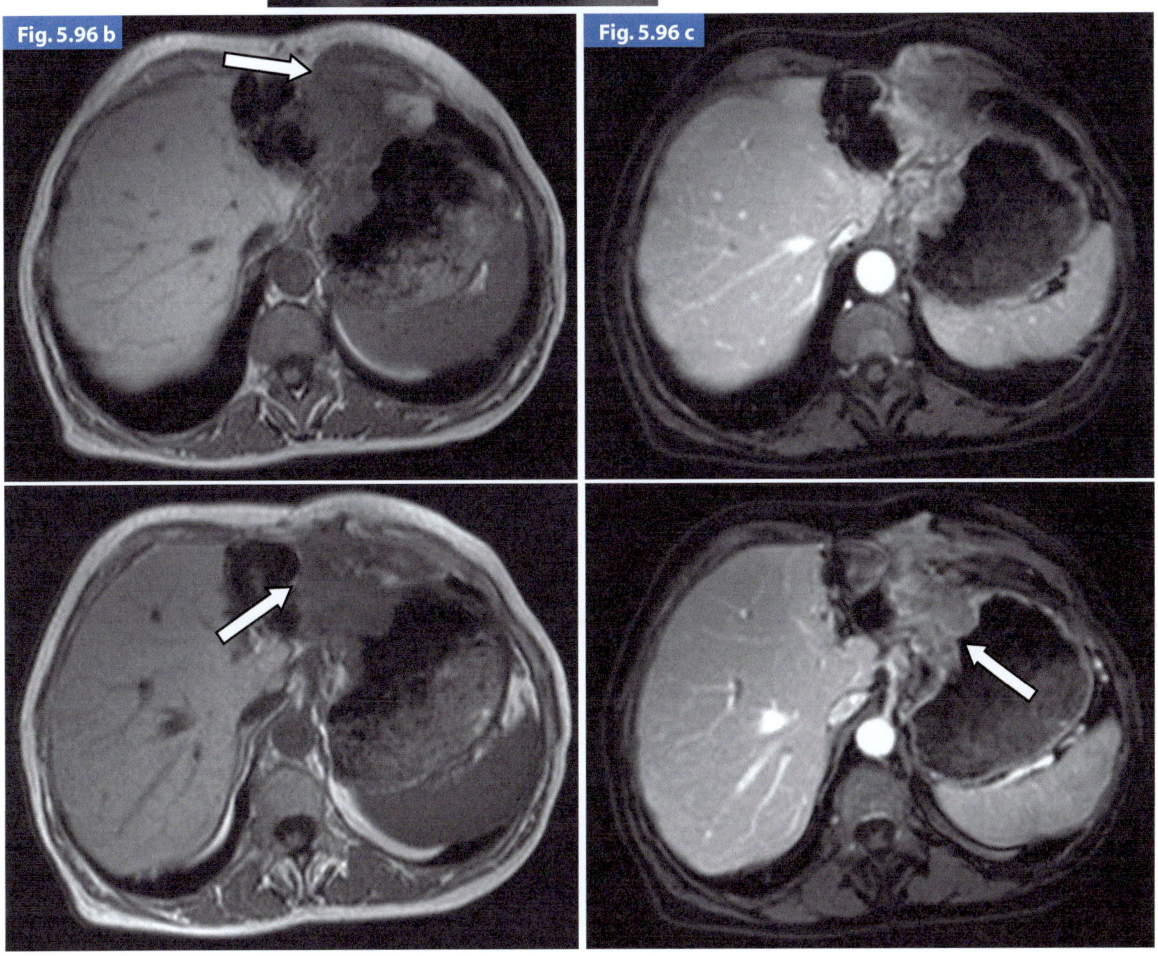

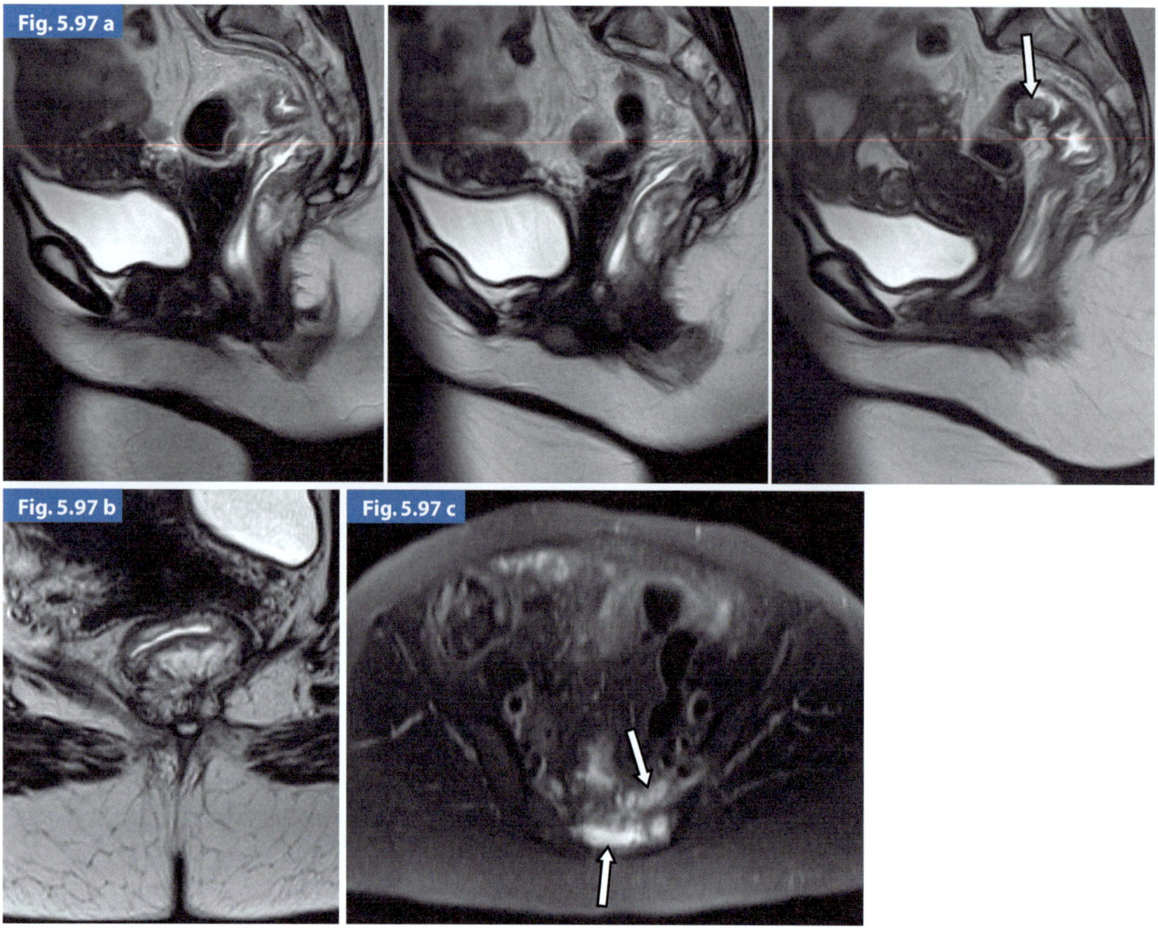

Fig. 5.97 Retrorectal metastasis of a mucinous adenocarcinoma of initially unknown primary origin. Patient history: Status after left ovarectomy and removal of tumorous tissue from the left pelvic sidewall and retrorectal space because of suspicion of teratoma. In contrast, histopathology diagnosed a metastasis of a mucinous adenocarcinoma with nerve sheath infiltration, R2 resection. During follow-up, the primary tumor site could not be identified over a period of 7 months. (**a**–**c**) MRI 7 months after initial surgery. On the sagittal (**a**) and axial (**b**) T2-TSE images, a signal-rich tumor highly indicative of metastasis from mucinous carcinoma is shown occupying the retrorectal space. The tumor infiltrates the rectal muscle layer and the submucosa. Additionally, there is detection of a small mass with high-signal foci located in the upper rectum (*arrow*). The axial (**c**) SMS TIRM image reveals infiltration of the sacral bone and left sacral nerves (*arrows*) at the site of previous surgery. (**d**, **e**) Control MRI 3 months later after diagnosis of metastasizing rectal cancer. The sagittal (**d**) and axial (**e**) T2-TSE images confirm progressive disease. Wall-penetrating, growing mucinous carcinoma of the upper rectum with wall-infiltrating retrorectal metastasis, which now involves all layers with an endoluminal portion (*asterisk*), is shown. Progressive tumor infiltration of left sacral nerves (example: S2, *arrow*) and progressive sacral bone involvement is also shown.

Fig. 5.97 d

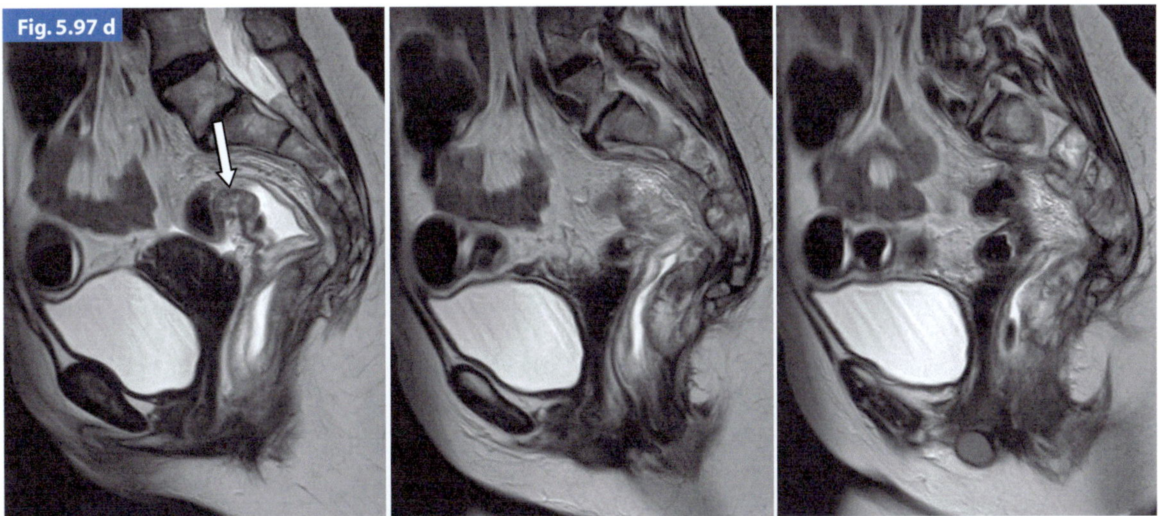

Fig. 5.97 e

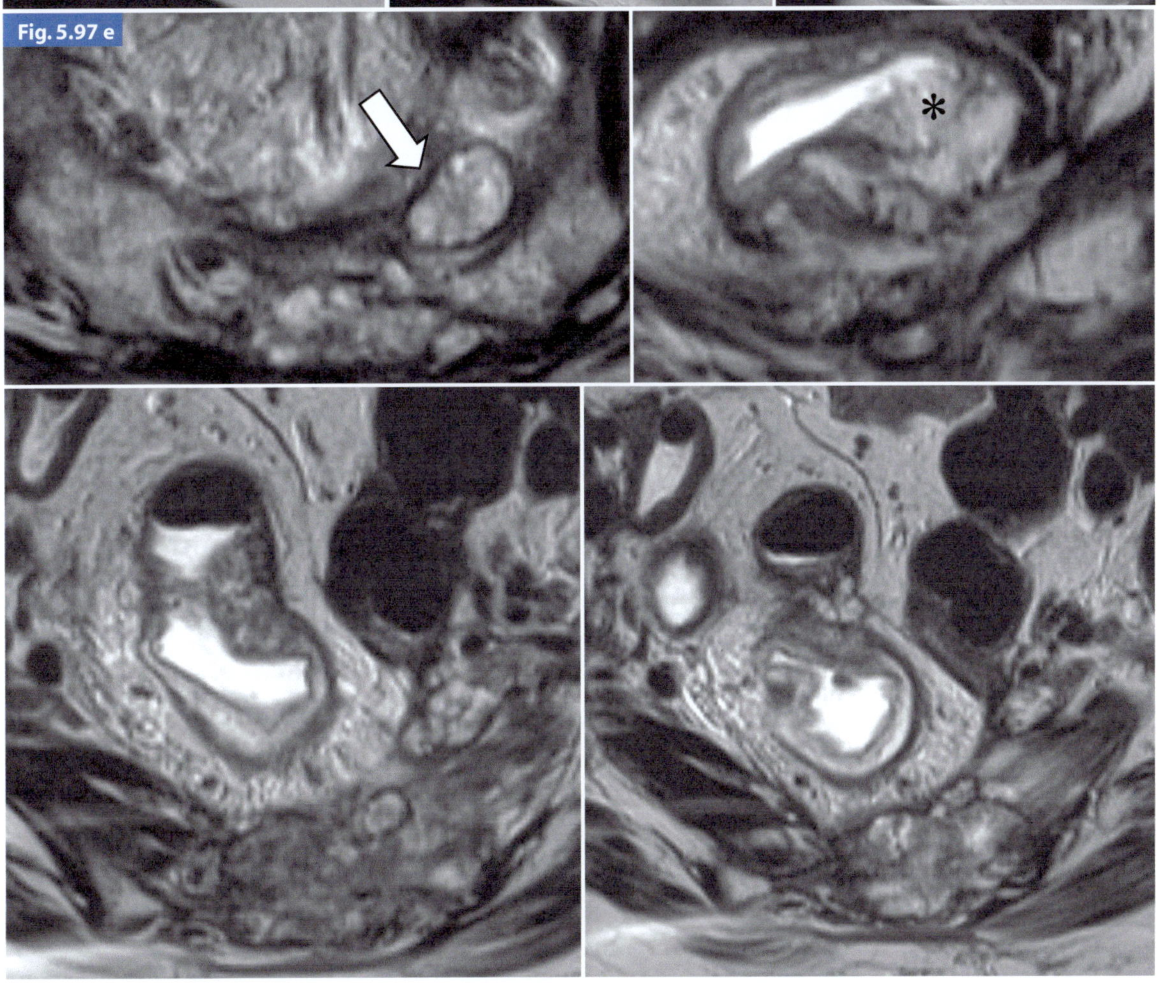

Fig. 5.98 Bone metastasis from rectal cancer. Sagittal (**a**) and axial (**b**) T2-TSE image and the corresponding axial (**c**) CE-FLASH 2D image show metastasis of the left acetabulum with soft-tissue infiltration.

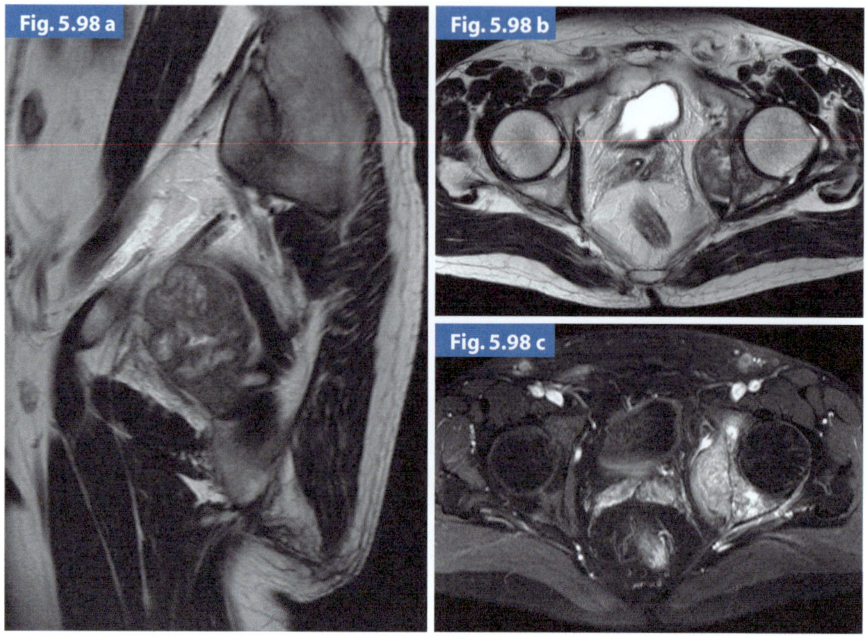

Fig. 5.99 Metastatic rectal cancer, wrist pain. Coronal (**a**) TIRM and (**b**) T1-TSE images show a metastasis to the left triquetral bone (*arrow*), confirmed by histopathology.

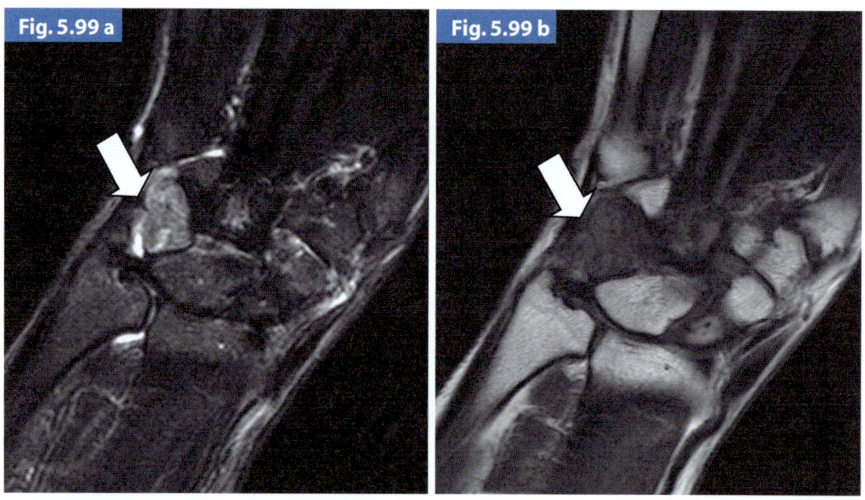

Fig. 5.100 Metastatic rectal cancer, shoulder pain. The coronal (**a**) TIRM and (**b**) CE-FLASH 2D images demonstrate extensive left scapular bone metastasis involving the coracoid process (*arrows*).

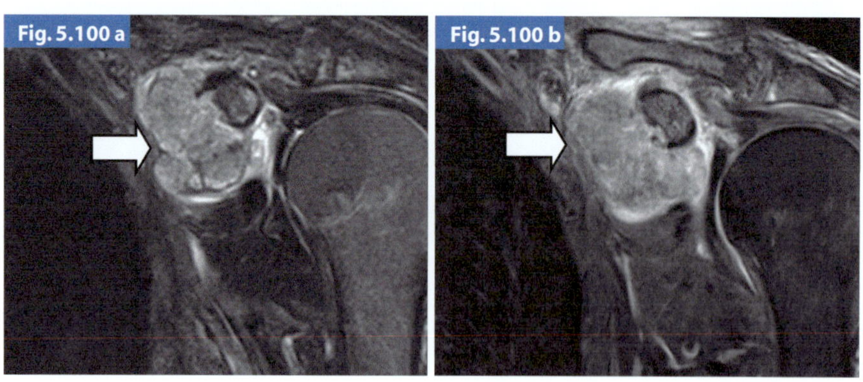

5.9 Differential Diagnosis of Rectal Cancer

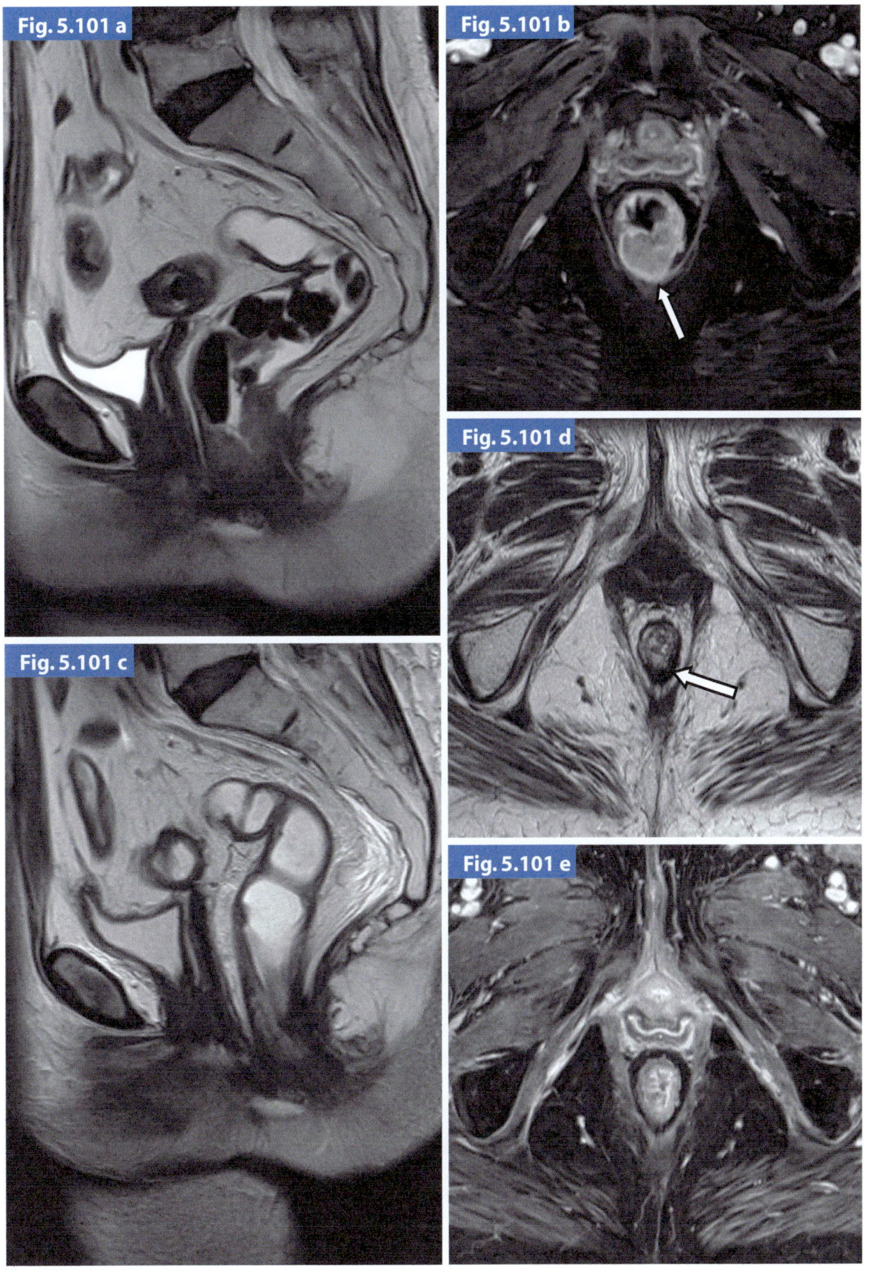

Fig. 5.101 Anal cancer prior to and after radiochemotherapy according to Nigro protocol. (**a**) On the initial sagittal T2-TSE image detection a tumor formation at the level of the anorectal junction. (**b**) The axial CE-FLASH 3D image shows tumor adherence to the levator muscle (*arrow*). On the sagittal (**c**) and axial (**d**) T2-TSE images and the corresponding axial (**e**) CE-FLASH 3D image obtained after radiochemotherapy, the tumor completely disappeared except for residual T2-dark-signal scar (*arrow*).

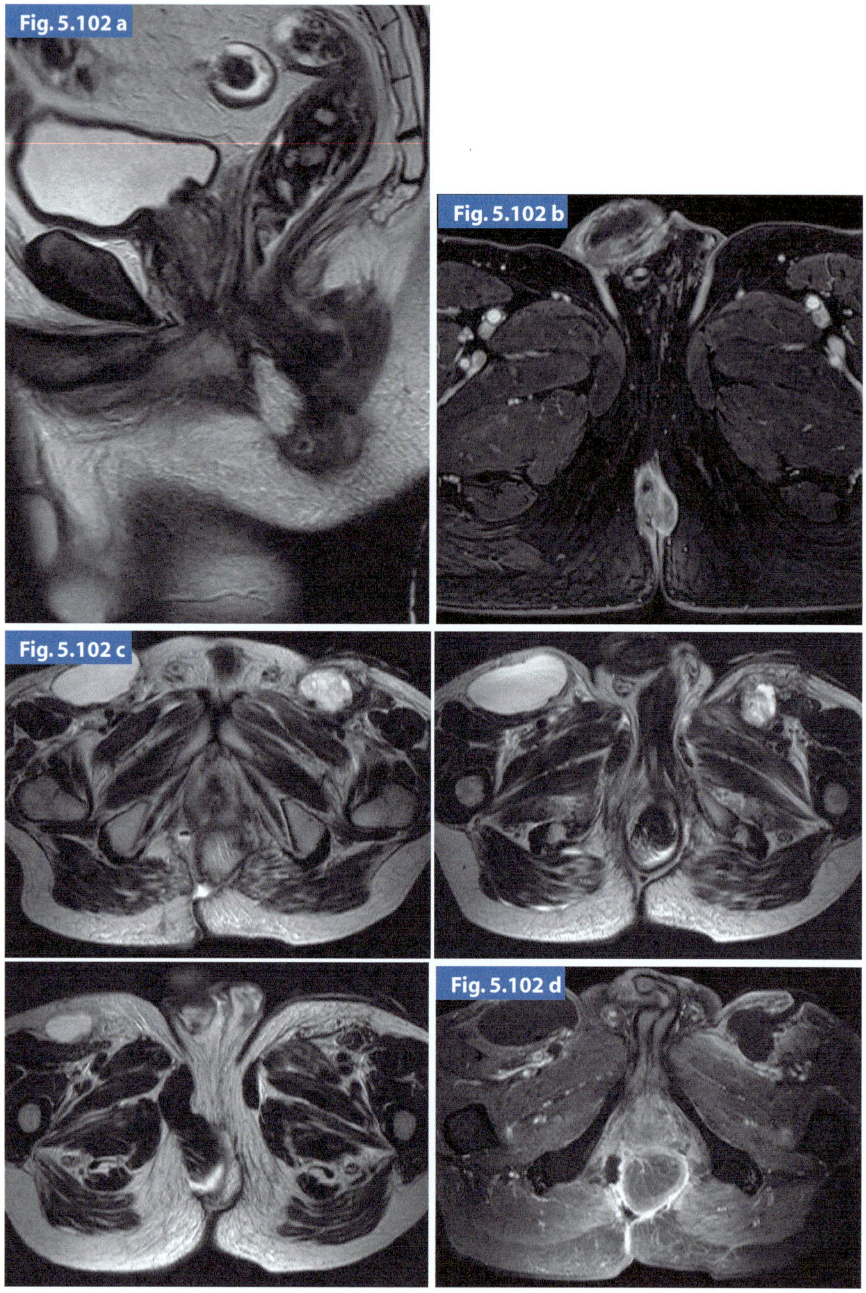

Fig. 5.102 Stage T2 anal cancer. (**a**, **b**) Pretreatment MRI. (**a**) On the sagittal T2-TSE image an irregular tumor formation is present in conjunction with the anal verge. (**b**) The axial CE-FLASH 3D image corroborates the finding of anal carcinoma measuring less than 5 cm in diameter, which is a T2 criterion. (**c**, **d**) Posttreatment MRI. The patient received radiochemotherapy according to Nigro protocol and groin lymph node dissection on both sides as well as gracilis flap closure of the perineum during the course of the disease. The axial T2-TSE images (**c**) and the corresponding axial (**d**) CE-FLASH 2D image demonstrate the gracilis flap, a postoperative lymphocele in the right groin, and an infected, open lymphocele in the left groin.The anal cancer was jugded as moderately differentiated squamous cell carcinoma, ypT2N3.

Fig. 5.103 a

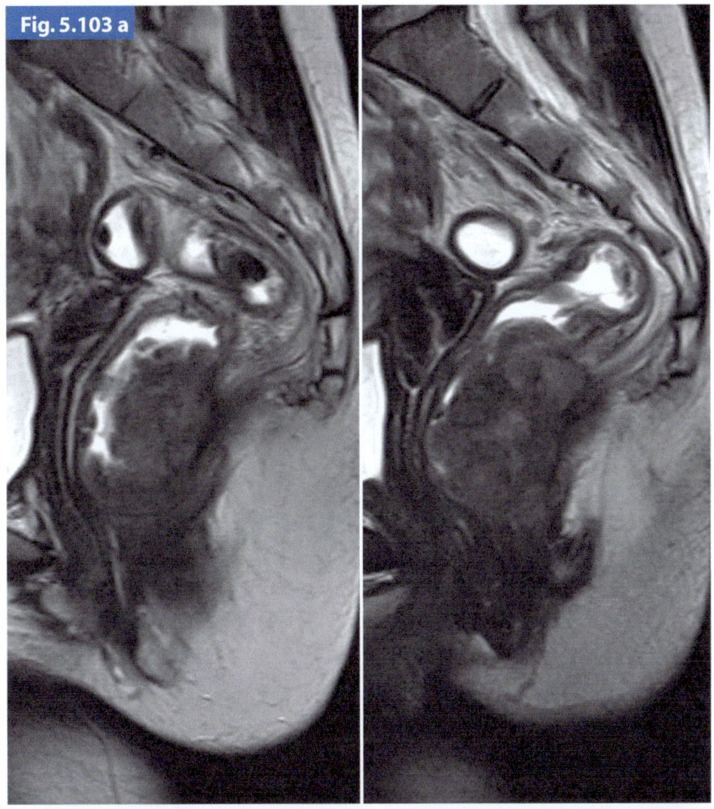

Fig. 5.103 b

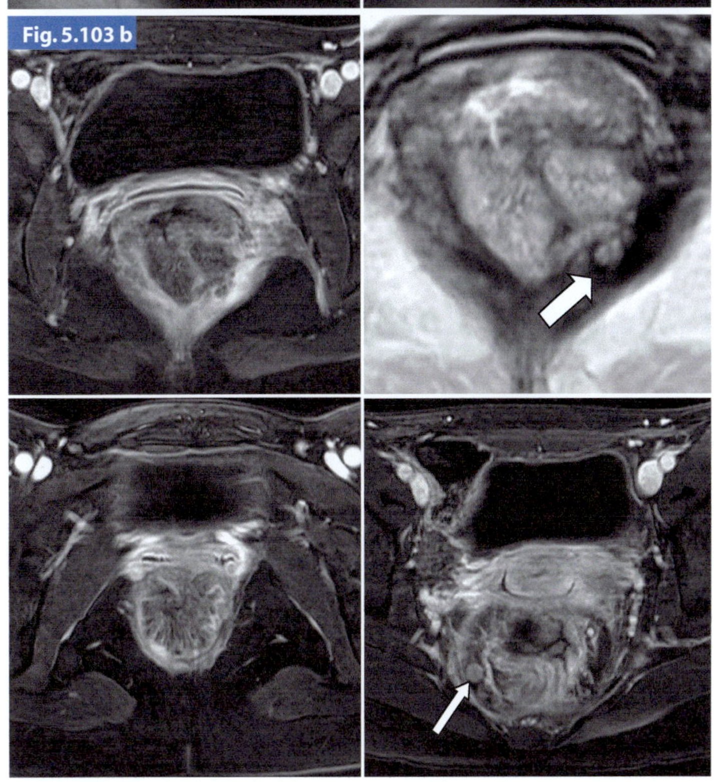

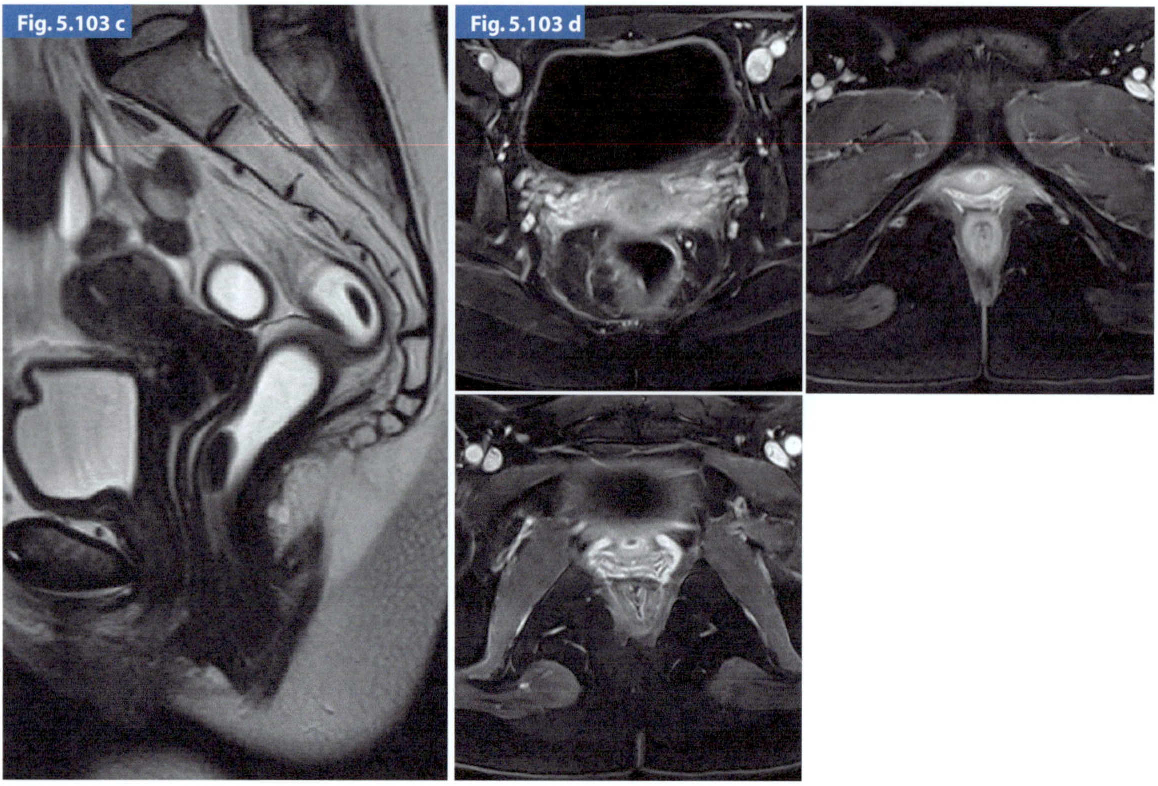

Fig. 5.103 Stage T3 anal cancer. (**a**, **b**) Pretreatment MRI. (**a**) Sagittal T2-TSE images illustrate a large mass affecting the anal channel, the lower rectum, and the mesorectal fat. (**b**) On the axial CE-VIBE 3D images, the circular growing tumor infiltrates the left levator ani muscle (*arrow* on the inverted image). Coexistent mesorectal lymph nodes suspicious of metastases (*small arrow*) are shown. The tumor was staged as cT4N1M0 rectal cancer. Interestingly, histopathology revealed moderately differentiated squamous cell carcinoma of the anal channel. The tumor was restaged as cT3N1 and the patient received radiochemotherapy according to Nigro protocol. (**c**, **d**) Follow-up MRI. The sagittal (**c**) and the axial (**d**) CE-VIBE 3D images demonstrate complete tumor response.

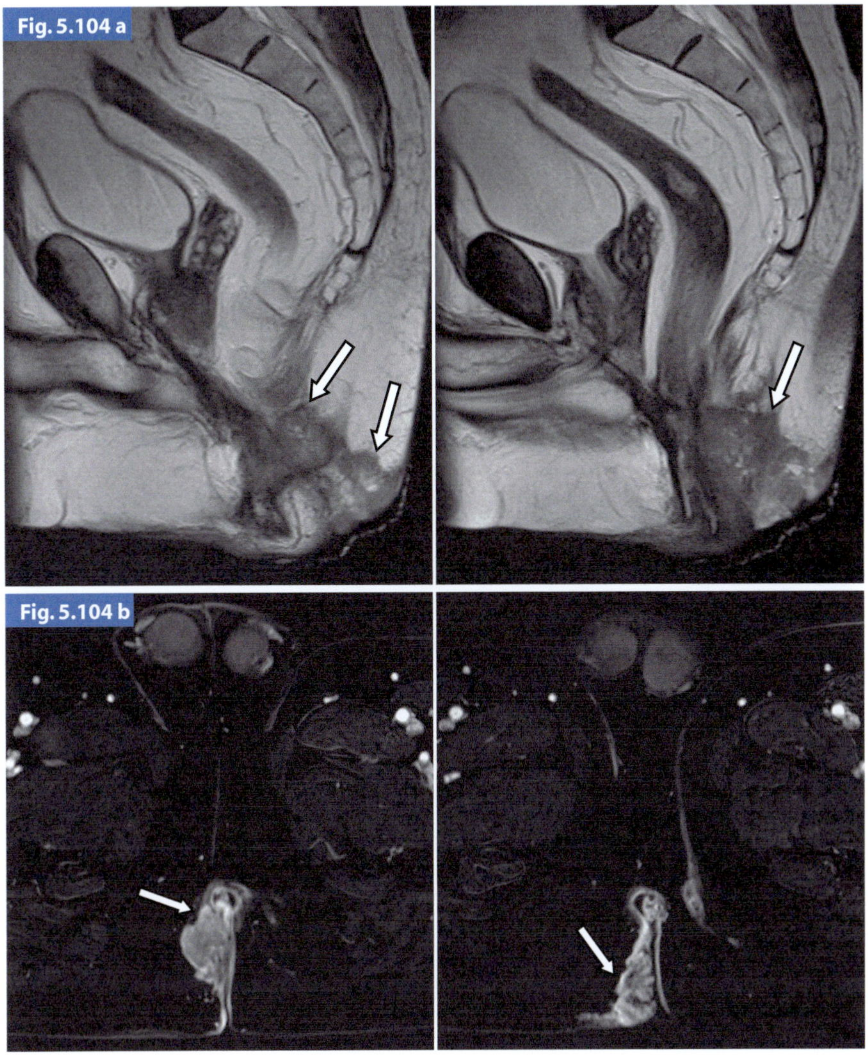

Fig. 5.104 Stage T3 anal cancer: course of the disease. Patient history: Crohn's disease since 1983 with longstanding anal fistulas, repetitive excisions of fistula tracks, and anal bleeding. (**a**, **b**) Pretreatment MRI, January 2006. (**a**) On the sagittal T2-TSE images, an ill-defined tumor formation in the region of the anus can be detected (*arrows*). (**b**) The subtracted axial CE-FLASH 3D images of indirect MR-fistulography reveal tumor involvement of the right posterior anal channel between 6- and 9-o'clock lithotomy positions with transspincteric extension to the rima ani (*arrows*). Abdominoperineal resection of the rectum was performed in February and histopathlogy diagnosed stage pT3N0 squamous cell carcinoma of the anal channel. Adjuvant radiochemotherapy was administered. Initial follow-up MRI, May 2006.

Fig. 5.104 c

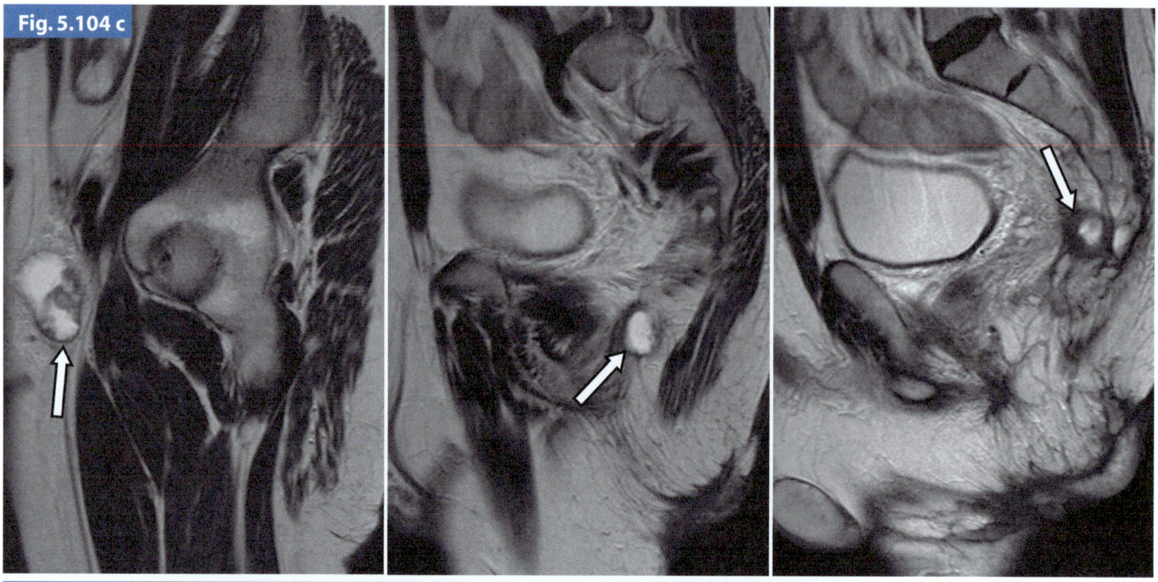

Fig. 5.104 d

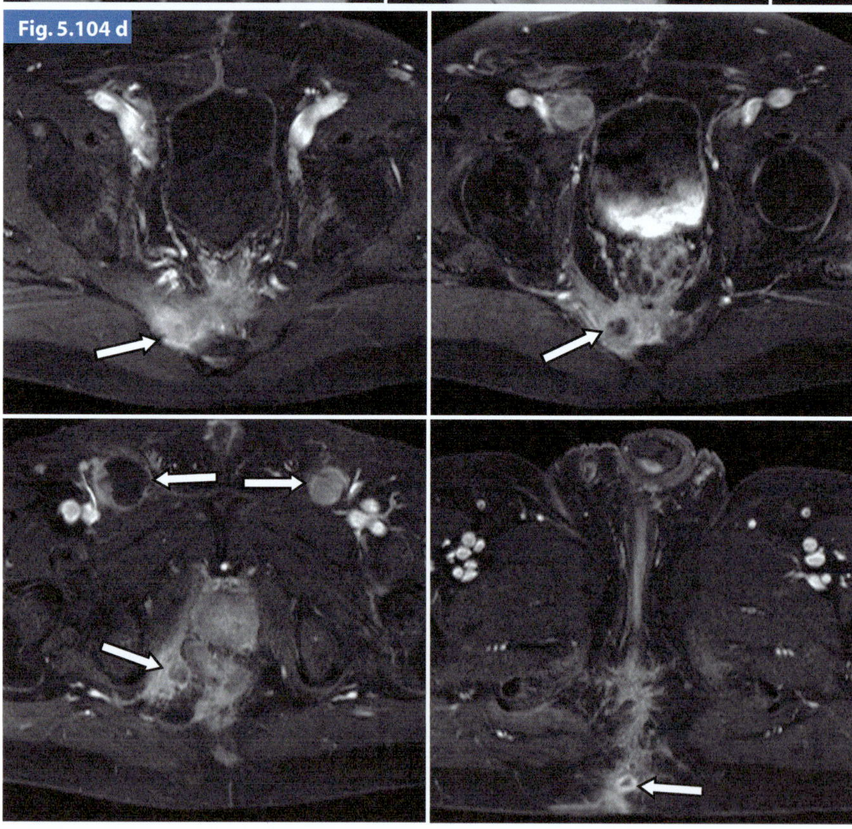

Fig. 5.104 (**c**, **d**) The sagittal T2-TSE (**c**) and axial fat-saturated CE-T1-TSE (**d**) images show inguinal, partially necrotic lymph node metastases (*arrows*) and cystic tumor nodules along the pelvic scar involving the right pelvic sidewall and the sacral bone (*arrows*).

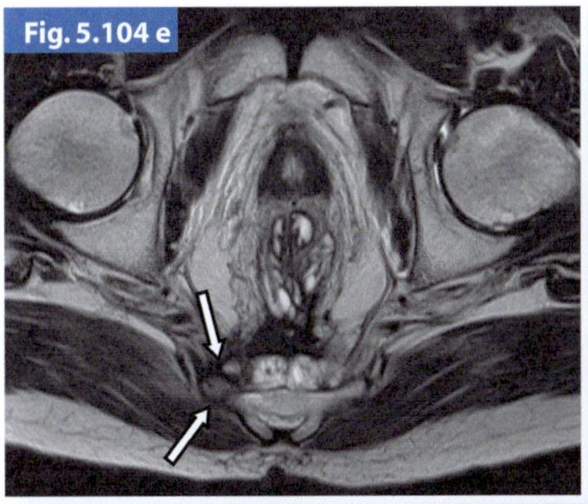

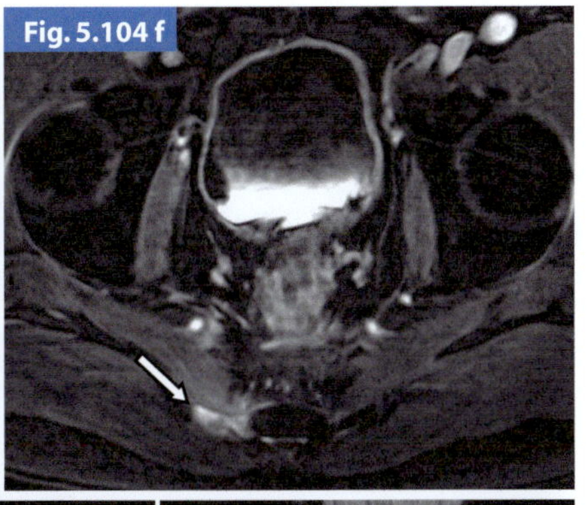

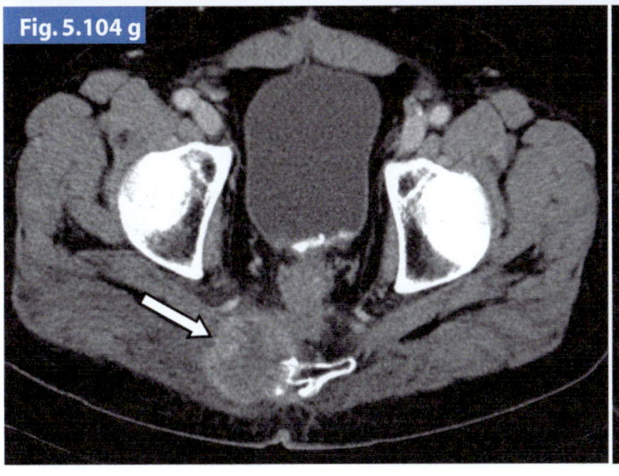

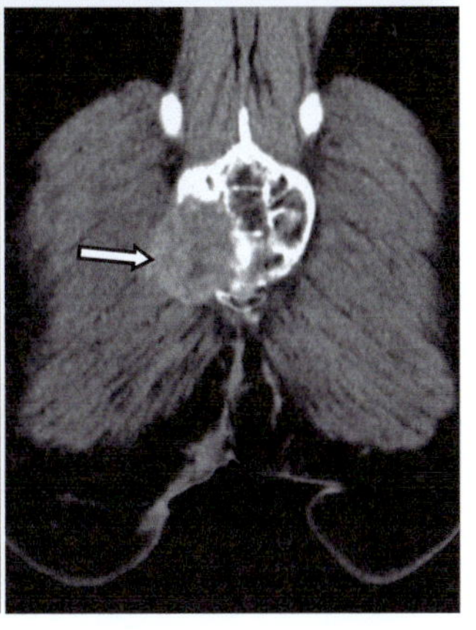

Fig. 5.104 Wide excision of the local recurrence and lymphonodectomy were performed, R1 situation. (**e**, **f**) Second follow-up MRI, October 2006. Again, the para-axial T2-TSE (**e**) and corresponding axial CE-VIBE (**f**) three-dimensional images demonstrate right sacral bone metastasis with surrounding soft-tissue infiltration (*arrows*). The patient refused further treatment but was readmitted 3 months later with right gluteal pain. (**g**) Abdominal MSCT, January 2007. Progressive right sacral bone metastasis (*arrows*), initially described by MRI

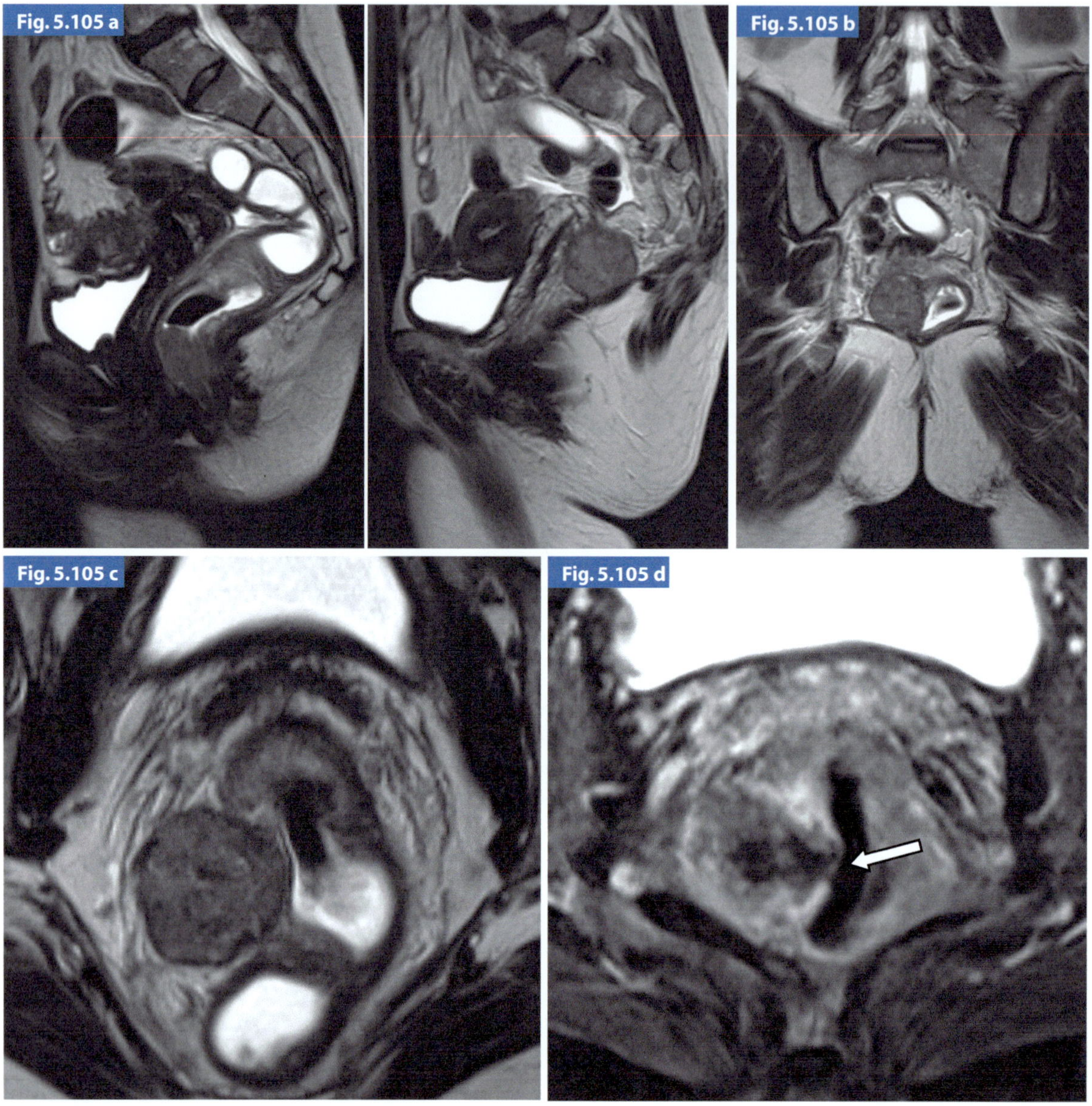

Fig. 5.105 Anal cancer. Sagittal (**a**) and coronal (**b**) T2-TSE images show a tumor arising from the anorectal junction and a lymph node metastasis in the mesorectum with adherence to the right levator ani muscle. On the para-axial T2-TSE image (**c**) and the corresponding axial CE-VIBE 3D image (**d**), the lymph node metastasis directly invades the rectal wall causing ulceration (*arrow*). Histopathologic examination of a biopsy confirmed the diagnosis of an invasive squmous cell carcinoma of the anus.

Fig. 5.106 Stage T4 anal cancer. (**a**) The sagittal T2-TSE image displays nodular tumor of the anal channel extending to the vagina (*arrows*). The axial T2-TSE image (**b**) and corresponding axial CE-VIBE 3D image (**c**) demonstrate an intravaginal tumor formation connecting with the anal channel at 12-o'clock lithotomy position (*arrows*). A sphincter defect between 11- and 1-o'clock lithotomy position is present (*arrows*). The histopathologic features were judged to be representative of a rare stage T4N0 adenocarcinoma of the anal channel.

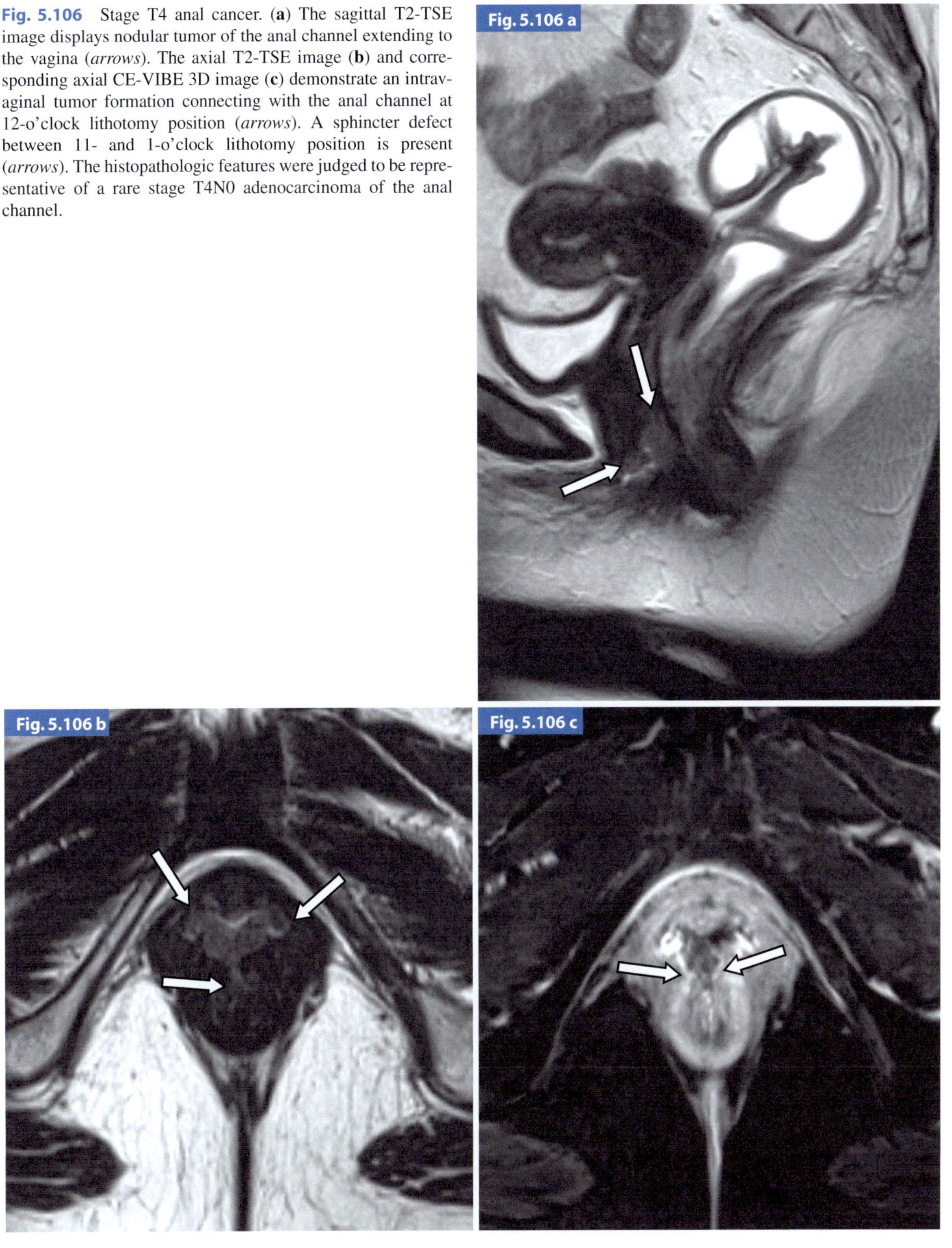

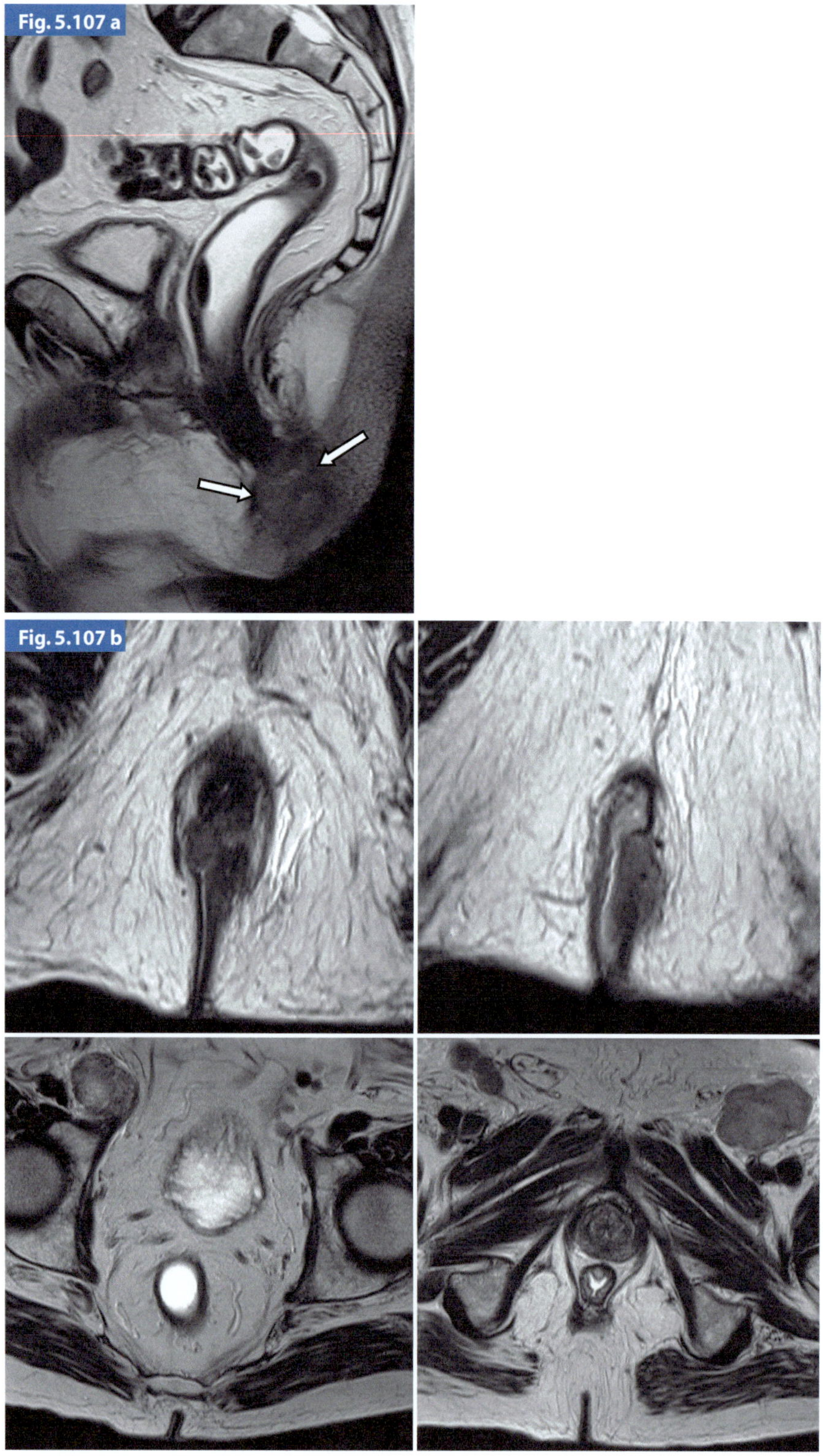

Fig. 5.107 Perianal Paget's disease associated with anal cancer. On the sagittal (**a**) and axial (**b**) T2-TSE images, an irregular perianal tumor can be detected involving the posterior commissure of the anus. Inguinal lymph node metastases are present on both sides.

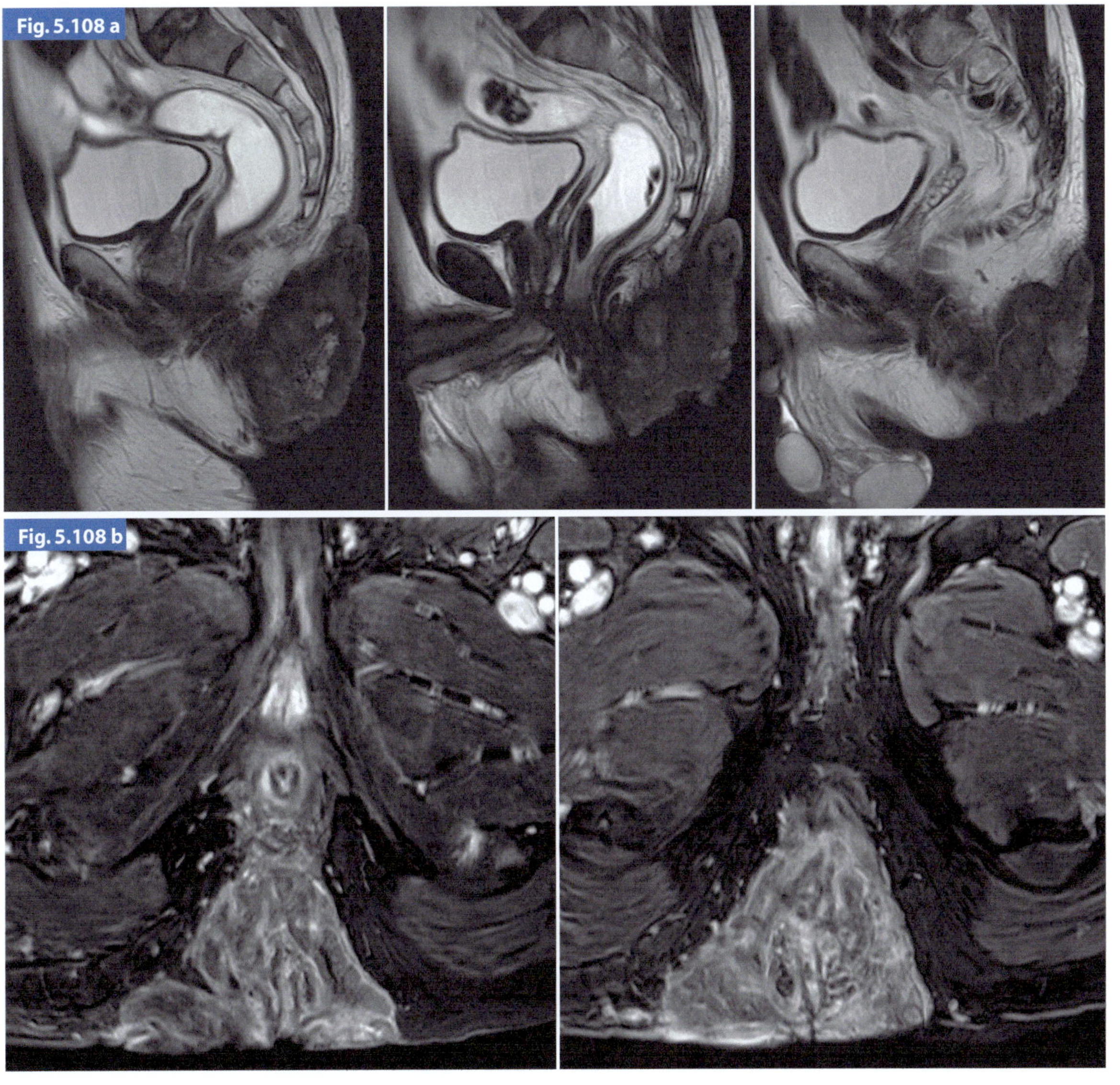

Fig. 5.108 Anorectal giant condyloma acuminatum (Buschke-Loewenstein tumor). (**a**) Sagittal T2-TSE images demonstrate irregular, intermediate to hypointense signal mass of per- and intra-anal distribution without rectal involvement. (**b**) On the axial CE-VIBE 3D images, the extensive tumor shows cauliflower-like appearance and invades the anal sphincter muscles on both sides. Histopathology revealed spots of verrucous carcinoma inside a Buschke-Loewenstein tumor.

Fig. 5.109 a

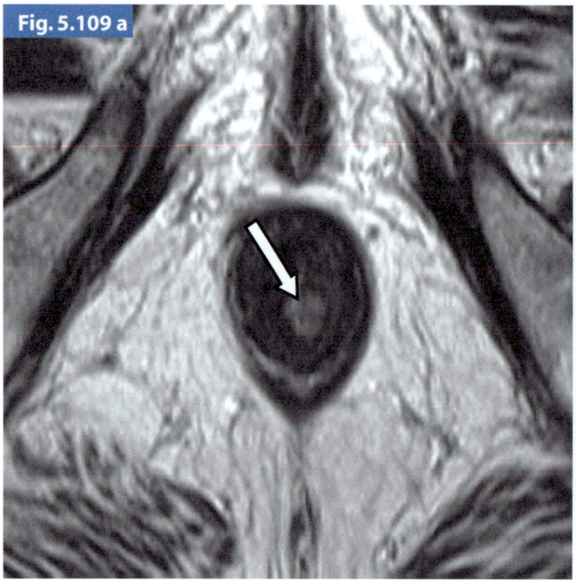

Fig. 5.109 b

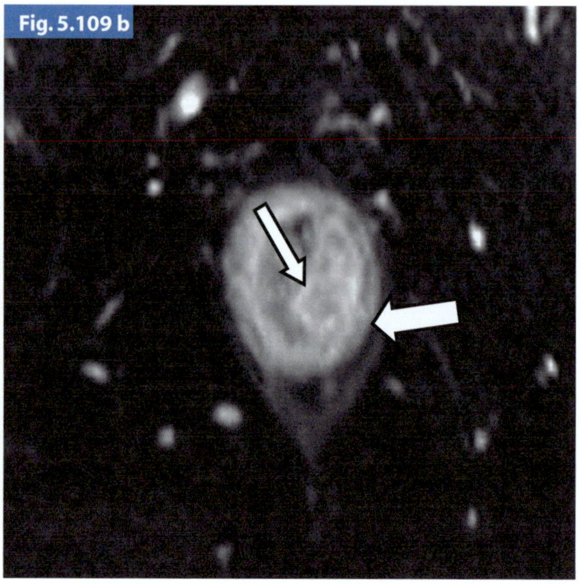

Fig. 5.109 Gastroenteropancreatic neuroendocrine tumor (GEP-NET) of the anal channel. (**a**) The axial T2-TSE image shows an intraanal small bright signal tumor nodule between 4- and 5-o'clock lithotomy position (*arrow*). On the corresponding axial (**b**) CE-FLASH 2D image unsharp delineation of the tumor which is of higher signal than the surrounding mucosa and submucosa of the anal channel (*small arrow*). Sharp differentiation of the margins of the internal sphincter muscle to the intersphincteric fat (*large arrow*) is shown. Based on these findings, the tumor was clinically staged as cT1N0. Local transanal tumor excision was performed and histopathology diagnosed stage pT1N0 GEP-NET of the anal channel.

Fig. 5.110 a

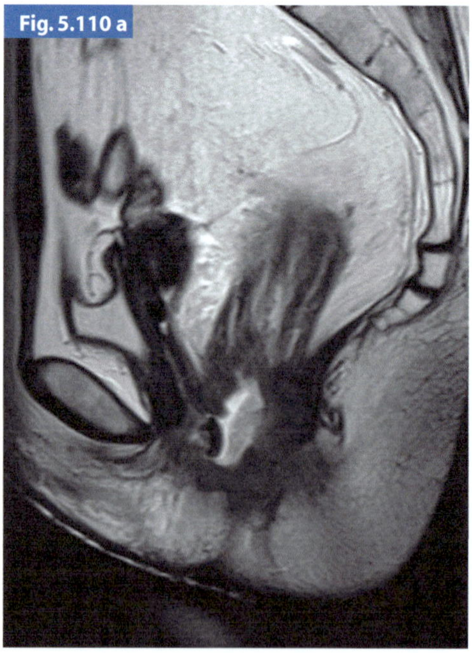

Fig. 5.110 Fistula cancer. Patient history: Crohn's disease since 1971 and a longstanding rectovaginal fistula. (**a**) Sagittal T2-TSE image shows a bizarre connection between the lower rectum, the anal channel, and the vagina resulting from a chronic rectovaginal fistula forming a common channel. Conspicuous thick-walled fistula rim. The fistula is completely filled with rectally administered water. (**b**) Axial T2-TSE images reveal circular rectal wall infiltration, infiltration of the anal channel and the vulva. (**c**) The corresponding axial CE-VIBE 3D images corroborate the findings. Biopsies were taken and histopathology diagnosed a squamous cell carcinoma arising from the rectovaginal fistula.

Fig. 5.110 b

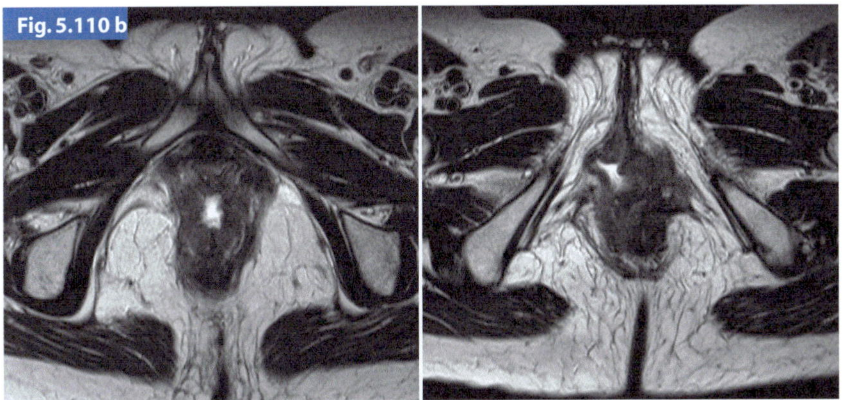

Fig. 5.110 c

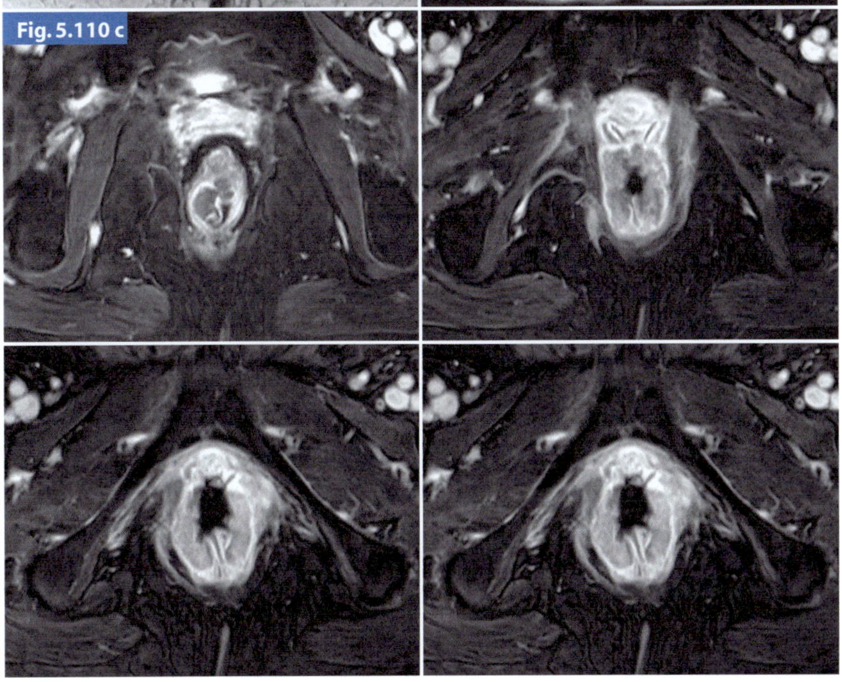

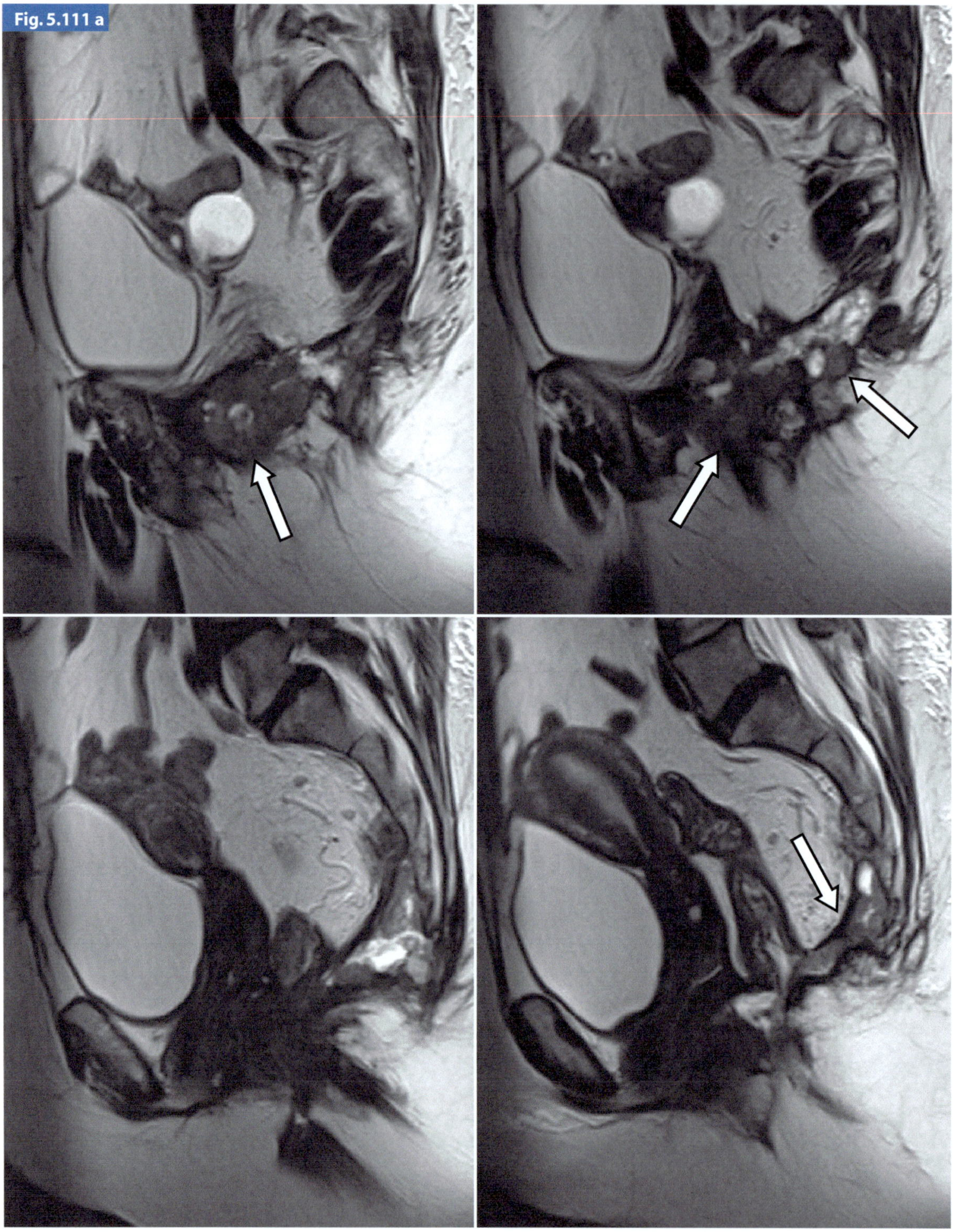

Fig. 5.111 a

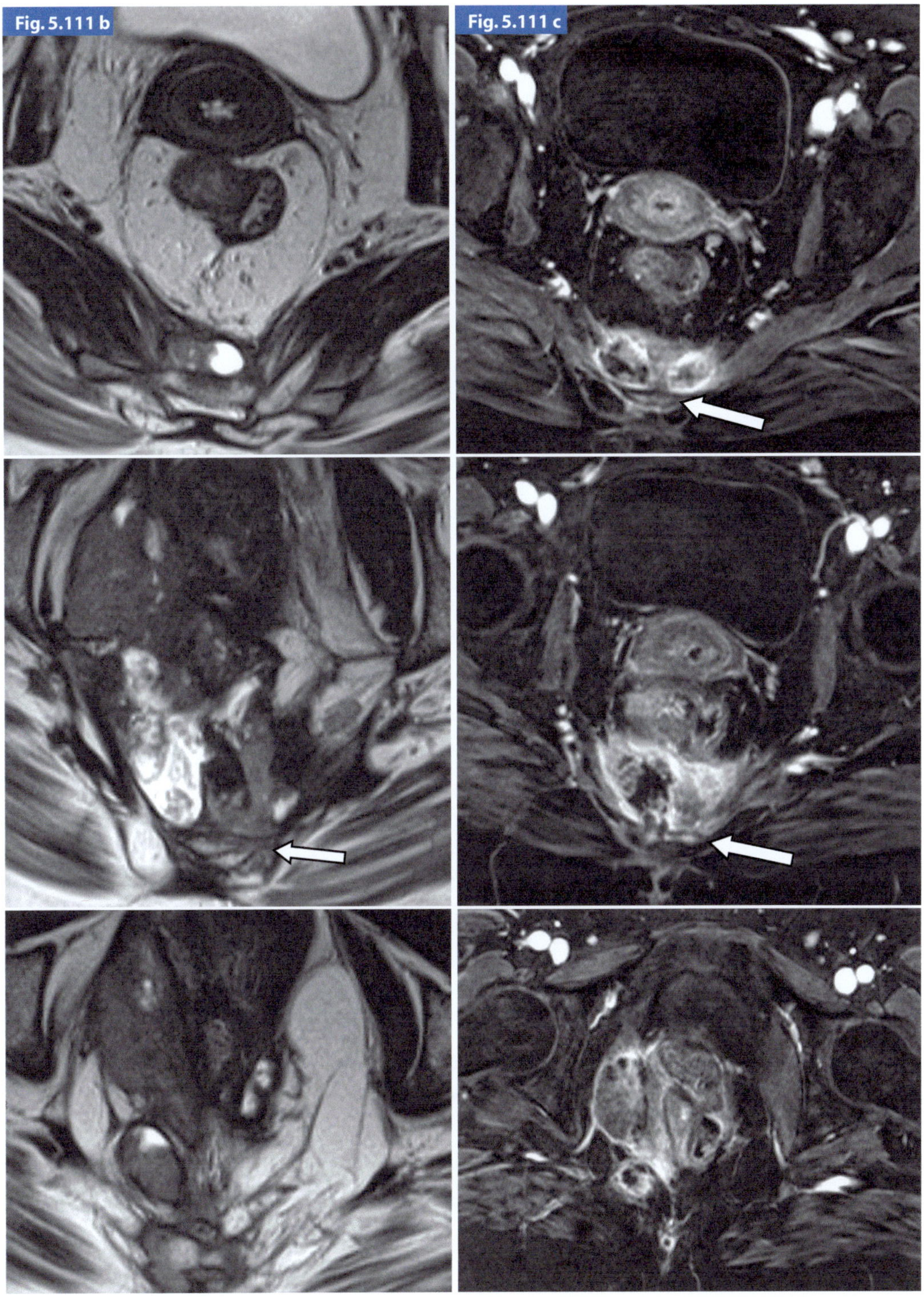

Fig. 5.111 Fistulizing anorectal Crohn's disease with fistula carcinoma. (**a**) Representative sagittal T2-TSE images obtained during the course of the disease. There is remarkably little fluid inside the widely ramified anorectal fistulas and known chronic abscesses. Instead, one can identify a replacement of the fluid-filled cavities by nodules with intermediate signal (*arrows*). The findings were corroborated by the corresponding axial (**b**) T2-TSE and (**c**) CE-VIBE 3D images derived from the same examination. Note the pathologic marrow signal of the coccygis as a result of tumor infiltration (*arrows*). The fistula margins and the rim of the right supralevatoric abscess exhibit strong contrat, whereas the tumor formations are hypovascular. The anal channel, vagina, and the right pelvic sidewall are connected via the histopathologically diagnosed fistula carcinoma.

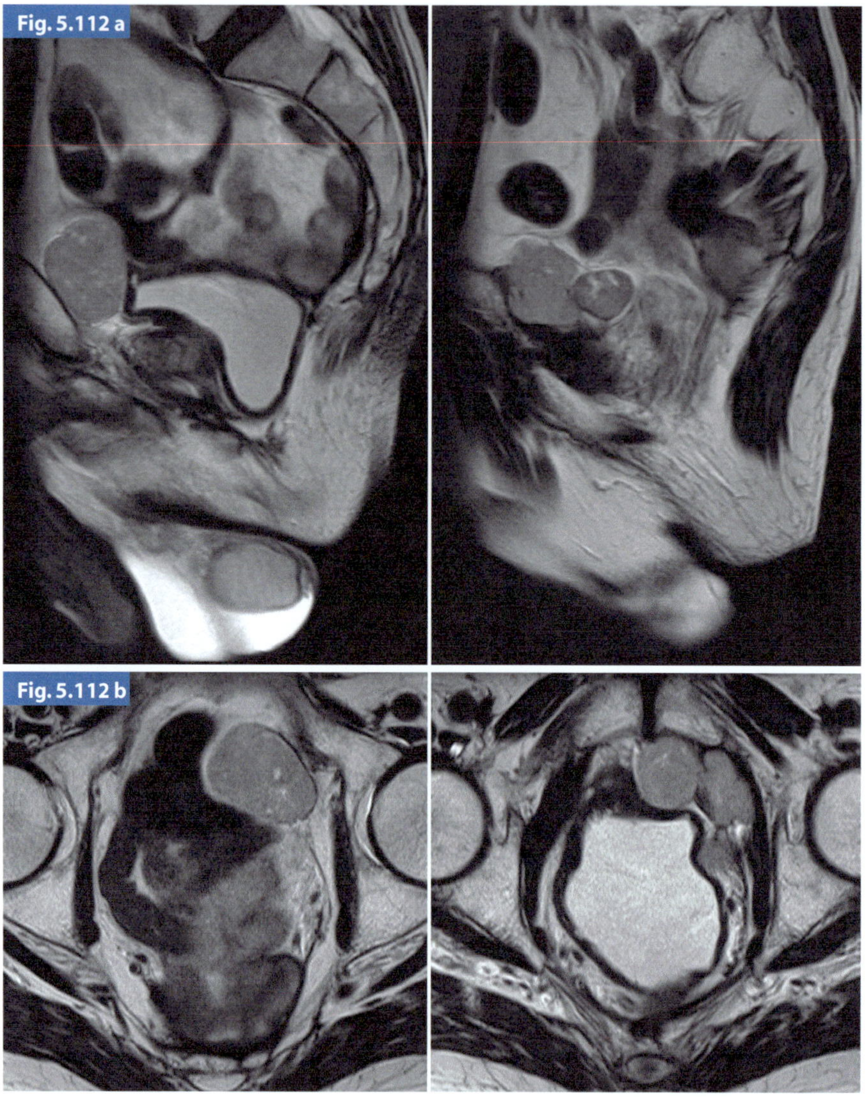

Fig. 5.112 Recurrent pelvic GIST. (**a**) Sagittal T2-TSE images show two sharply delineated pelvic sidewall tumors located in the fatty tissue around the urinary bladder. (**b**) On the axial T2-TSE images, the tumor nodules exhibit a capsula, and no signs of metastases to the pubic bone, the bladder, or the internal obturator muscle. Histopathology diagnosed recurrent pelvic GIST.

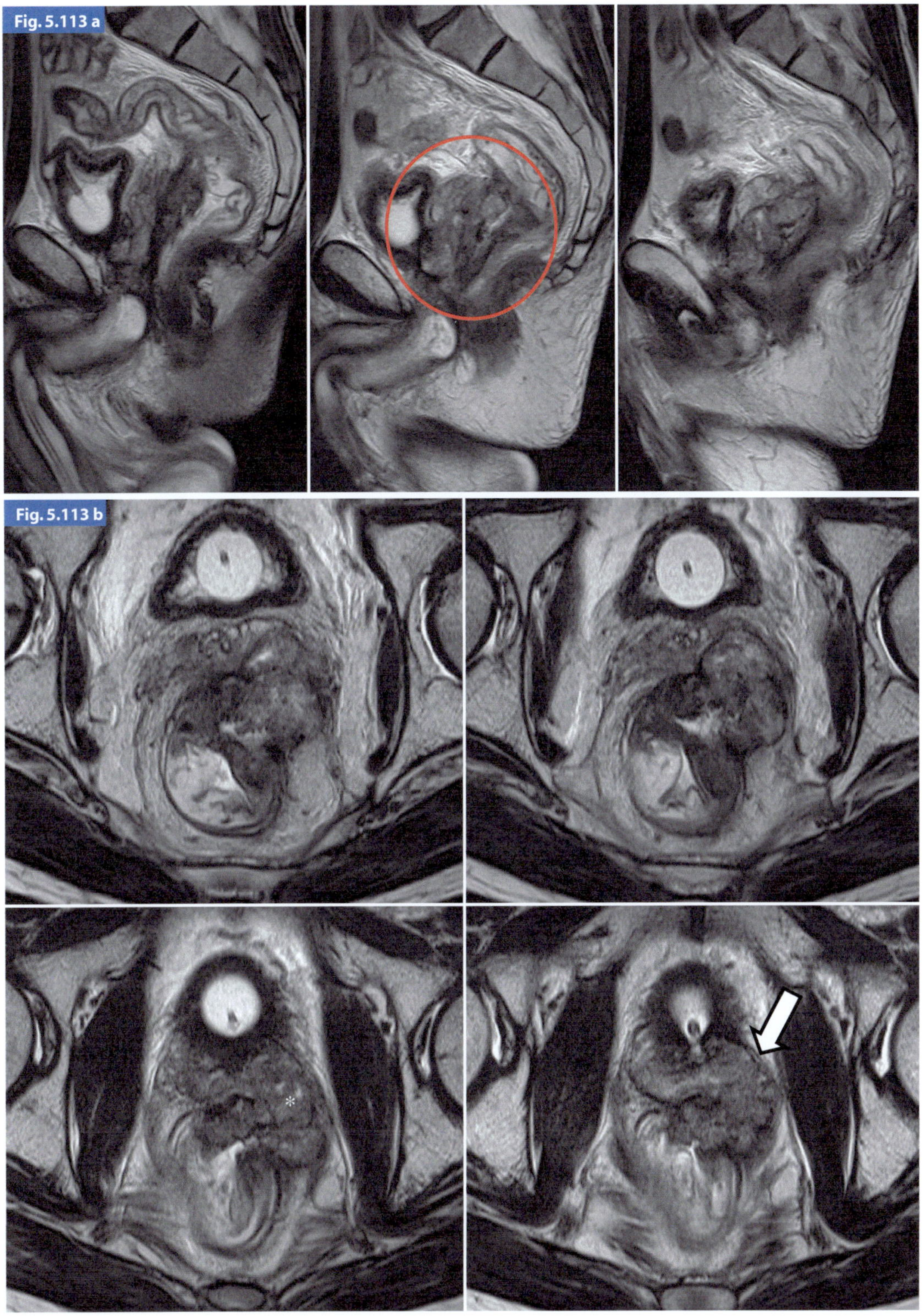

Fig. 5.113 Invasive rectal GIST. (**a**) Sagittal T2-TSE images reveal an ill-defined mixed signal intensity mass, which is located between the rectum, prostate, and seminal vesicles. (**b**) Axial T2-TSE images show an ulcerative tumor originating from the rectum between 9- and 5-o'clock lithotomy positions, which involves all wall layers. The tumor extends to the mesorectum, penetrates the Deonvilliers' fascia, and invades the prostate (*asterisk*, *arrow*) and seminal vesicles.

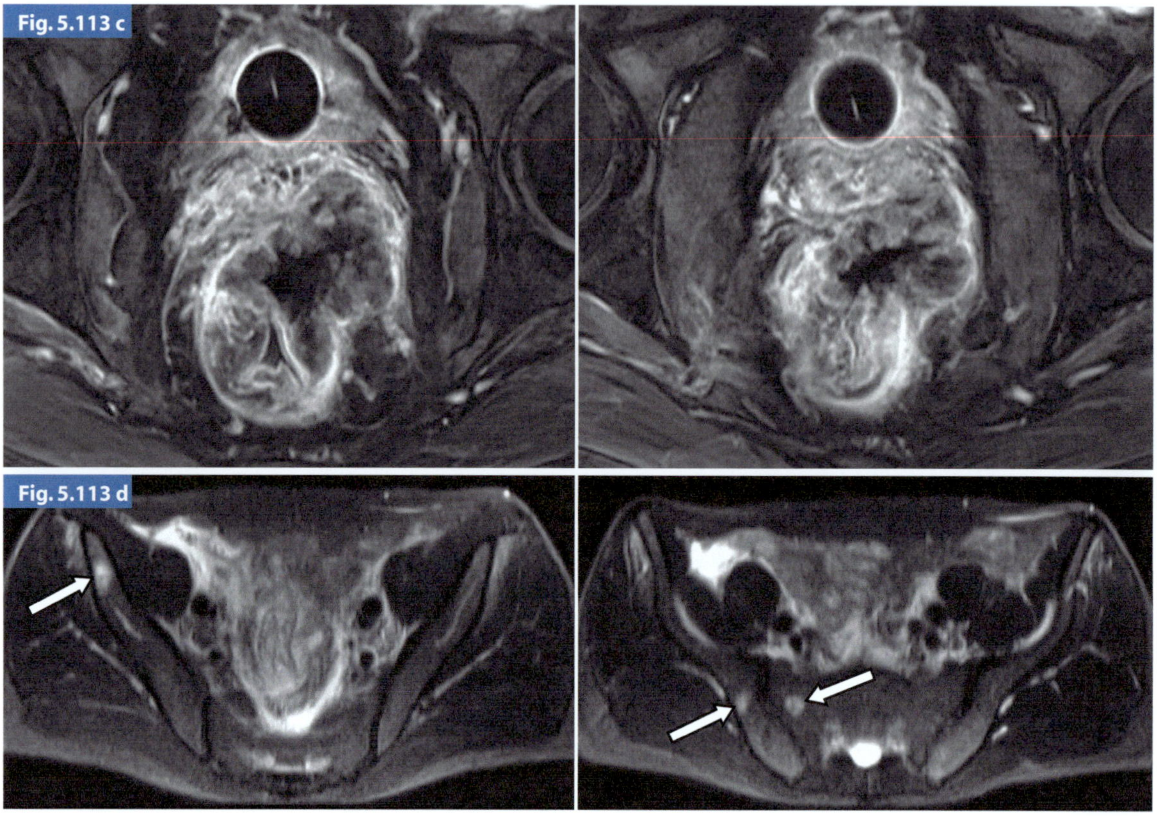

Fig. 5.113 (**c**) Axial CE-VIBE 3D images demonstrate the patterns of contrast-enhancement of the tumor bed. On the axial (**d**) TIRM images derived from the SMS moving-table examination differentiation of three pelvic bone metastases (*arrows*).

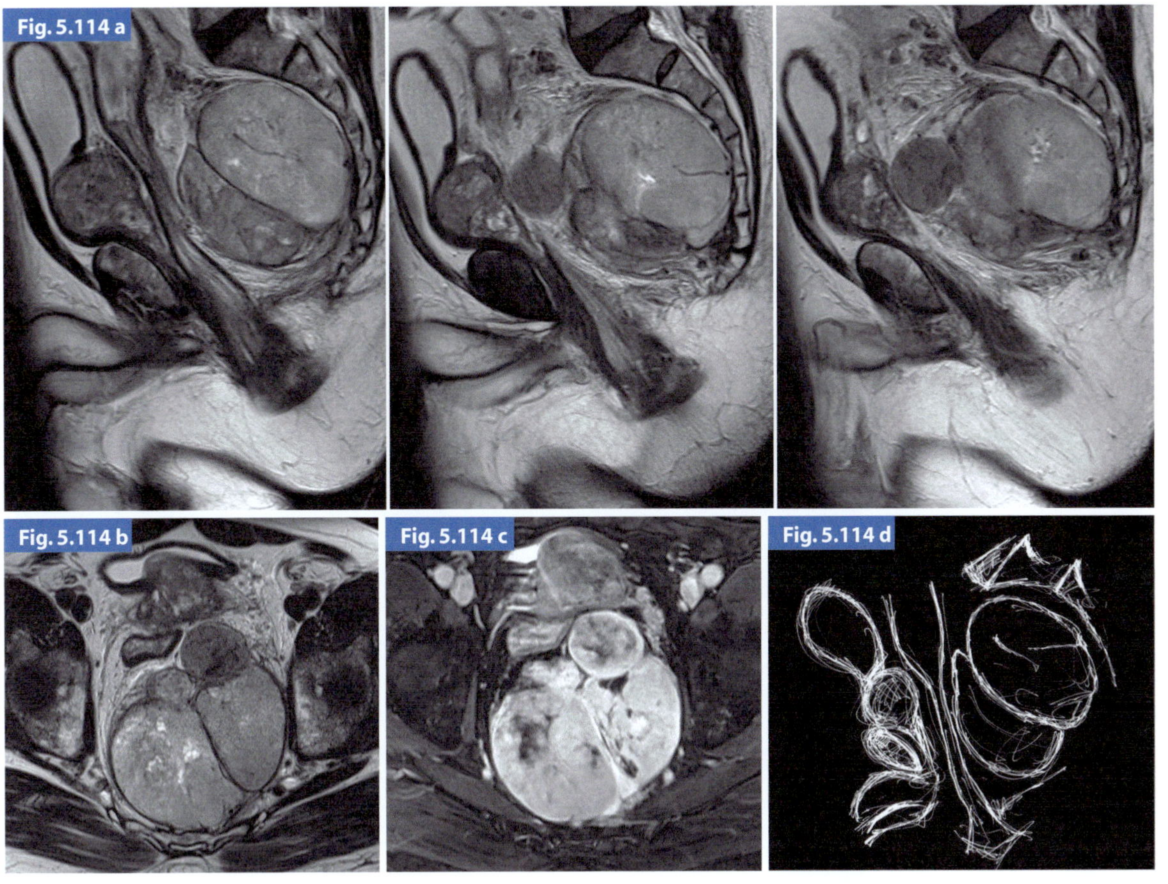

Fig. 5.114 Mesorectal GIST. (**a**) The sagittal T2-TSE images reveal a tumor mass occupying the mesorectal fat by displacing the rectum. The tumor comprises several nodules surrounded by a hypointense capsula. On the corresponding axial, T2-TSE (**b**) and CE-VIBE (**c**) three-dimensional images necrotic foci can be observed. The nodules strongly enhance after gadolinium. No signs of rectal or pelvic wall infiltration. Histopathology confirmed the diagnosis of a mesorectal GIST without lymph node metastases. (**d**) Ink drawing: Mesorectal GIST.

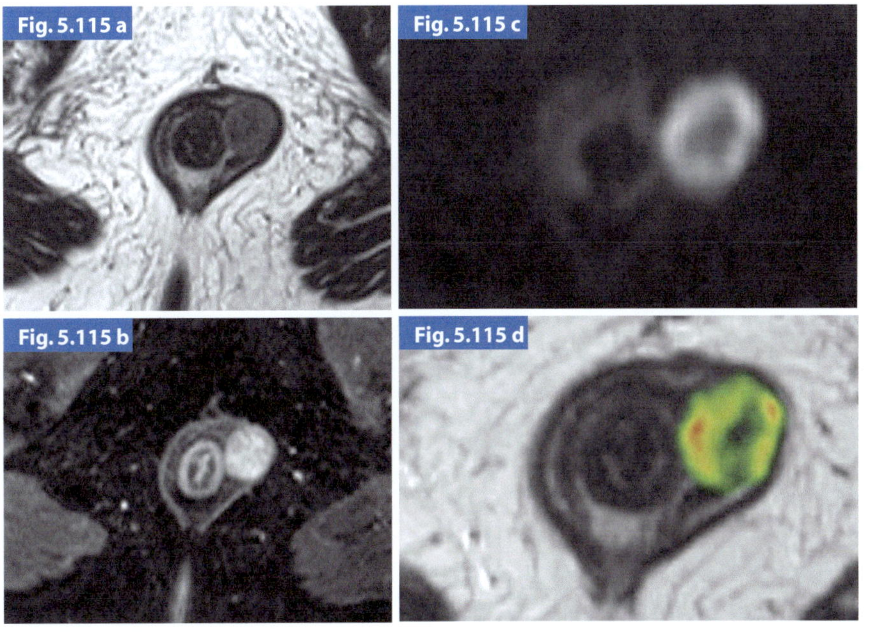

Fig. 5.115 Anal GIST. (**a**) The axial T2-TSE image display a sharply delineated round tumor within the intersphincteric fat at 3 o'clock lithotomy position expanding the left external sphincter muscle.(**b**) A homogeneous contrast agent uptake is shown for the lesion on the corresponding axial CE-VIBE 3D image. (**c**) The DWI image (b-value 750 s/mm^2) demonstrates high signal within the tumor. (**d**) Corresponding image fusion of the DWI image and the axial T2-TSE image using a color scale is shown. The tumor was surgically removed and histopathology revealed anal GIST.

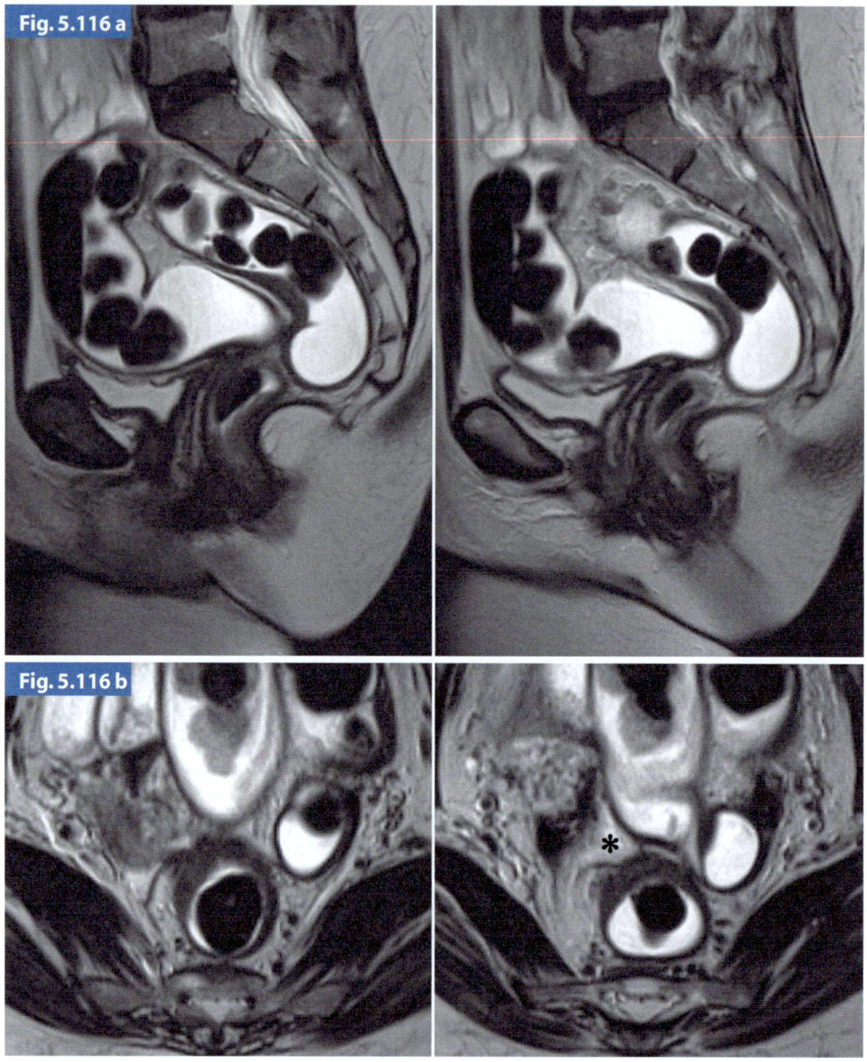

Fig. 5.116 Metastatic breast cancer. (**a**) On the sagittal T2-TSE images, conspicuous thickening of the anterior wall of the midrectum is shown. (**b**) Axial T2-TSE images display thickening of the peritoneal reflection with small amounts of ascites (*asterisk*) and rectal tumor formation between 8- and 3-o'clock lithotomy position indicate peritoneal carcinosis with rectal wall ingrowth, confirmed by histopathology.

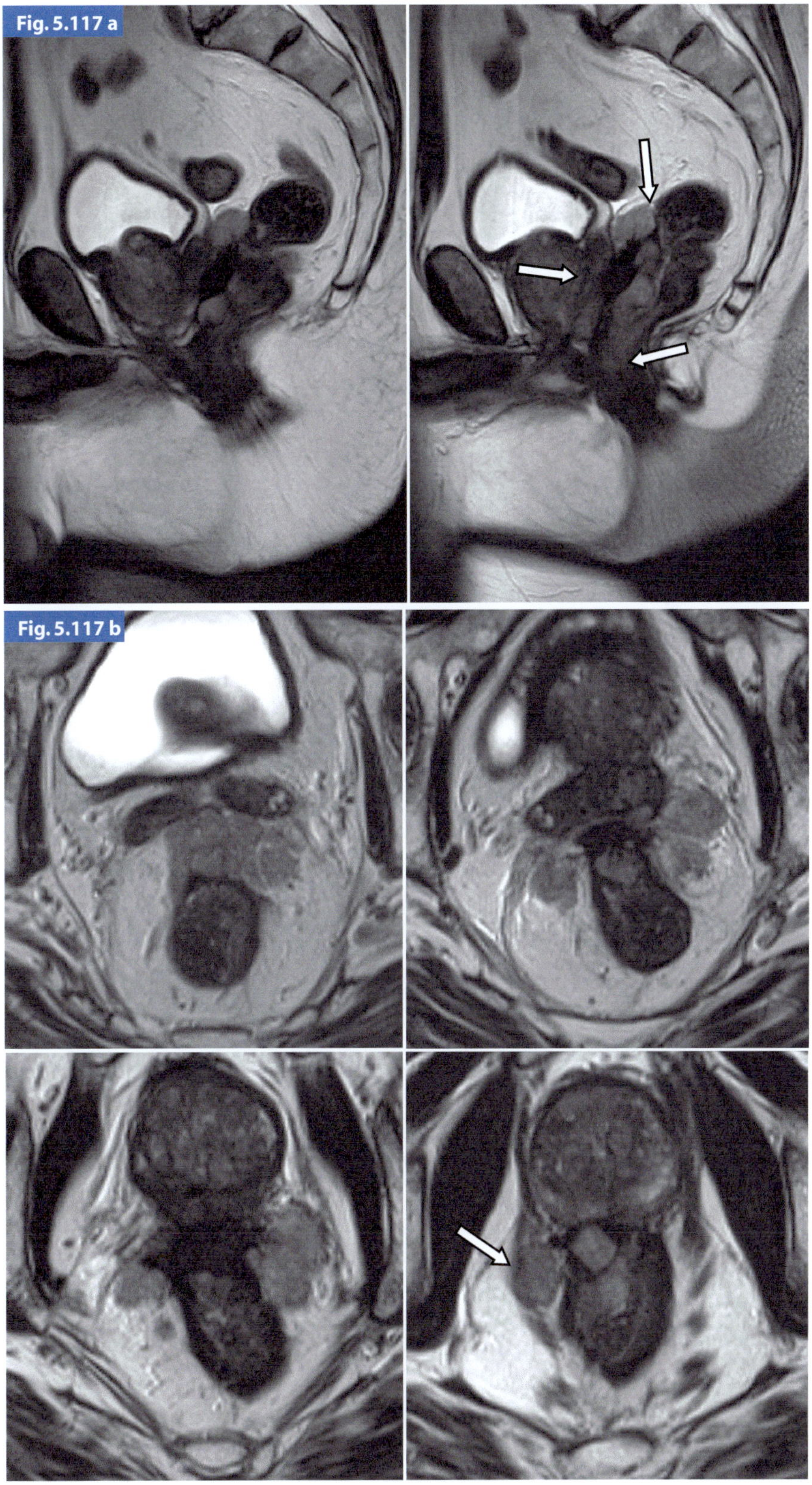

Fig. 5.117 Stage T4 prostate cancer mimicking rectal tumor. (**a**) The sagittal T2-TSE images show extensive tumor formation involving the prostate, seminal vesicles, mesorectum, anterior rectal wall, and anorectal junction. (**b**) The tumor has a low- to intermediate-signal intensity on the para-axial T2-TSE images and infiltrates the right levator ani muscle (*arrow*).

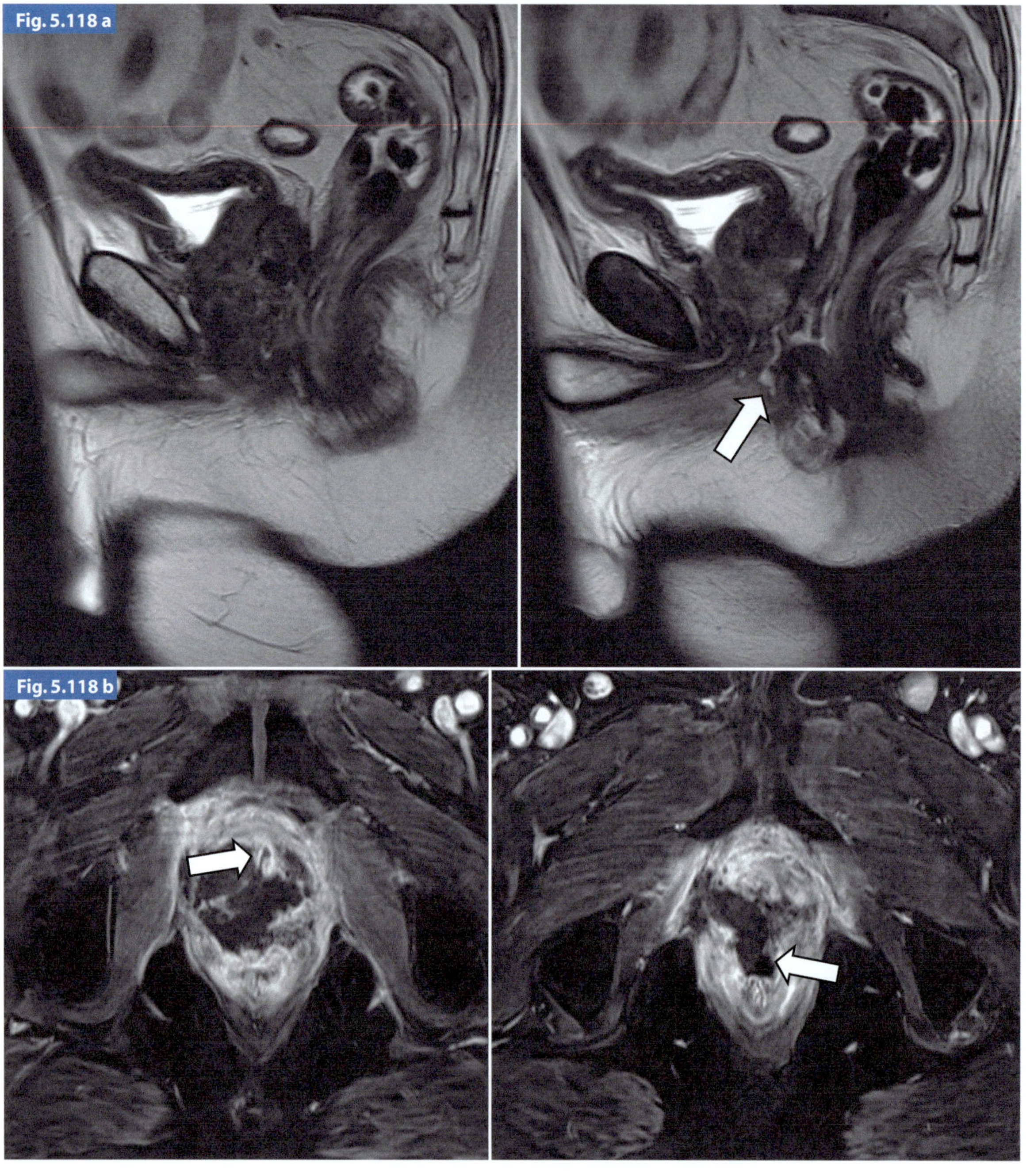

Fig. 5.118 Prostate cancer and subsequent squamous cell carcinoma of the urinary bladder: course of disease. Sagittal (**a**) T2-TSE and axial (**b**) CE-VIBE 3D images before pelvic exenteration resulting from T4 prostate cancer with inavsion of the bladder and the rectum. The tumor is hypovascular and of very low-signal intensity on the VIBE images. Note the fistula between tumor, rectum, urethra, and penile root (*arrows*).

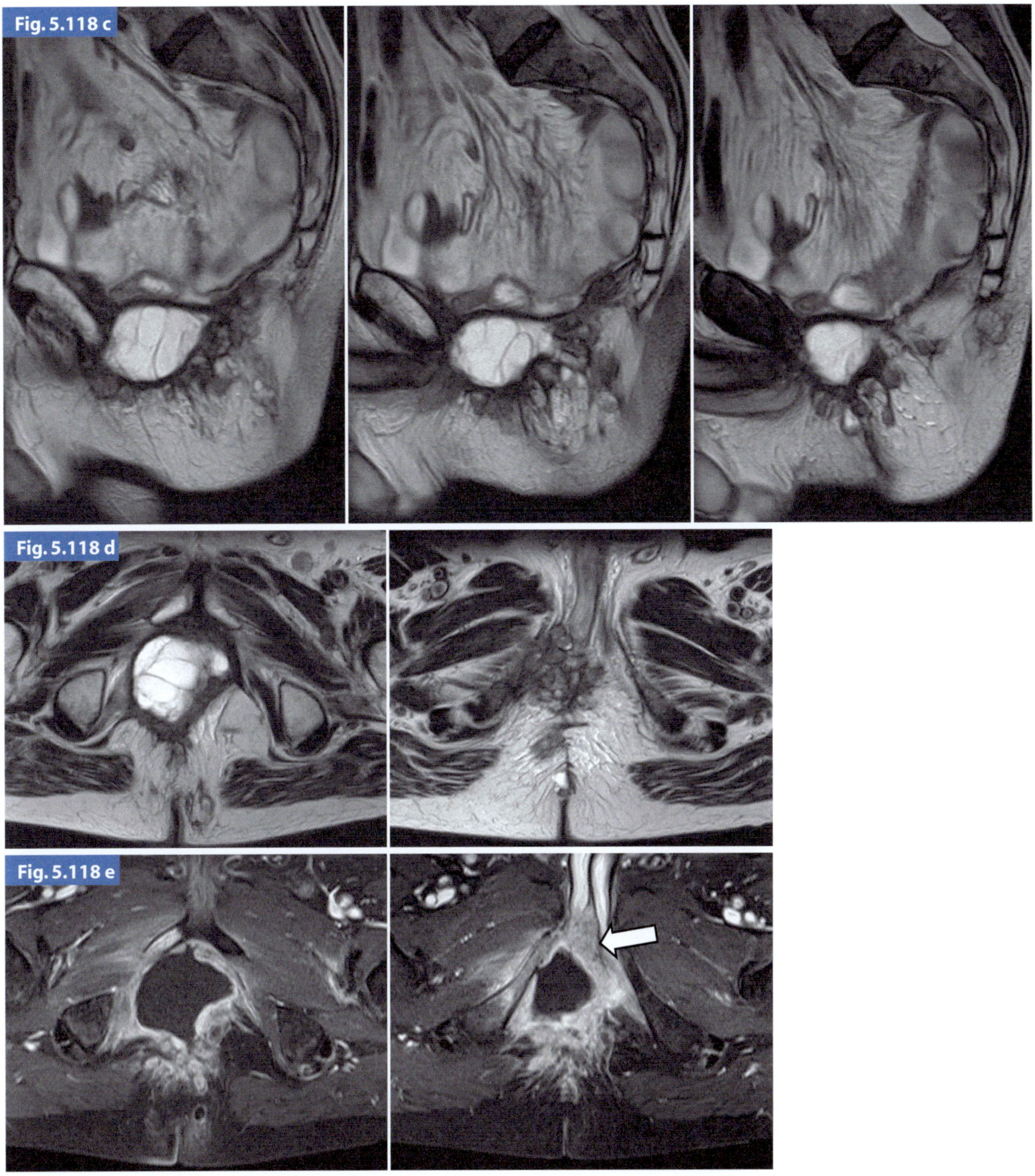

Fig. 5.118 Sagittal (**c**) and axial (**d**) T2-TSE and axial (**e**) CE-FLASH 2D images following surgery reveal pelvic abscess formation with surrounding foci of recurrent squamous cell carcinoma of the bladder. The abscess originated from peritoneal carcinosis of the ileum with perforation and fistula. Osteomyelitis of the right inferior pubic ramus can be seen on the FLASH images along with infiltration of the penile root (*arrow*) sagittal.

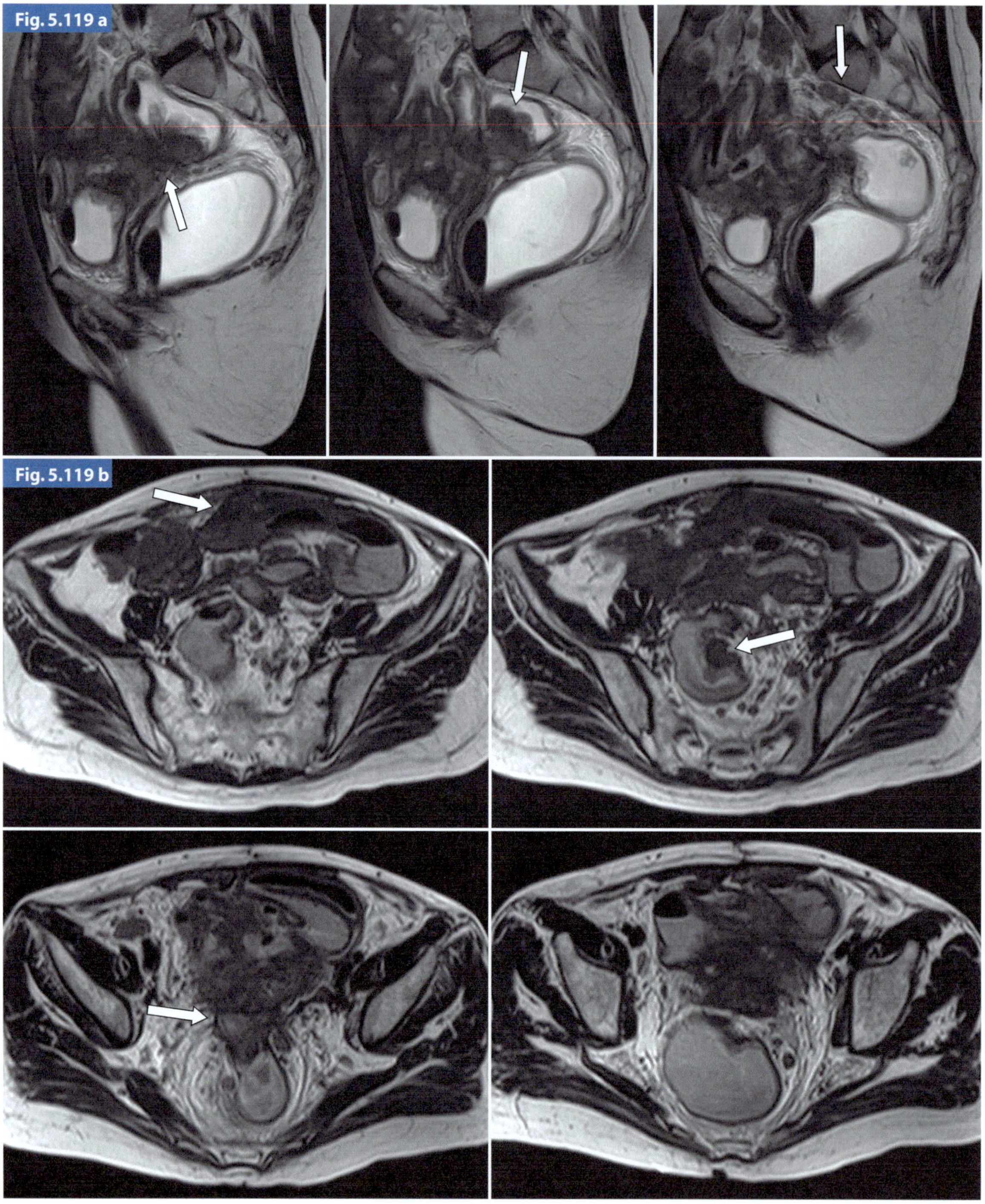

Fig. 5.119 Recurrent ovarian cancer. Patient history: Status after ovarectomy resulting from stage pT3N0M0 G3 ovarian cancer with adjuvant chemotherapy, local recurrence with extensive reoperation and concomittant chemotherapy, second recurrence. Advanced local tumor recurrence originating from the vaginal stump with infiltration and obstruction of the rectosigmoid shown on the sagittal (**a**) and axial (**b**) T2-TSE images. Widespread peritoneal carcinosis forming a conglomerate tumor that involves the sigmoid colon, the cecum, and the ileum was also present along with signs of perileus. Additional retroperitoneal and mesenterial nodal disease is noted (*arrows*).

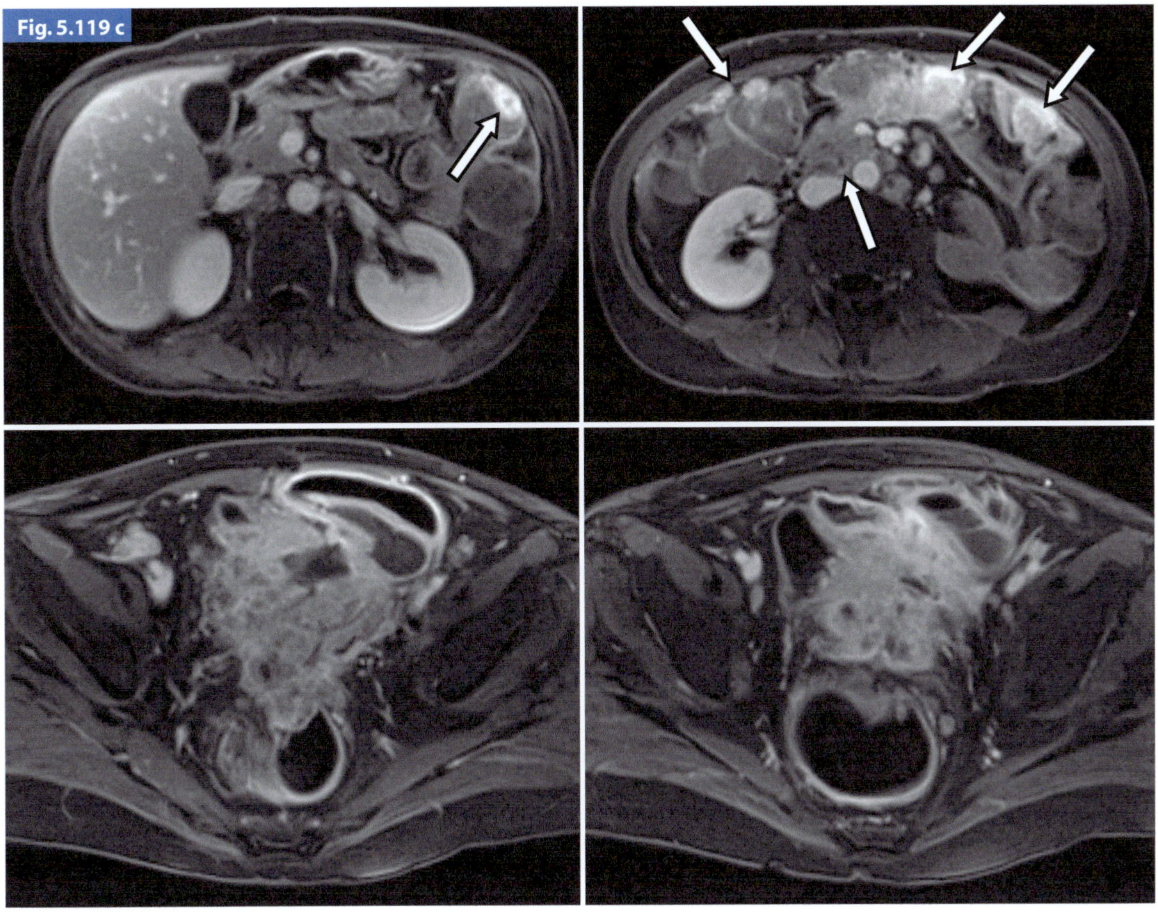

Fig. 5.119 (**c**) On the axial CE-FLASH 2D images from SMS moving-table M-staging omental, peritoneal, and lymph node metastases can be observed (*arrows*).

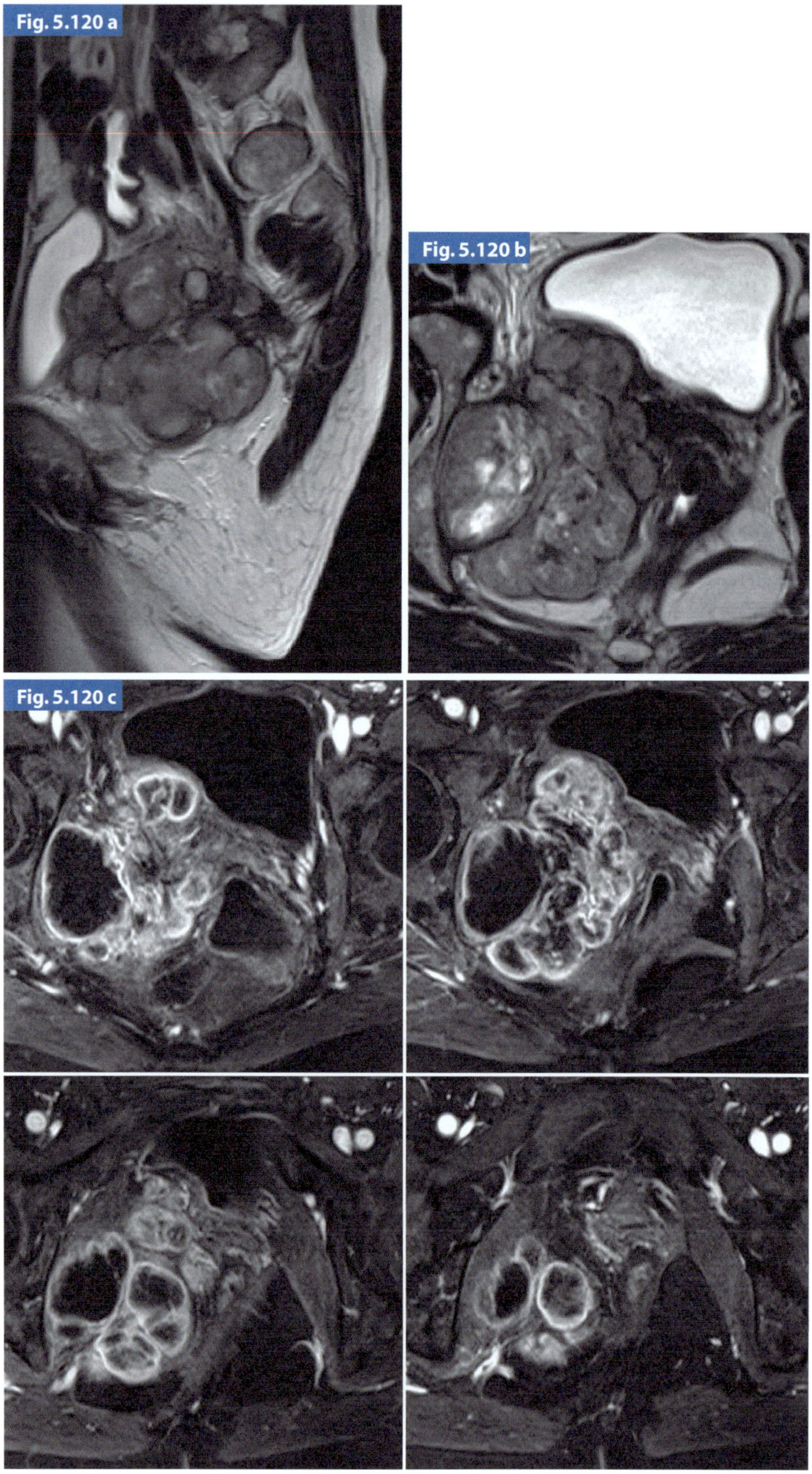

Fig. 5.120 Recurrent leiomyosarcoma of the uterus. Patient history: Status after hysterectomy and partial vaginal resection with reconstruction. Postoperative chemoradiation. Extensive right pelvic side-wall recurrence is demonstrated one the sagittal (**a**) and axial (**b**) T2-TSE images. The polynodular tumor is surrounded by a hypointense capsule. The bladder wall and the vaginal stump are infiltrated; additionally, there is contact with the anorectal junction. (**c**) The recurrence displays areas of necrosis which appear hypointense on the axial CE-VIBE 3D images, whereas other parts of the tumor show marked contrat, indicating viability. Invasion of the right internal obturator muscle and the ipsilateral ischiorectal fossa is shown. The signal behavior of the pelvic bone is normal without any signs of infiltration.

Fig. 5.120 d

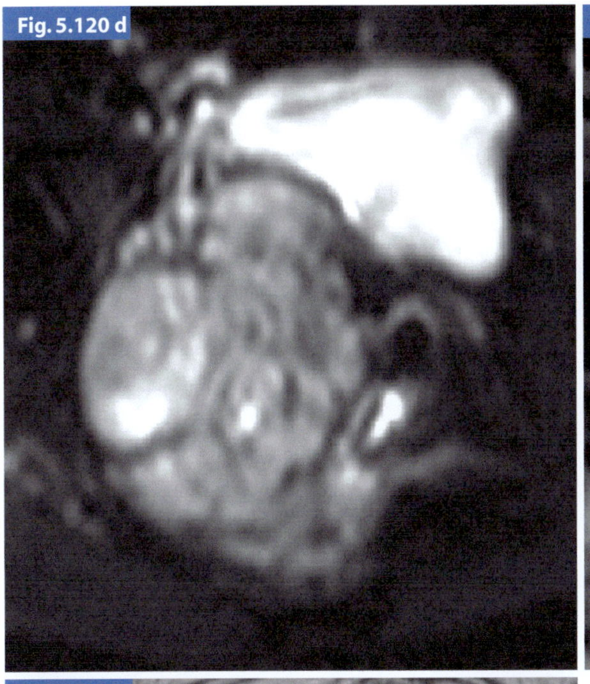

Fig. 5.120 e

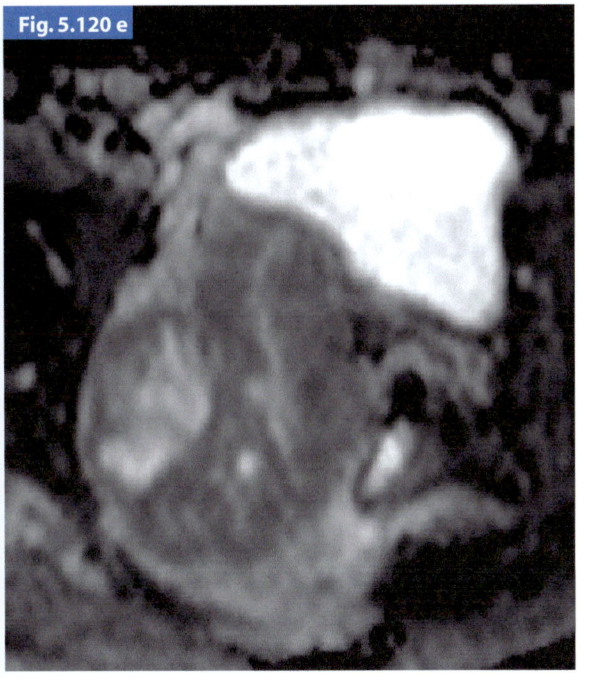

Fig. 5.120 f

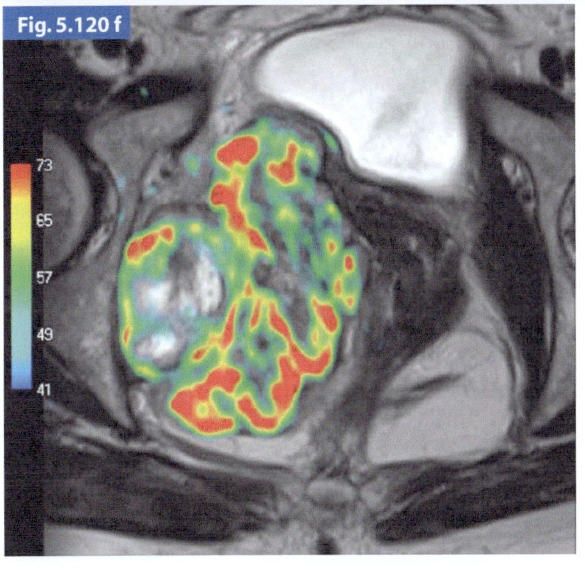

Fig. 5.120 The DWI (**d**) image (b-value of 500) and the corresponding ADC map (**e**) confirm the findings displaying a partly necrotic tumor recurrence. The necrotic area shows high signal on both images, in contrast to viable tumor displaying lowsignal on the ADC map. (**f**) Image fusion of DWI and a representative axial T2-TSE slice summarizes the above mentioned characteristics of the recurrent tumor.

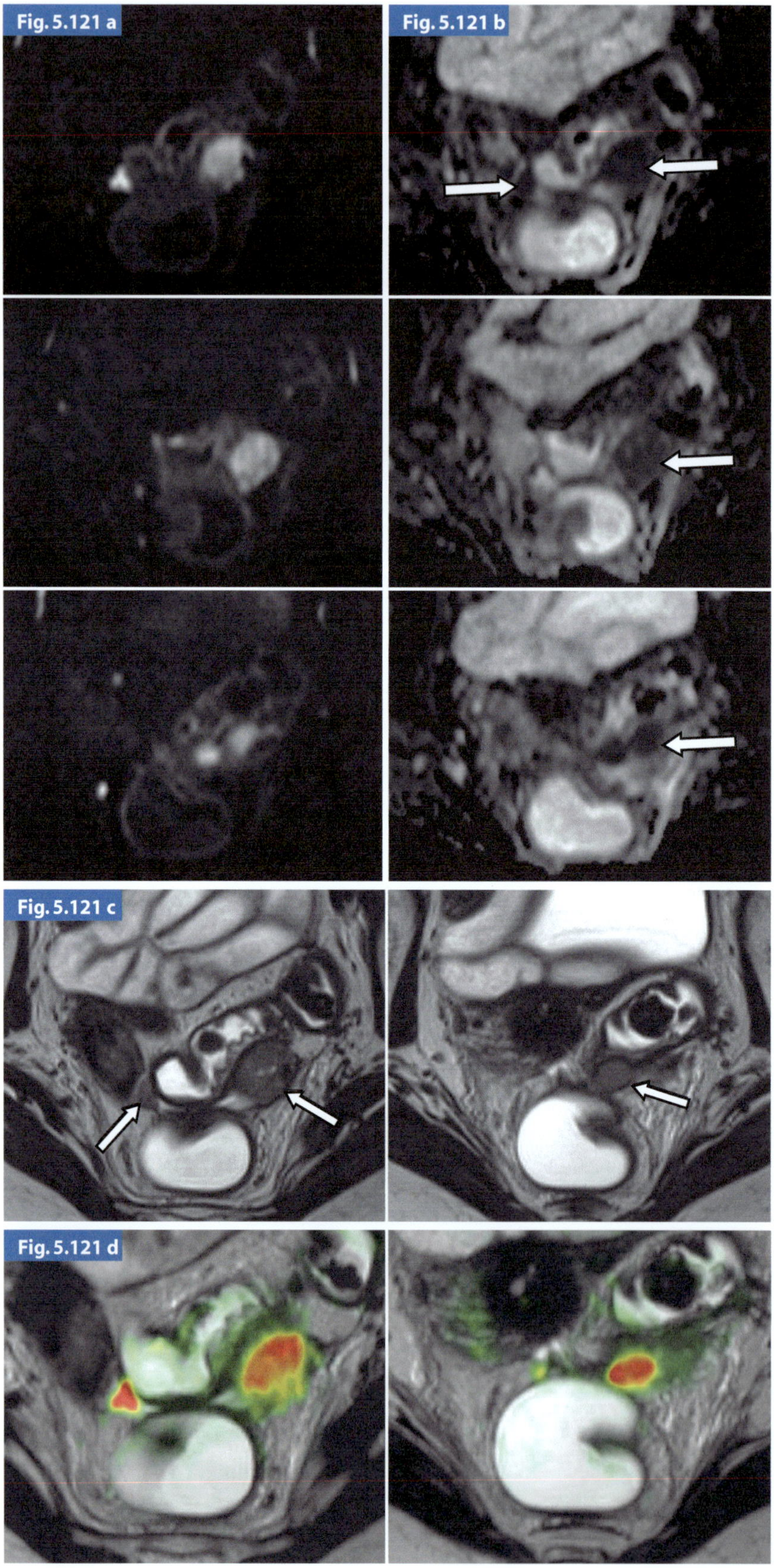

Fig. 5.121 Reccurent ovarian cancer. DWI (**a**) images (b = 750 s/mm^2) and corresponding ADC maps (**b**) depict three tumor nodules adjacent to the rectal wall. The nodules show high-signal intensity on DWI images indicative of restricted diffusion, whereas these tumors exhibit low-signal intensity on the corresponding ADC maps suggestive of high cellularity (*arrows*). Para-axial (**c**) T2-TSE images and corresponding image fusion of T2-TSE and DWI (**d**, *color coded*). The tumors display intermediate signal intensity on the T2-weighted images. The left-sided tumor invades the wall of the rectosigmoid; note the thickening of the submucosa in the area of the tumor infiltration. Patient history: Status after hysterectomy and ovarectomy with adjuvant chemotherapy. Relaparotomy was performed 11 months following initial surgery; biopsies were taken from the pelvic tumor nodules, the mesenteric and iliac lymph nodes, and anterior resection of the rectum was performed. Histopathologic examination revealed peritoneal and nodal metastases from serous ovarian cancer. The MR diagnosis of peritoneal carcinosis involving the rectosigmoid was confirmed.

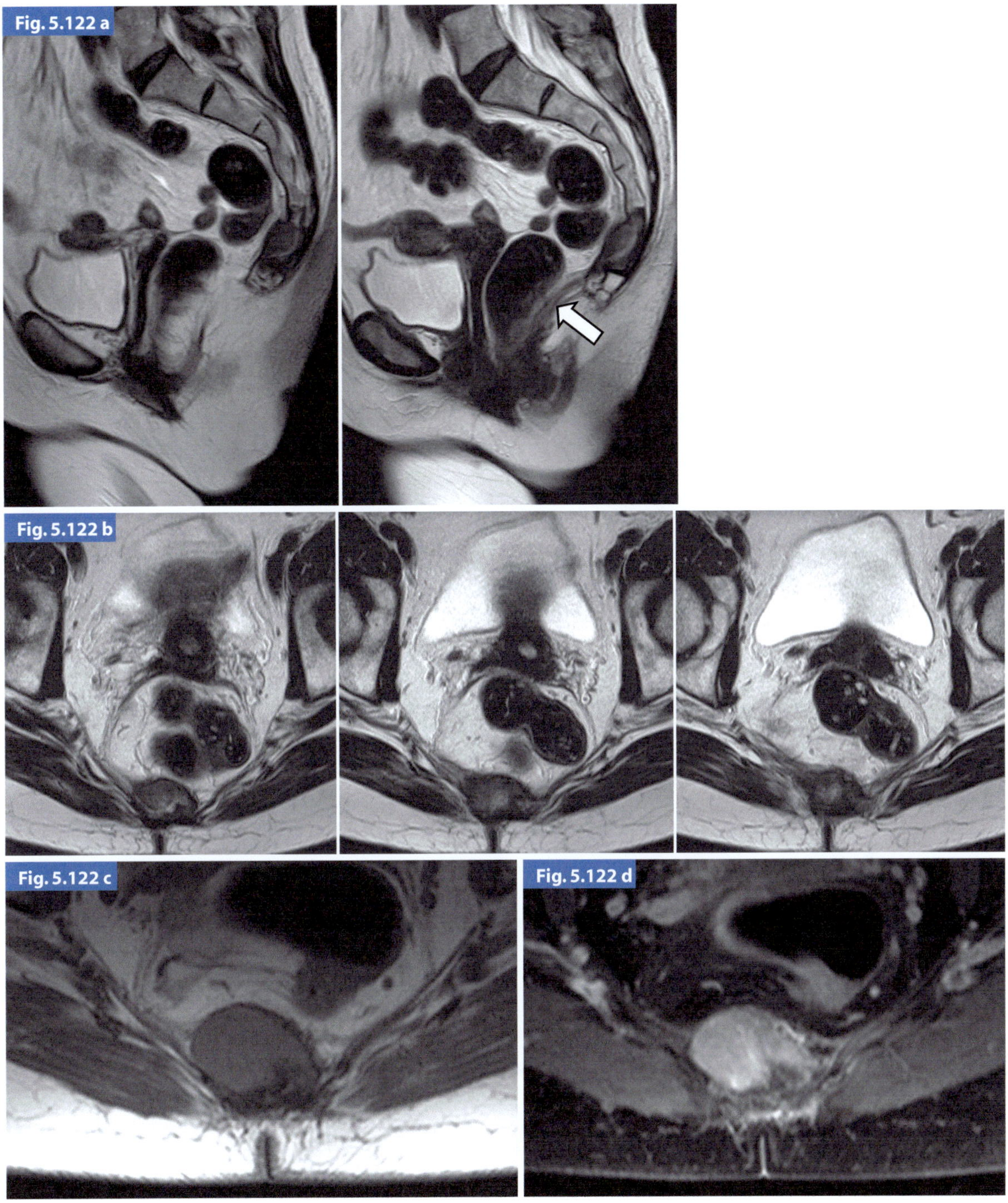

Fig. 5.122 Malignant transformation of a tailgut cyst. (**a**) On the sagittal T2-TSE images, delimitation of a retrorectal mass that infiltrates the fifth sacral segment and the coccygis. Additionally, the Waldeyer's fascia is thickened (*arrow*). (**b**) The corresponding axial images reveal signal inhomogeneities, within the tumor. In summary, the tumor origin remains unclear. In a previous examination, the mass seemed to have a hypointense capsule on T1 (**c**) and spots of contrast enhancement (**d**). The central uniform high-signal on T1 resembled a protein-rich cyst. Histopathologic review of the specimen led to the infrequent diagnosis of a neuroendocrine carcinoma developed in a tailgut cyst

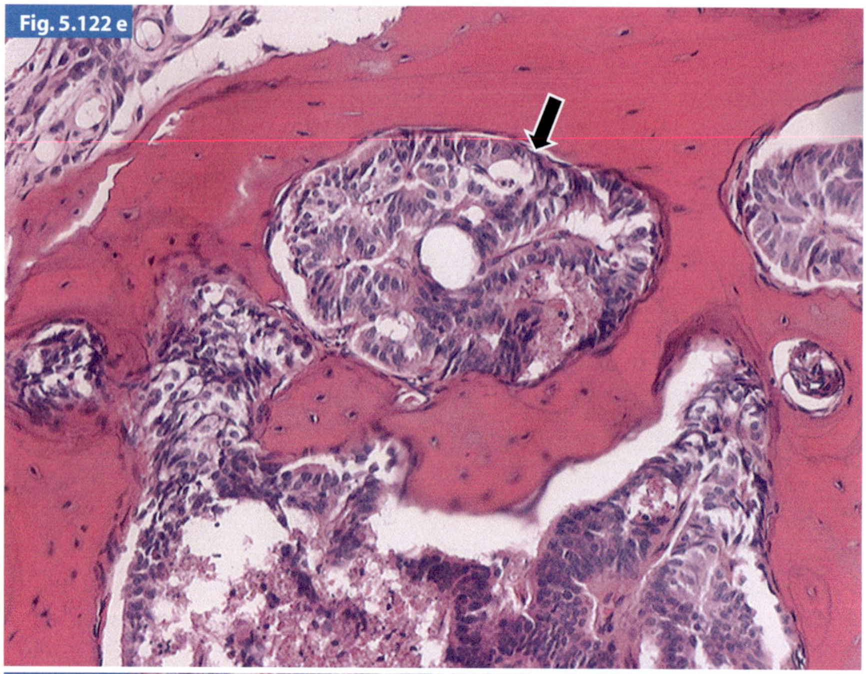

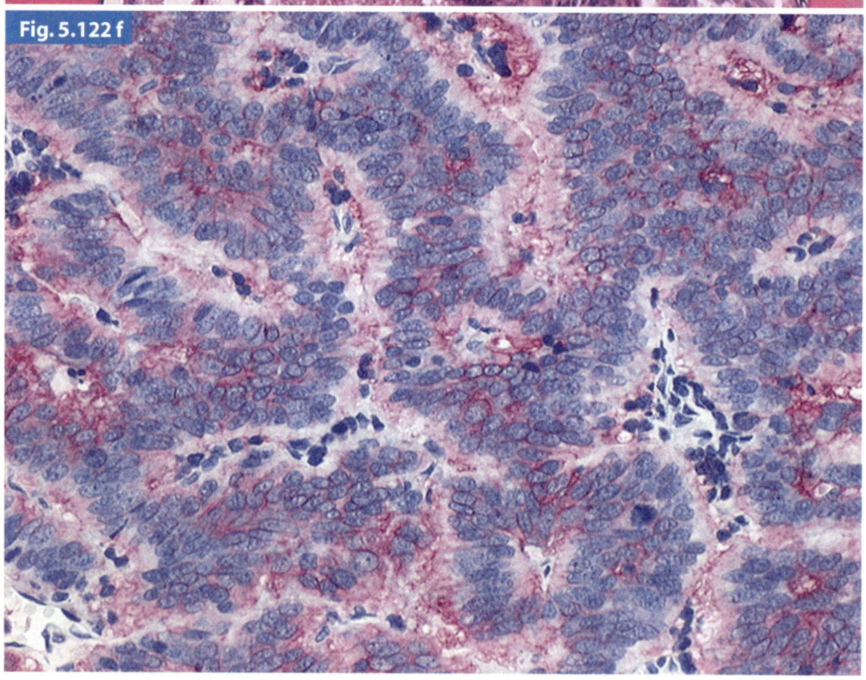

Fig. 5.122 (**e**, **f**). Histopathologic specimen of the patient: inclusions of a neuroendocrine carcinoma within the sacral bone (*arrow* in **e**, H&E, ×10) confirmed by Somatostatin IHC (F, ×20).

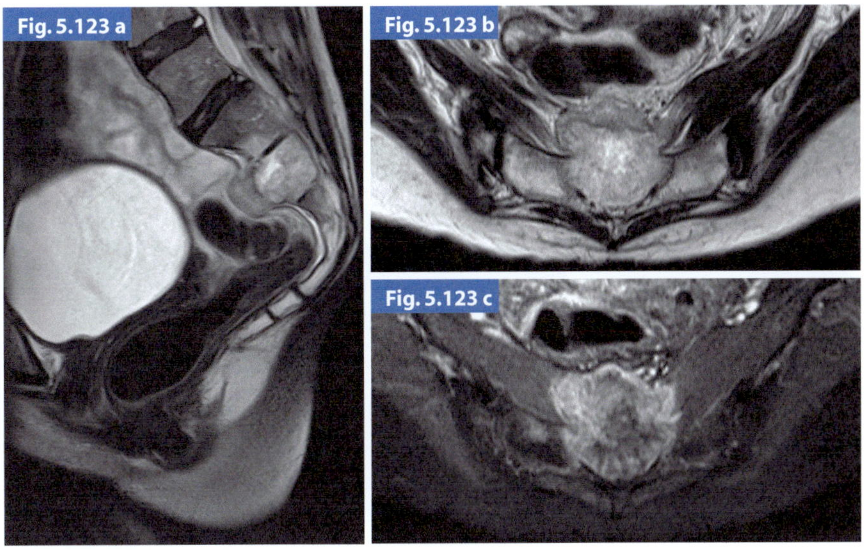

Fig. 5.123 Metastasizing malignant peripheral nerve sheath tumor. Sagittal (**a**), axial T2-TSE image (**b**), and axial fat-saturated CE-T1-TSE image (**c**) demonstrate sacral bone metastasis involving the S1, S2, and S3 segments.

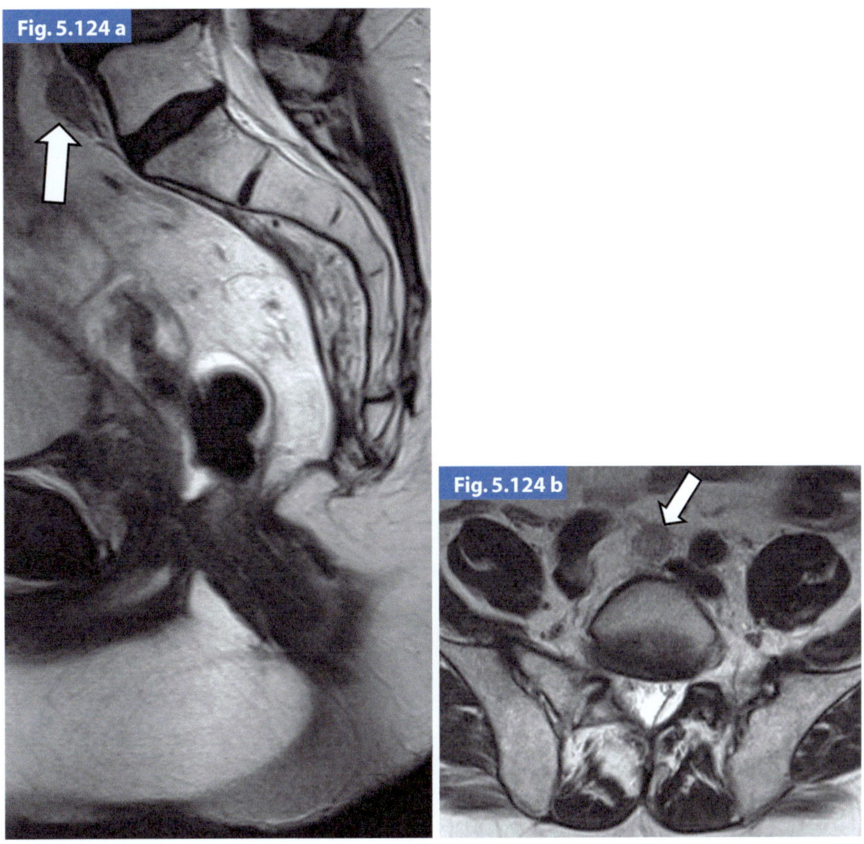

Fig. 5.124 Differential diagnosis of lymph node metastasis. Sagittal (**a**) T2-TSE image and the corresponding axial (**b**) T2-TSE image show a retroperitoneal node with intermediate-signal intensity at the level of the aortic bifurcation as a hint to nodal metastasis during follow-up after rectal cancer surgery (*arrow*). The pathologic work-up resulted in the diagnosis of a nerve sheath tumor, which was an unexpected finding and for this reason an interesting differential diagnosis.

5.10 Postsurgical Anatomy

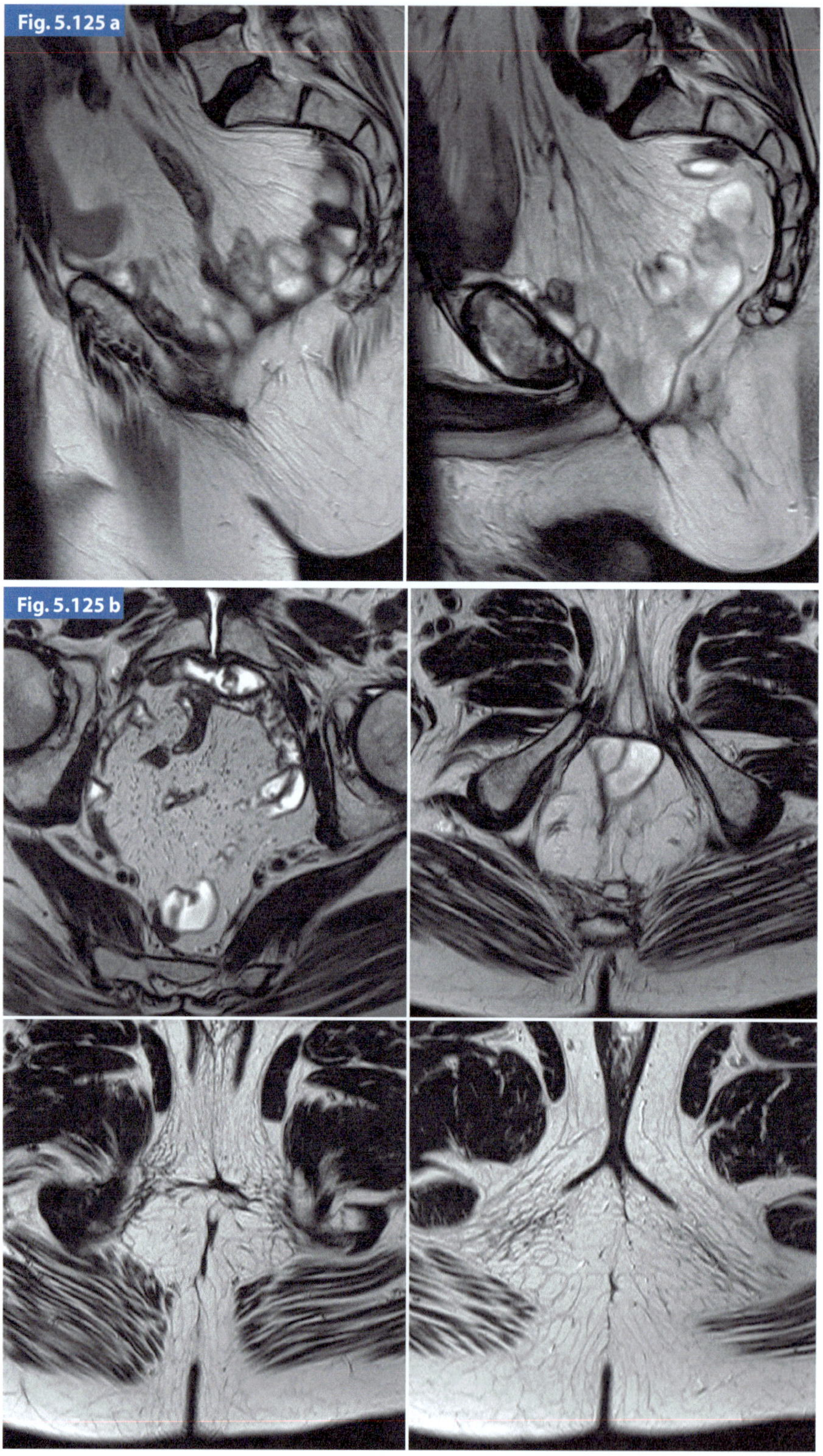

Fig. 5.125 Normal status after abdominoperineal rectal resection. T2-weighted sagittal (**a**) and para-axial (**b**) views of the pelvis showing normal anatomy following abdominoperineal resection.

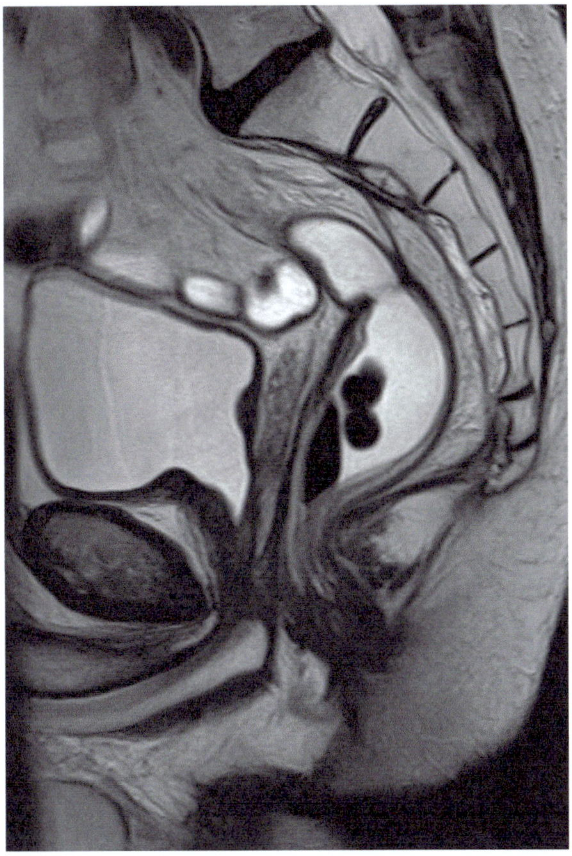

Fig. 5.126 Normal anastomosis. Sagittal T2-TSE image shows normal end-to-end descendorectostomy.

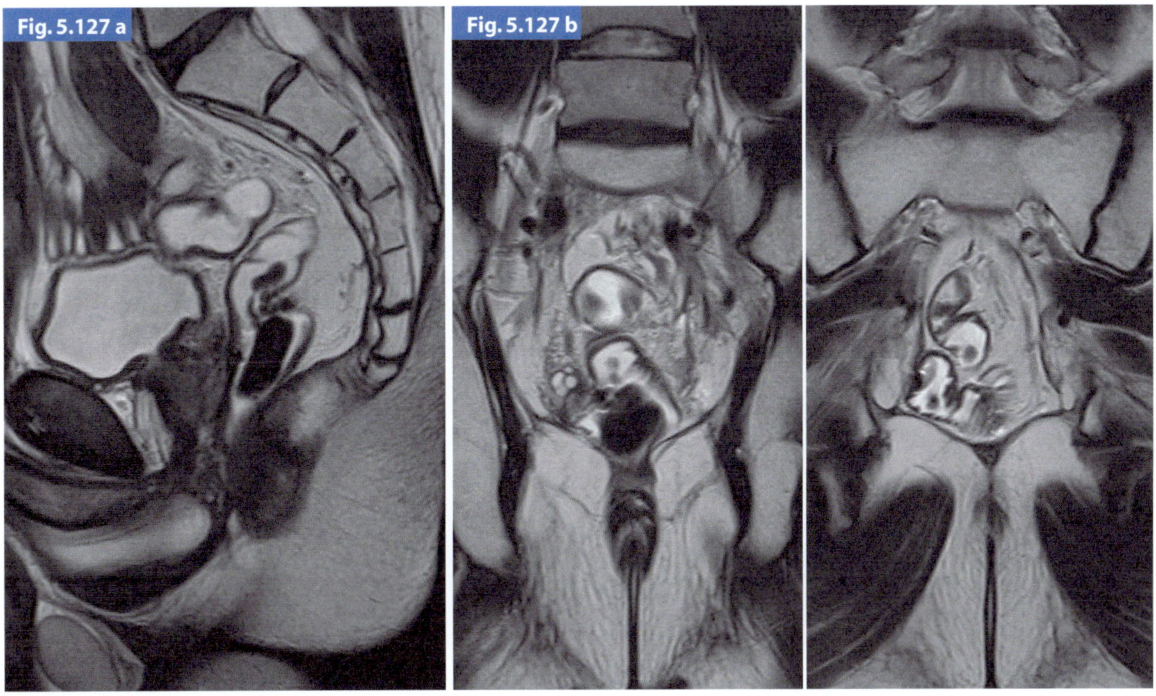

Fig. 5.127 Normal anastomosis. Sagittal (**a**) and coronal (**b**) T2-TSE images of a posttreatment examination reveal normal J-pouch anastomosis.

Fig. 5.128 a

Fig. 5.128 b

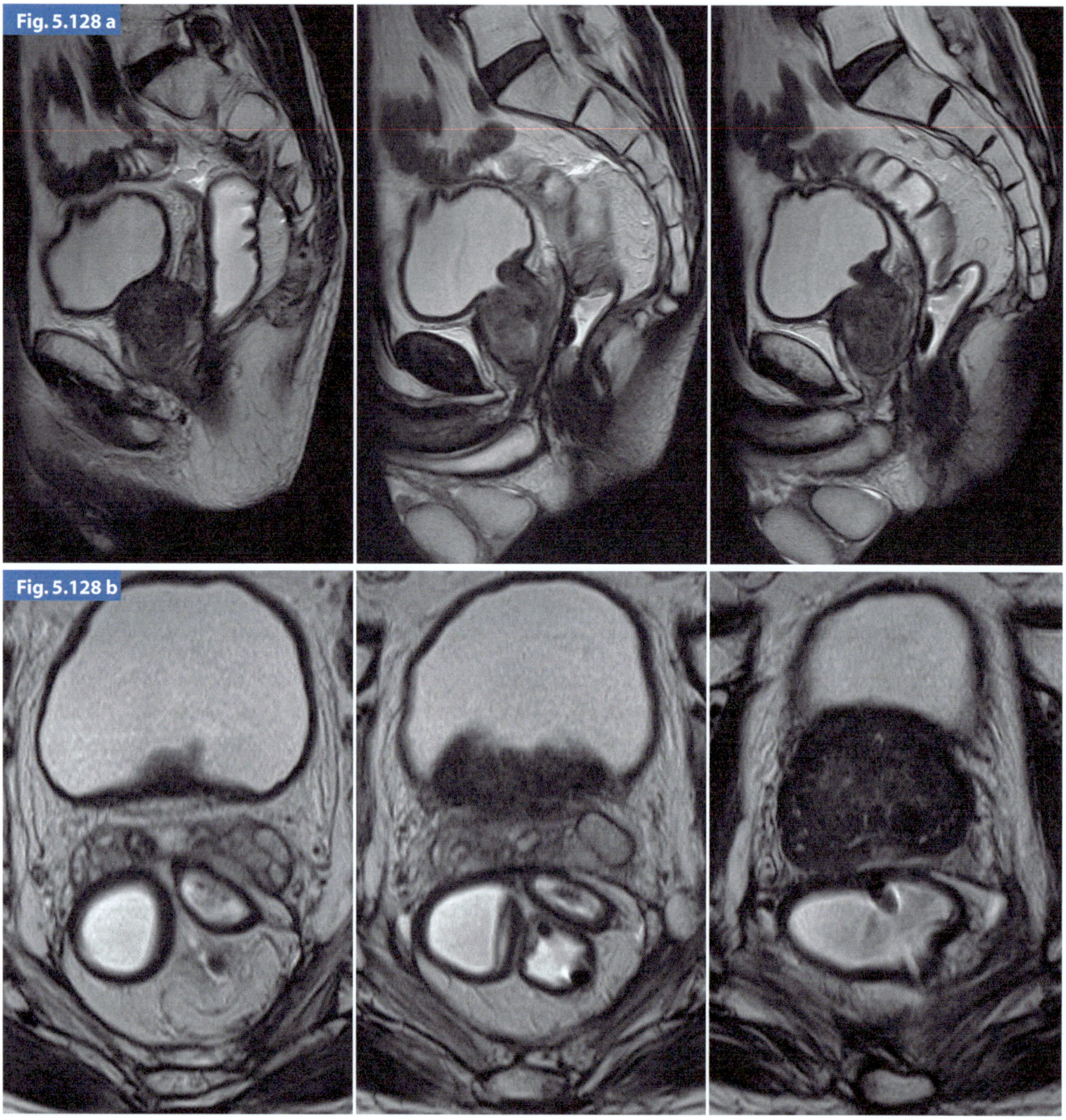

Fig. 5.128 Example of a J-pouch anastomosis after low anterior resection. (**a**) Sagittal T2-TSE images. (**b**) Axial T2-TSE images.

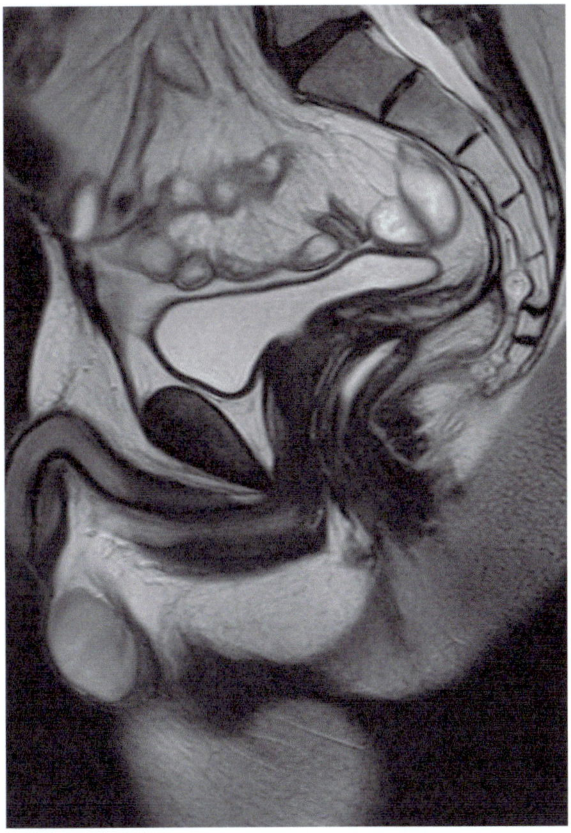

Fig. 5.129 Short rectal stump after low anterior resection of the rectum and Hartmann procedure as a result ot pT3N0 rectal cancer shown on the sagittal T2-TSE image.

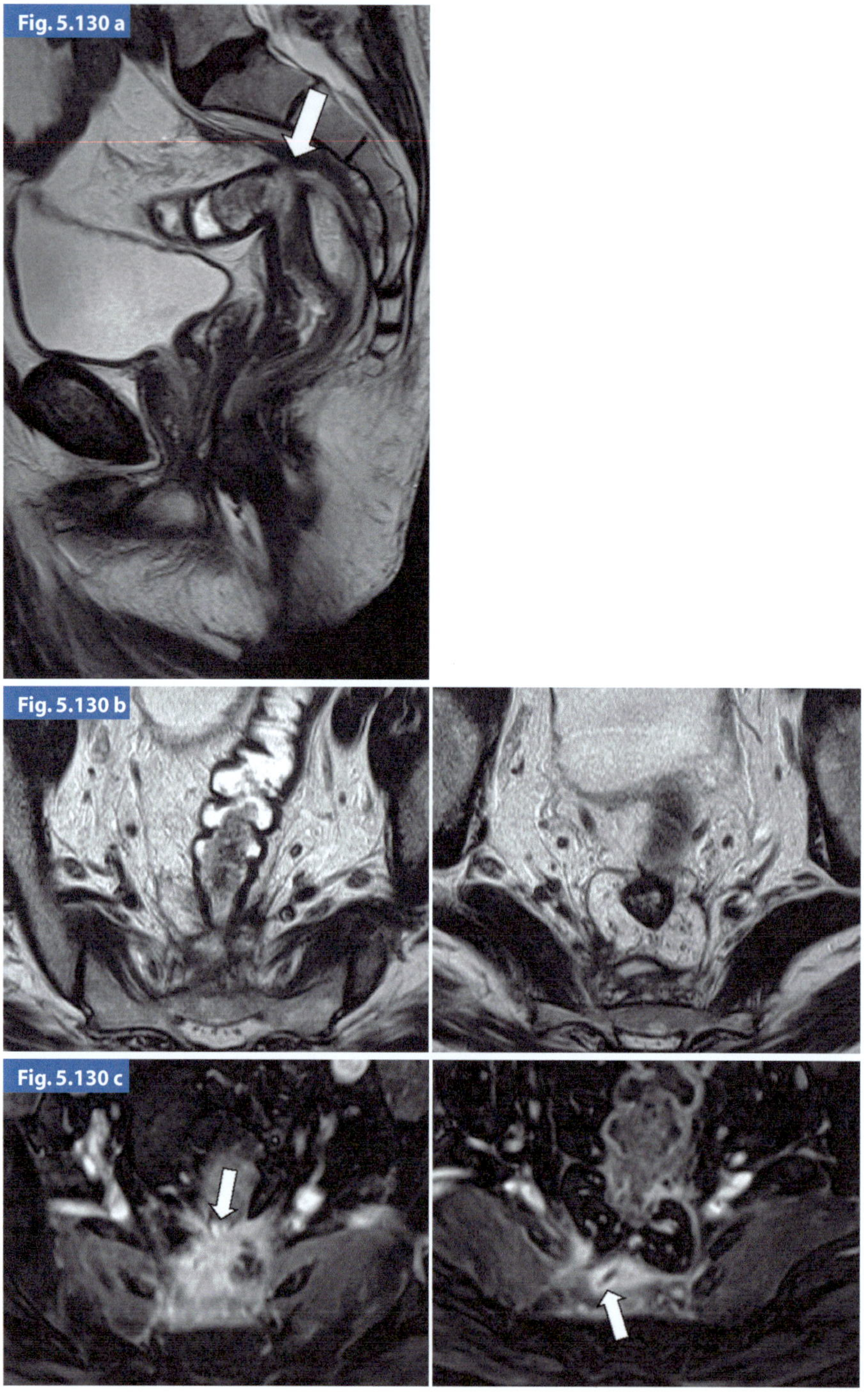

Fig. 5.130 Course of anastomotic leakage: Sagittal (**a**) and axial (**b**) T2-TSE images, axial CE-FLASH 3D images (**c**). Differentiation of post-anastomotic rectal stenosis and anastomotic leak following descendorectostomy with discharge of rectally applied water into a presacral blind ending fistula (*arrow*). The inflamed granulation tissue surrounding the anastomosis and the fistula channel shows substantial contrat (*arrows*).

Fig. 5.130 (**d,e**) After widening of the anastomotic stenosis and conservative treatment, the fistula healed leaving a dark signal-intensity scar demonstrated on the sagittal (**d**)T2-TSE image (*arrow*). A small poly-shaped mass can be identified on the axial (**e**) T2-TSE image mimicking endoluminal tumor recurrence (*arrow*). This tissue formation turned out to be a granuloma.

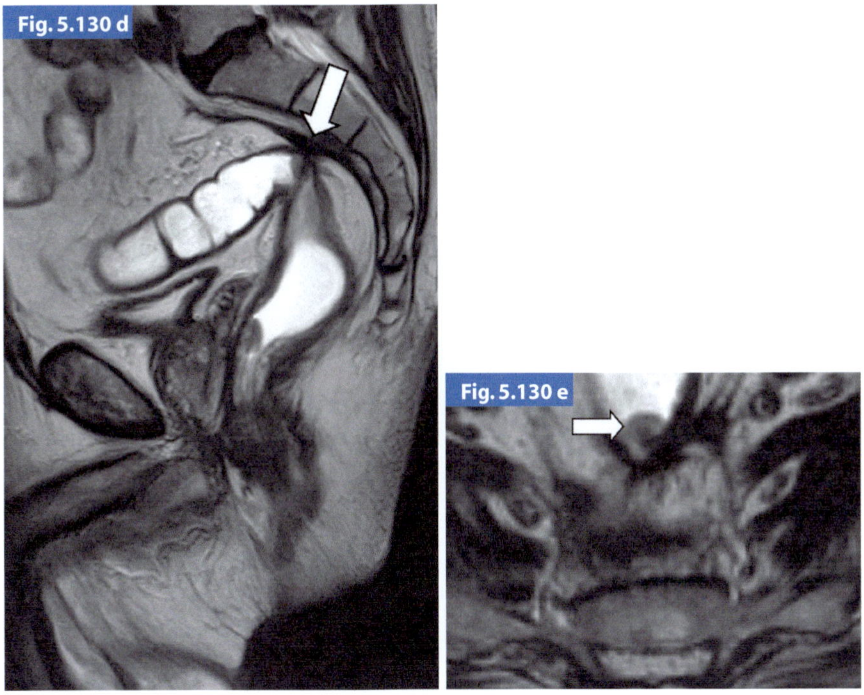

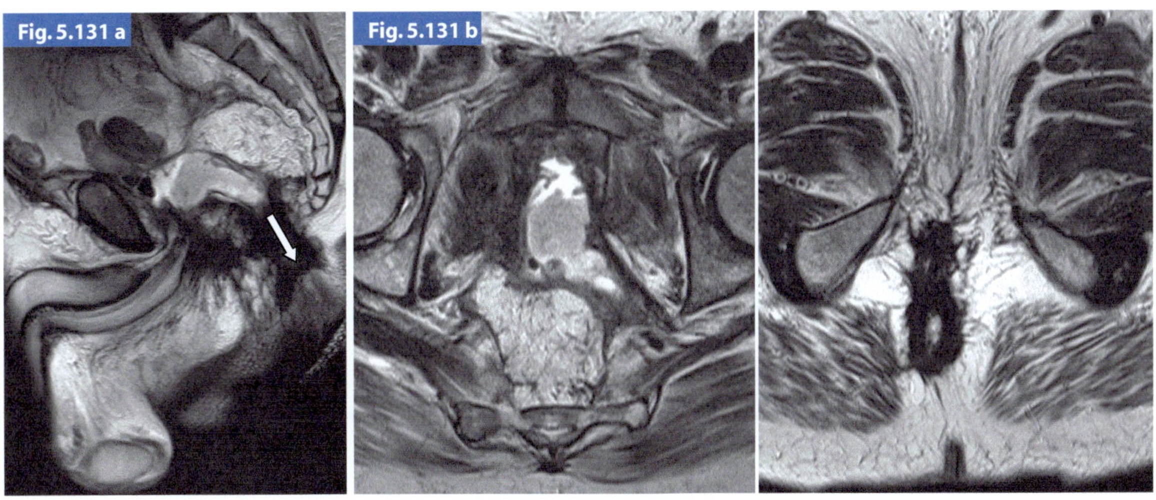

Fig. 5.131 Abscess and fistula after pelvic exenteration. Patient history: pT3N0M0 G2 rectal cancer was diagnosed following neoadjuvant radiochemotherapy and pelvic exenteration. Wound healing disturbance. The sagittal (**a**) and axial (**b**) T2-TSE images reveal pelvic abscess formation with draining perineal fistula (*arrow*).

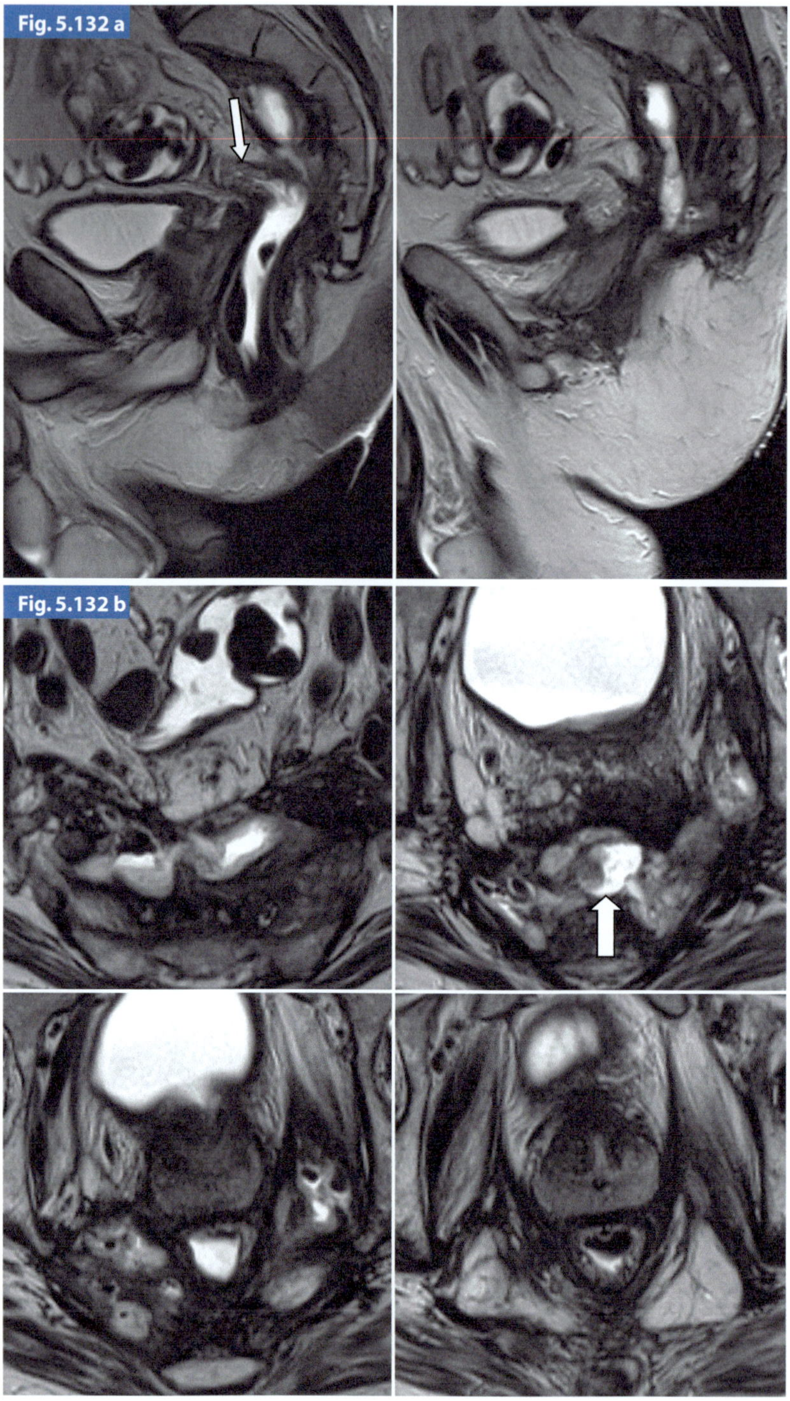

Fig. 5.132 Patient history: Status after deep anterior resection of the rectum due to moderately differentiated adenocarcinoma, pT3N0M0. Persistent anal pain on defecation 4 years after surgery. (**a**) The sagittal T2-TSE images reveal bowel wall edema above the level of the anastomosis (*arrow*). Entry of rectally applied water into the presacral scar as a result of an anastomotic leak. (**b**) Para-axial T2-TSE images show an extensive abscess formation with air-fluid levels involving the left obturator muscle. The anastomotic leakage is located at the 6-o'clock lithotomy position (*arrow*).

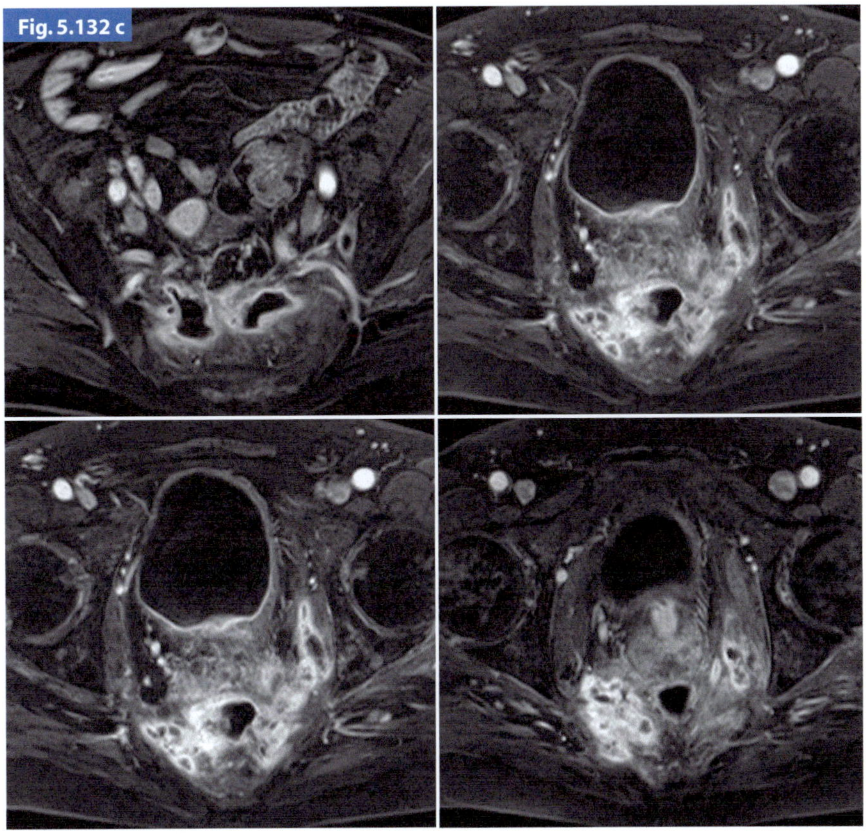

Fig. 5.132 (**c**) On the corresponding axial CE-VIBE 3D images, the ramified abscess formations are surrounded by a hypervascular rim of inflammatory granulation tissue.

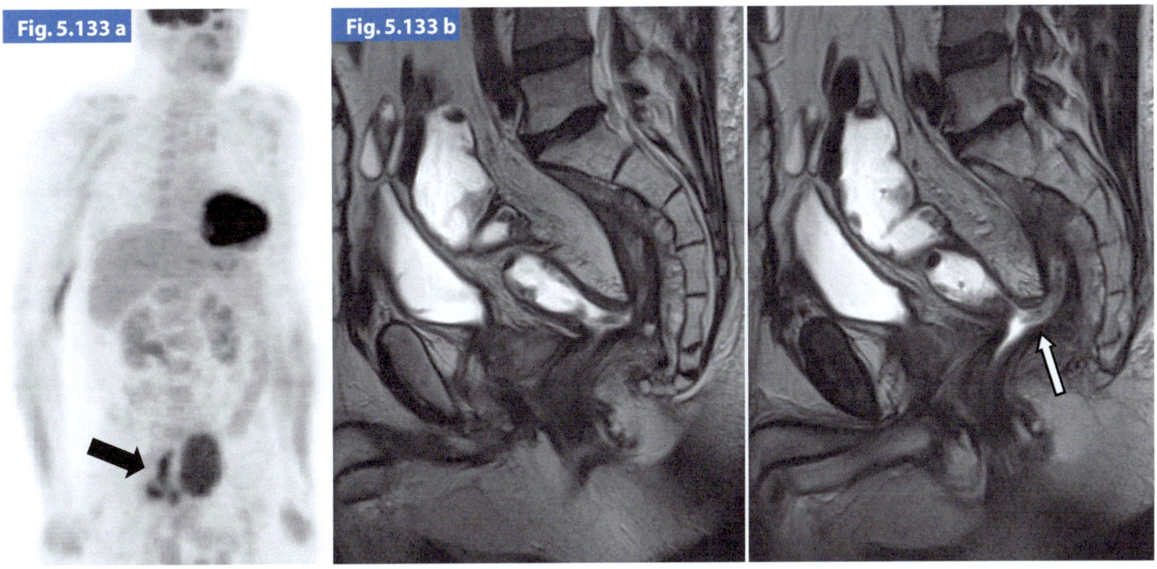

Fig. 5.133 Anastomotic leak mimicking local recurrence. (**a**) Follow-up FDG-PET examination diagnosed a local recurrence after J-pouch anastomosis resulting from stage ypT3N0 rectal cancer (*arrow*). (**b**) In contrast sagittal T2-TSE images derived from subsequently performed pelvic MRI reveal anastomotic leak with fistula track, which proceeds into the presacral scar causing chronic inflammation (*arrow*). No signs of luminal or extraluminal local recurrence is shown.

MIX
Papier aus verantwortungsvollen Quellen
Paper from responsible sources
FSC® C105338

If you have any concerns about our products,
you can contact us on
ProductSafety@springernature.com

In case Publisher is established outside the EU,
the EU authorized representative is:
Springer Nature Customer Service Center GmbH
Europaplatz 3, 69115 Heidelberg, Germany

Printed by Libri Plureos GmbH
in Hamburg, Germany